# Adverse Reactions to Food

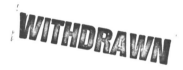

Also published by Blackwell Science

**Obesity**
The Report of the
British Nutrition Foundation Taskforce
0-632-05298-8

# Adverse Reactions to Food

## The Report of a British Nutrition Foundation Task Force

### Edited by Dr Judith Buttriss

*b*

**Blackwell
Science**

Published by Blackwell Science
for the British Nutrition Foundation

© 2002 by
Blackwell Science Ltd
Editorial Offices:
Osney Mead, Oxford OX2 0EL
25 John Street, London WC1N 2BS
23 Ainslie Place, Edinburgh EH3 6AJ
350 Main Street, Malden
    MA 02148 5018, USA
54 University Street, Carlton
    Victoria 3053, Australia
10, rue Casimir Delavigne
    75006 Paris, France

Other Editorial Offices:

Blackwell Wissenschafts-Verlag GmbH
Kurfürstendamm 57
10707 Berlin, Germany

Blackwell Science KK
MG Kodenmacho Building
7–10 Kodenmacho Nihombashi
Chuo-ku, Tokyo 104, Japan

Iowa State University Press
A Blackwell Science Company
2121 S State Avenue
Ames, Iowa 50014-8300, USA

First published 2002

Set in 9.5/11.5 Times
by DP Photosetting, Aylesbury, Bucks
Printed and bound in Great Britain by
The Alden Press, Northampton and Oxford

DISTRIBUTORS

Marston Book Services Ltd
PO Box 269
Abingdon
Oxon OX14 4YN
(*Orders:* Tel: 01235 465500
         Fax: 01235 465555)

USA and Canada
Iowa State University Press
A Blackwell Science Company
2121 S. State Avenue
Ames, Iowa 50014-8300
(*Orders:* Tel: 800-862-6657
         Fax: 515-292-3348
         Web: www.isupress.com
         email: orders@isupress.com)

Australia
Blackwell Science Pty Ltd
54 University Street
Carlton, Victoria 3053
(*Orders:* Tel: 03 9347 0300
         Fax: 03 9347 5001)

A catalogue record for this title
is available from the British Library

ISBN 0-632-05547-2

Library of Congress
Cataloging-in-Publication Data
Adverse reactions to food: the report of a British nutrition foundation task force/edited by Judith Buttriss.
      p. cm.
Includes bibliographical references and index.
ISBN 0-632-05547-2 (paper)
   1. Food allergy.   2. Malabsorption syndromes.
3. Food—Toxicology.   4. Nutritionally induced diseases.
I. Buttriss, Judith.

RC596 .A455 2001
616.97′5—dc21
                                        2001043328

For further information on Blackwell Science, visit our website: www.blackwell-science.com

# Contents

*This report is the collective work of all the members of the Task Force.
Authors of the first draft of each chapter are given below.*

**13  Immunomodulation of Food Allergies**                                    **165**
*Dr Gideon Lack*

**14  Conclusions of the Task Force**                                    **170**

# Foreword

The Task Force was invited by the Council of the British Nutrition Foundation to review, analyse, report and make recommendations on adverse reactions to food. The subject is an important one as about 20% of people consider that they are intolerant or 'allergic' to particular foodstuffs. The true prevalence of food allergy is probably no more than 1–2% of children and less than 1% of adults. However, for some of these individuals the condition may be life-threatening, as with peanut allergy and for others, the long-term failure to diagnose a condition such as coeliac disease can be very serious indeed. In addition, the use of unnecessary dietary restrictions, some quite bizarre, can be harmful in themselves, lead to malnutrition, be unpleasant and interfere with living generally.

The report uses the phrase 'adverse reactions to food' to describe a range of different types of responses to food, in particular food intolerance including food allergy, food aversion and food poisoning. This classification of terms is consistent with current practice in the UK and is valuable when so many different professionals are involved with the problems. There are of course other classifications.

The Task Force is completely independent. The members are all experts in their fields and between them cover a range of topics from feeding infants to manufacturing practices. The report is aimed at a wide variety of professionals who are not necessarily experts in this field or familiar with all the details. It has been written in such a way that the main key points are very helpful and recognise that some of the complex immunology and biochemistry may not be of value to all its readers.

The members of the Task Force have contributed so much of their time and expertise to this Report and I am most grateful to them all. The support provided by the Secretariat has been outstanding and I thank them most sincerely.

Barbara Clayton

# Terms of Reference

The Task Force was invited by the Council of the British Nutrition Foundation to:

(1) Review the present state of knowledge of the causes, consequences, prevention and treatment of adverse reactions to food, in particular food intolerance.

(2) Prepare a report and, should it see fit, draw conclusions, make recommendations and identify areas for future research.

# British Nutrition Foundation Adverse Reactions to Food Task Force Membership

## Chair:
Professor Dame Barbara Clayton, Honorary Research Professor in Metabolism, The Medical School, Southampton General Hospital, Tremona Road, Southampton, SO16 6YD

## Members:

**Dr Philip Calder**
Reader in Human Nutrition
Institute of Human Nutrition
University of Southampton
Bassett Crescent East
Southampton, SO16 7PX

**Professor Timothy David**
Professor of Child Health and
    Paediatrics
Booth Hall Children's Hospital
Charlestown Road
Blackley
Manchester M9 7AA

**Dr Graham Devereux**
Senior Registrar in Thoracic
    Medicine
Chest Clinic C
Aberdeen Royal Infirmary
Foresterhill
Aberdeen AB25 2ZN

**Dr Julia Ellis**
Senior Research Fellow
Department of Gastroenterology
Rayne Institute (Kings College
    London)
St. Thomas' Hospital
Lambeth Palace Road
London SE1 7EH

**Ms Johanna Hignett**
Group Nutritionist
Specialist Nutrition
Nestlé UK
St George's House
Croydon
Surrey CR9 1NR

**Professor Mike Kemeney**
Head of Department of
    Immunology
Rayne Institute
123 Coldharbour Lane
London SE5 9NW

**Professor Ian Kimber**
Head of Research, Health
    Assessment and
    Environmental Safety
Syngenta Central Toxicology
    Laboratory
Alderley Park
Macclesfield
Cheshire SK10 4TJ

**Dr Riitta Korpela**
    (corresponding)
Manager in Nutrition Research
Valio Ltd
PO Box 30
FIN-00039 VALIO
Finland

**Dr Gideon Lack**
Consultant in Paediatric Allergy
    and Immunology
Ground Floor
Salton House
St Mary's Hospital
Praed Street
London W2 1NY

**Professor Maurice Lessof**
London University Emeritus
  Professor of Medicine
8 John Spencer Square
London N1 2LZ

**Dr Anita MacDonald**
Head of Dietetic Services
Department of Nutrition and
  Dietetics
Birmingham Children's Hospital
  Trust
Steelhouse Lane
Birmingham B4 6NH

**Professor Stephan Strobel**
Vice Dean
Consultant Paediatric
  Immunologist
Institute of Child Health
30 Guilford Street
London WC1N 1EH

## Observers:

**Dr Christopher E. Fisher**
Joint Food Safety and Standards
  Group
Ministry of Agriculture
Fisheries and Food (until March
  2000)

**Dr Esther Heller**
Food Standards Agency
Aviation House
125 Kingsway
London WC2B 6NH (from
  March 2000)

**Dr Lisa Jackson**
Branch Head Nutrition
Food Standards Agency
Aviation House
125 Kingsway
London WC2B 6NH (from April
  2000)

**Dr Timothy Marrs**
Senior Medical Officer
Food Standards Agency
Aviation House
125 Kingsway
London WC2B 6NH

**Dr Sheela Reddy**
Dept of Health (until January
  2000)
Skipton House
80 London Road
London SE1 6LW

**Professor Martin Wiseman**
Dept of Health (until June 1999)
Skipton House
80 London Road
London SE1 6LW

## Contributors:

**Professor Ian Clarke**
Head of Cell and Molecular
  Medicine
School of Medicine
Southampton General Hospital
Tremona Road
Southampton SO16 6YD

**Professor Michael Farthing**
Dean of Medical Faculty
University of Glasgow
University Avenue
Glasgow G12 8QQ

**Professor John Walker-Smith**
Professor in Paediatric
  Gastroenterology
Royal Free and University
  College Medical School
Rowland Hill Street
London NW3 2PF

## Editor:

**Dr Judith Buttriss**
Science Director
British Nutrition Foundation
High Holborn House
52–54 High Holborn
London WC1V 6RQ

## Secretariat:

**Dr Sarah Schenker**
Nutrition Scientist
British Nutrition Foundation
High Holborn House
52–54 High Holborn
London WC1V 6RQ

**Paula Heath**
Science Secretary
British Nutrition Foundation
High Holborn House
52–54 High Holborn
London WC1V 6RQ

**Maxine Ide**
Science Secretary
British Nutrition Foundation
High Holborn House
52–54 High Holborn
London WC1V 6RQ

---

The British Nutrition Foundation Task Force would like to thank the copyright holders acknowledged in the text for permission to reproduce data and figures in this book.

# 1
# Introduction and Definitions

## 1.1 Introduction

In this Task Force report, the phrase *Adverse Reactions to Food* is used as the umbrella term to describe a range of different types of responses to food, in particular *food intolerance*, *food aversion* and *food poisoning* (Fig. 1.1). A brief description of food aversion and food poisoning is given here (Sections 1.3 and 1.4), but the main focus of the report is food intolerance, in its various manifestations. The report has been compiled in such a way as to enable readers to dip in and out of sections, and the discussion of some topics is more technical than others, which is reflected to some extent in the differences in style between the chapters.

The classification of terms used by the Task Force is based on current practice in the UK and is derived from a classification scheme published in a joint report from the Royal College of Physicians and the British Nutrition Foundation in 1984. However, other valid classification schemes exist. For example, the advisory report to government on adverse reactions to food, *Adverse Reactions to Food and Food Ingredients*, prepared by a Working Group of the Committee on Toxicity of Chemicals in Food, Consumer Products and the Environment (COT) and published in 2000 (Food Standards Agency, 2000), uses a different classification (Appendix A) modified slightly from the categorisation and definitions of the European Academy of Allergy and Clinical Immunology (Bruijnzeel-Koomen *et al.*, 1995), which begins by describing adverse reactions to food as toxic or non-toxic. The main difference between the BNF Task Force's classification and that of COT is that the latter uses the term 'intolerance' to describe only non-allergic, non-toxic adverse reactions, whereas the BNF Task Force's definition uses 'intolerance' as an umbrella term for allergic and non-allergic reactions, as is common practice in the UK. Another classification, which is different again, is used in the USA (Anderson & Sogn, 1984). It is important to note that the terminologies used in this Task Force report are working definitions, selected to provide a structure to the report.

One way of distinguishing food intolerance and food poisoning is to consider the former as a characteristic of the individual and the latter as that of food. The emphasis of this Task Force report is on reproducible adverse reactions to specific foods or food ingredients, rather than focusing on responses to contaminants (food poisoning) or psychological reactions (food aversion) that cannot be repro-

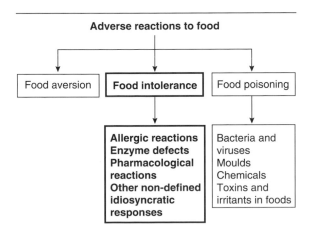

**Fig. 1.1** Definitions of terms.

duced when the food/food ingredient is given in a disguised or covert manner to the subject.

The chapters in this report are divided into various sections. The initial chapters consider the immune system, how nutrition influences immune functions, the epidemiology of food intolerance, non-immunological food intolerance and current thinking about sensitisation in early life. These are followed by information on specific forms of food intolerance, diagnosis and treatment. The final part of the report considers consumer issues, such as labelling of allergens and efforts of manufacturers to reduce cross-contamination with allergens, and considers the potential for desensitisation of atopic individuals.

## 1.2 Food intolerance

Food intolerance is the term used in this report to describe a range of responses to food, including allergic reactions, adverse reactions resulting from enzyme deficiencies, pharmacological effects and other non-defined idiosyncratic responses.

All of the adverse reactions categorised under this heading share one specific characteristic, they are reproducible adverse responses to a specific food or food ingredient.

Estimates of the true prevalence of total food intolerance in the general population suggest that no more than 5–8% of children and 1–2% of adults are affected. Among children, the prevalence of proven IgE mediated allergy is thought to be of the order of 1–2%, and less than 1% in adults (typically 0.2–0.5%). On the other hand, as many as 20% of people perceive themselves to be intolerant (or 'allergic') (Chapter 4).

### 1.2.1 Allergic reactions

#### *(i) IgE mediated reactions*

Allergic reactions with immunoglobulin (Ig) involvement are immediate, can be severe, and are mediated by IgE antibodies, which trigger mast cells (and other cells) to release inflammatory products. Details about the immune processes involved can be found in Chapter 2.

- The mast cells are present below the surface of the skin and in the membranes lining the nose,

respiratory tract, eyes, intestine and other mucosal sites.

- Histamine and other pro-inflammatory substances, which are released from mast cells, cause symptoms such as rhinitis, asthma, eczema, dilation of blood vessels and flushing, swelling (*e.g.* of the lips) and difficulty in breathing.
- These allergic reactions are usually localised to one or two organs of the body.

Allergic reactions to food (Chapter 6) vary considerably in their severity and the discomfort they cause, but the majority are not life-threatening. However, anaphylactic reactions can be very severe and even fatal.

- The term anaphylaxis is now mainly applied to severe reactions of rapid onset, often accompanied by a fall in blood pressure and severe shock.
- Peanuts are well known for causing this type of extreme reaction.
- Other foods that are known occasionally to cause a severe (IgE-mediated) reaction include nuts, seeds, eggs, milk and shellfish.

Genetic factors are considered to be of particular importance in the development of IgE-mediated reactions. Atopy is the term used to describe a situation where there is a predisposition to the production of IgE antibodies and development of allergic disease.

- The prevalence of IgE mediated allergy to food is higher in young children than adults, and most children with sensitisation to eggs or milk spontaneously recover in 12–24 months.
- However, sensitisation to peanut protein typically is more persistent.
- The prevalence of proven IgE-mediated food allergy in young children is of the order of 1–2%, and it is less than 1% in adults (typically 0.2–0.5%). (The prevalence of food intolerance in general is of the order of 5–8% in children and 1–2% in adults.)
- Children with IgE-mediated reactions often react to more than one food and high levels of IgE antibodies to common food proteins, such as ones present in eggs and cows' milk, are often predictive of later allergy to inhalants such as house dust and pollen.

- It is generally accepted that inhalant allergies have increased in prevalence, but the swiftness with which the apparent change has come about precludes a change in the gene pool being responsible. The same may have also occurred for food allergies, but this is currently less clear (see Chapter 4).
- Food allergy does not commonly develop for the first time in adults. An exception is a reaction to shellfish; this tends to develop in older people rather than children. Oral allergy syndrome is normally (but not exclusively) seen in subjects (children and adults) who have an allergy to common inhaled allergens, *e.g.* those that result in hay fever (Chapter 6).

Detailed information about IgE mediated allergy can be found in Chapter 6.

### *(ii) Non-IgE-mediated reactions*

These reactions are delayed and complex (details can be found in Chapter 7). Coeliac disease is the best defined example of this form of response (Chapter 9).

- Coeliac disease involves a sensitivity to gluten and appears to be mediated by the cells of the immune system.
- Most experts agree that coeliac disease is a non-IgE mediated reaction brought about in genetically susceptible individuals by exposure to the gluten fraction of wheat and other related cereal grains (Chapter 9).

Delayed reactions to food may take several hours or even days to develop. Reactions to cows' milk are often delayed and the majority of these are not accompanied by detectable IgE antibodies (see Chapter 7).

### 1.2.2 Enzymic reactions

The most common intolerance linked to an insufficiency of an enzyme is lactose intolerance (also known as lactose maldigestion) (Chapter 8).

- Before it can be absorbed and utilised by the body as fuel, lactose (the sugar in milk) has to be broken down to its two component sugars, glucose and galactose.
- This requires the enzyme lactase.
- If lactase is produced in insufficient quantities, some of the lactose can pass undigested into the large intestine causing symptoms such as diarrhoea and flatulence. The symptoms result from bacterial fermentation of lactose in the colon and associated osmotic effects.

On occasions, other enzyme deficiencies (*e.g.* inborn errors of metabolism) can result in an inability to handle specific forms of dietary carbohydrate (such as galactose and sucrose) or dietary protein components (such as phenylalanine and methionine), and hence cause inability to metabolise components from particular foods. These conditions are very rare (Scriver *et al.*, 2001).

### 1.2.3 Pharmacological reactions

There are many food components that can produce a pharmacological effect. These effects are usually insignificant in clinical terms unless the substance is consumed in very large quantities, *e.g.* caffeine amongst heavy consumers.

Also sometimes responsible for this type of reaction is the group of substances known as vasoamines, which includes histamine and tyramine (Baldwin, 1997; Bodmer *et al.*, 1999; Food Standards Agency, 2000).

- These are normal constituents in a variety of foods such as some cheeses, *e.g.* Blue Roquefort and Parmesan (histamine) and matured cheeses (tyramine), hard-cured sausages, *e.g.* salami, pickled fish, chocolate, bananas, citrus fruits, marmite and wine.
- It is often stated that some foods have a histamine releasing action, *e.g.* strawberries, tomatoes and chocolate.
- Histamine-induced symptoms are similar to those found with IgE-mediated food allergy (section 1.2.1*i*).
- The two conditions can be distinguished by the relatively large amount of the substance needed to trigger a histamine-induced reaction, in contrast to the small quantity needed to trigger an immediate (IgE) allergic reaction.

### 1.2.4 Other non-defined idiosyncratic responses

From time to time, cases of food intolerance occur that cannot be attributed to any of the mechanisms described in the previous sections. These can be categorised as non-defined idiosyncratic responses in that they fulfil the definition of a food intolerance (are reproducible and relate to a characteristic of the individual rather than of the food).

For example, some foods contain toxins or substances that can irritate the lining of the intestine of some individuals (Chapter 7).

- Examples of natural toxins include protease inhibitors in legumes, cyclopeptides and muscarine in mushrooms, and oxalates in spinach and rhubarb. A comprehensive list of naturally occurring food toxicants can be found in the report from the Committee on Toxicity of Chemicals in Food, Consumer Products and the Environment (COT) (Food Standards Agency, 2000).
- The effect of spices and chilli on the gut mucosa, known as intestinal hurry, is sometimes mistaken for food intolerance.

## 1.3 Food aversion

*This subject is dealt with in a little more detail, as it will not be addressed again in this report.*

### 1.3.1 Food avoidance

Dislike and subsequent avoidance of various foods (sometimes referred to as 'faddiness') is commonplace and is referred to as **food avoidance**. Although true food intolerances do exist in some cases, food avoidance is frequently the result of a decision made by an individual based on food preferences (*i.e.* a matter of choice), rather than because the food is associated with specific and reproducible symptoms when consumed by that person (defined as food intolerance). For example, many children and adolescents, and some adults, refuse certain vegetables; this is usually because they dislike the taste or texture rather than because they have a food intolerance, even when the individual describes the reason for avoiding the food as 'allergy'. The extremes of this type of behaviour

manifest as the eating disorders anorexia nervosa and bulimia nervosa.

In the psychology literature, **food aversion** tends to have a very specific meaning in that it is used to describe aversions to 'tastes' that have become associated with sickness, nausea and gastro-intestinal discomfort (Bernstein, 1994). This results in the individual developing a 'distaste' for the food (often despite their knowledge that the food is not harmful and did not cause the illness). This is also called **conditioned taste aversion** (CTA), and is distinguished from more general food avoidance, *i.e.* avoidance due to ethical, religious or other reasons, such as food phobia in anorexia nervosa. **Psychological food intolerance** is the clinical manifestation of an adverse physical or psychological reaction caused not by the food itself but by emotions associated with the food or with the act of eating food. In summary:

- Food aversion may be associated with symptoms that are similar to those associated with true food intolerances. Such reactions are in fact psychosomatic and do not occur when the food or food ingredient is administered in a disguised form.
- Anecdotally, in some cases the bodily reaction can even be reproduced by the mere suggestion that a particular food has been consumed.
- In some individuals, food aversion can manifest itself as hyperventilation syndrome in response to the food. In such cases, being faced with the food the individual hyperventilates to the extent that they suffer severe symptoms and may even lose consciousness (Chapter 6, Section 6.3.1).
- A variant of this form of avoidance has been dubbed 'food intolerance by proxy'. This has become increasingly recognised in children (Warner & Hathaway, 1984). It occurs when an individual's family is unable to accept the symptoms and behaviour of the person except in terms of a physical illness. The belief that the problem is attributable to an 'allergy' is continuously reinforced within the family but there is no evidence of a physical intolerance on double blind challenge.

In addition to the circumstances described above, some individuals routinely avoid specific foods because they believe that they are responsible for suboptimal health. The media has popularised the idea that a food might be responsible for commonplace symptoms, such as tiredness, indigestion or fullness after a meal, nausea, difficulty in sleeping, depression, palpitations and breathlessness; and claims have been made that a variety of physical and psychological symptoms are a result of 'food allergy'. Such claims are not new. In 1983, Pearson and colleagues published results of a study in which they sought objective evidence of food hypersensitivity. They used exclusion diets and provocation tests in 23 patients who attributed a wide variety of symptoms to food allergy. Hypersensitivity was confirmed in just four subjects, each of whom presented with typical atopic symptoms. None of these had psychiatric symptoms, but a high incidence of psychiatric disorder was found in the remaining 19 patients whose belief that they had a food allergy could not be confirmed. In another study by the same researchers (Bentley *et al.*, 1983), inclusion of psychotherapy as part of the treatment in a controlled study of 50 patients with symptoms of irritable bowel syndrome resulted in significantly greater improvement. Again this should not be interpreted to mean that all those who claim to be intolerant to a food (as opposed to simply not liking it), but are subsequently shown not to react to a double blind challenge with that food, are suffering from some form of psychiatric disorder. It may be that the 'food does not agree with them' as a result of a yet to be defined idiosyncratic response.

## 1.4 Food poisoning

*This subject is dealt with in a little more detail as it will not be addressed again in this report.*

The term food poisoning has been defined by the Advisory Committee on the Microbiological Safety of Food (1993) as 'any disease of an infectious or toxic nature caused by, or thought to be caused by, the consumption of food or water'. Consumption of contaminated food may give rise to bacterial, protozoal, viral or helminthic infections, or to poisoning caused by toxins present in the food before ingestion.

A wide range of agents can give rise to food poisoning. In Europe and North America, by far the most common causes of food poisoning are microorganisms, in particular bacteria and viruses.

The involvement of other agents, such as parasites, toxins naturally present in foods and chemicals, will vary according to country, diet of the population, level of hygiene in food production and storage and the sophistication of the food technologies employed.

The symptoms of food poisoning can be diverse and the presenting symptoms, together with the incubation period, often point to the diagnosis. The most common symptoms include nausea, vomiting and diarrhoea, with or without fever. Some agents may give rise to symptoms other than gastroenteritis, such as jaundice or effects on the nervous system. In severe cases and with particular agents there may be more serious effects, such as septicaemia or renal failure.

### 1.4.1 Chemical food poisoning

- In the UK, chemical food poisoning is very uncommon and probably not responsible for more than 1% of all food poisoning episodes, although it is recognised to occur more commonly elsewhere in the world.
- Acute chemical food poisoning may occur as the result of accidental contamination of food, *e.g.* residues from produce previously treated with insecticides, fungicides or herbicides; or from animals treated with veterinary drugs or feed additives.
- Cumulative chemical food poisoning results from consumption of foods and liquids regularly in contact with a contamination source, *e.g.* pipework or cooking utensils.
- The main characteristic of chemical food poisoning is often vomiting within a few minutes to half an hour of ingestion of the food. Recovery is usually rapid, although with some poisons there may be a high case-fatality rate.

Some foods, both of plant or animal origin, are poisonous to human beings because they contain naturally occurring toxins. These include:

- undercooked red kidney beans (which contain a lectin) and puffer fish (which contain tetrodotoxin)
- toadstools
- cereals infected with the fungus *Claviceps purpurea* (ergot) that forms the poison responsible

for ergotism (a disease resulting from consumption of bread made from flour contaminated with ergot)
- poorly stored peanuts contaminated with aflatoxin
- incorrectly stored scombroid fish. Scombroid fish (*e.g.* mackerel and tuna), which are rich in histidine, become toxic largely as a result of breakdown of histidine to histamine by their own natural microbial flora, during poor storage.

Other foods can become toxic as a result of contamination with chemical poisons produced by organisms (*e.g.* algae) upon which they feed. For example, mussels, scallops and some fish, which have fed on marine dinoflagellates (*e.g. Alexandrium tamarensis*), may be capable of causing various forms of shellfish poisoning (*e.g.* paralytic, neurotoxic, diarrhoeal and amnesic shellfish poisoning) although the shellfish themselves are unharmed. Ciguatera poisoning (*e.g. Gambierdiscus toxicus*), caused by a similar mechanism, is generally found specifically in warmer latitudes.

### 1.4.2 Foodborne bacterial gastroenteritis

The term bacterial gastroenteritis is usually restricted to the acute gastroenteritis caused by the presence in food of bacteria or bacterial toxins. Onset of symptoms can occur within a few hours of food ingestion to up to a week or more later. This form of food poisoning can be subdivided into three basic types according to the mode of action of the bacteria responsible:

- **Infection type food poisoning** results from the multiplication *in vivo* of bacteria ingested with the food, *e.g. Salmonella* spp. or *Vibrio parahaemolyticus*. The dose of organisms required to initiate infection must be large enough to enable sufficient organisms to pass through the acid region of the stomach and reach the intestine, where they set up their infection. Classically, the infectious dose for this type of organism has been considered to be large ($10^6$ or more per g). However, infections may result from a low dose of bacteria if the organism is resistant to gastric acid, if gastric acidity is reduced, or if the food has a protective effect on the bacteria present as the food passes through the stomach, *e.g.* if it is

high in fat or has a high buffering capacity. Thus, occasional outbreaks of salmonella infection have resulted from foods such as chocolate and cheese containing levels of <100 salmonella bacteria per g of food.
- **Toxin type food poisoning** results from the ingestion of food in which a toxin has already been formed due to microbial growth in the food. Examples of this type include *Staphylococcus aureus* (enterotoxin), *Bacillus cereus* (emetic toxin) and *Clostridium botulinum* (neurotoxin). Typically, though not in all cases, the organisms need to multiply to levels exceeding $10^5$ organisms per g of food in order for sufficient toxin to be produced to cause illness. The emetic toxins, which act on the vomiting centre and also cause diarrhoea, produce symptoms fairly rapidly, within a few hours of consumption of the food, whereas the neurotoxins take longer to act.
- **Intermediate type food poisoning** results from the release of enterotoxin from bacteria that do not readily produce the toxin in food but which do so in the bowel, *e.g. Clostridium perfringens*.

### *(i) Incidence*

It is difficult to assess the true incidence of bacterial gastroenteritis in the UK. When food is contaminated with potentially pathogenic organisms, the risk of gastroenteritis is generally small unless the organisms are able to grow. However, some organisms have a very low infective dose and multiplication in the food vehicle is not required to produce illness. See the Public Health Laboratory website www.phls.co.uk for up-to-date information on UK cases.

- *Campylobacter* is the most common cause of bacterial gastroenteritis in the UK and the incidence of campylobacter infection has been steadily increasing over the last 10 years, and reached over 60 000 cases per year in 1999. The infective dose is relatively low but campylobacter does not multiply in food and, although food is thought to be an important vehicle for sporadic cases, foodborne outbreaks are relatively uncommon. *Salmonella* is the next most common cause of bacterial gastroenteritis, with case numbers more than doubling in the last 20 years, reaching a peak in 1997 of 36 000 cases. However, the number of cases has subsequently plummeted to under 20 000 cases in 1999.

- The third major bacterial pathogen is verotoxin-producing *Eschericha coli* (VTEC). Over 1000 cases were documented in 1999.

### 1.4.3 Food vehicles

#### (i) Eggs and poultry

- In recent years, the epidemiological pattern of human salmonella infection has been dominated by outbreaks associated with eggs and poultry, implicated in 41% and 26%, respectively, of recent incidents (although many other foods may be a vehicle for these bacteria).
- Salmonella on egg shells can contaminate egg contents by migration through the shell and associated membranes when the shell is damaged, when a warm newly laid egg comes into contact with faecal matter or as a result of a combination of these events. Salmonella may also thrive if the broken egg, having come into contact with a contaminated shell, is then stored in the raw state at ambient temperature. Some strains of salmonella may also be present in the oviducts of chickens and can result in contamination of the egg itself during egg production.
- Poultry meat can also be a source of *Campylobacter* if not cooked properly or if, when raw, it is allowed to cross-contaminate cooked or ready-to-eat foods.

#### (ii) Slow cooked meats

- *Clostridium perfringens* is widely distributed in a variety of foods, particularly meat, poultry and their products.
- Spores of *Clostridium perfringens* survive cooking and germinate to form vegetative cells that multiply rapidly under optimal growth temperatures of 43–47°C (slow cooking).
- Outbreaks are caused by meat and poultry dishes that have been cooked hours in advance and then cooled slowly or allowed to stand at room temperature and inadequately reheated before serving.

#### (iii) Cold meats

- The *Eschericha coli* O157-H7 (VTEC) outbreak in Scotland in 1997 resulted from the transfer of the bacteria from raw meat to cold cooked meats. Raw minced meat can also be a vehicle for VTEC and so should be thoroughly cooked and should not be allowed to come into contact with cooked meats or other ready-to-eat foods.
- Cold ham, meat pies and chicken account for 70% of *Staphylococcus aureus* gastroenteritis outbreaks in the UK.
- In outbreaks of gastroenteritis resulting from *Staphylococcus aureus,* human beings are most commonly implicated as the source of the infection. It is usually the food handler (15% of the population carry enterotoxigenic strains of the organism) who contaminates the food, and under favourable conditions the staphylococcus will multiply and produce enterotoxin in the product.

#### (iv) Rice

- Approximately 85% of outbreaks of the emetic syndrome of *Bacillus cereus* gastroenteritis (distinct from the diarrhoeal syndrome) have been associated with boiled or fried rice.
- Outbreaks can be attributed to the practice of preparing rice too far in advance of serving. The endospores of certain strains found on raw rice, survive boiling; they then germinate under favourable conditions, such as being held for long periods at room temperature before being reheated.

#### (v) Spices

- Outbreaks of the diarrhoeal syndrome of *Bacillus cereus* gastroenteritis are often attributed to widespread culinary use of spices, heavily contaminated with *Bacillus cereus*, and unsatisfactory hygiene.
- *Salmonella* contamination of spices has also given rise to outbreaks.
- In the UK, irradiation of spices is permitted under licence, although this is not commonly practised. Use of irradiation would in fact destroy these bacteria.

Prevention of most types of bacterial gastroenteritis hinges upon avoidance of contamination of foods during production and processing, and the practice of good hygiene. This requires education of those involved in the preparation, processing and service of food, both commercially and in the home.

### 1.4.4 Foodborne viral gastroenteritis

Four main virus families are associated with human gastroenteritis: rotaviruses, enteric adenoviruses, caliciviruses and astroviruses. However, most of these viruses do not grow well (and in some cases they do not grow at all) in cell culture. The caliciviruses are the only group of viruses consistently associated with foodborne gastroenteritis. The caliciviruses are named after characteristic cup-shaped structures seen on the virion surface by direct negative stain electron microscopy. Within the calicivirus family there are two genera associated with human disease. The so-called classic caliciviruses or Sapporo-like viruses display a typical calicivirus morphology, they are predominantly associated with paediatric disease and are only a minor cause of gastroenteritis. In sharp contrast, the small round structured viruses (SRSVs) or Norwalk-like viruses (NLVs) are the major agents of foodborne gastroenteritis. The fastidious nature of these viruses means that there is no cell culture system for virus isolation, hence knowledge and understanding of these viruses lags significantly behind that of the other enteric viruses. It is a widely held view that the incidence of enteric disease caused by SRSVs exceeds that of all other pathogens.

### i Small round structured viruses

Illness caused by SRSVs occurs in widespread epidemics, often in winter, and has a high secondary attack rate. Although mainly transmitted directly from person to person, SRSVs are also the major viral cause of water and foodborne gastroenteritis. In relation to the latter, illness is frequently linked to the consumption of raw or undercooked molluscan shellfish (*e.g.* raw oysters). Bivalve molluscs concentrate SRSVs by filtration from sewage contaminated water. Consumption of such contaminated shellfish in other countries has given rise to very large outbreaks involving thousands or even tens of thousands of individuals. Food may also become contaminated by viruses shed from infected food handlers, giving rise to large outbreaks. It is important to note that the SRSVs do not replicate in food (even in live molluscs), however even the slightest trace of contamination is enough to cause infection because these viruses are some of the most infectious agents known. In summary:

- Volunteer studies have established the extremely infectious nature of these viruses with as few as 10 virions required.
- These viruses have emerged as the most important cause of epidemic non-bacterial gastroenteritis.
- UK national surveillance and diagnosis by electron microscopy have recently shown that SRSVs are a more common cause of infective gastroenteritis than *Salmonella* spp.
- Outbreaks have winter seasonality and all age groups are affected. They often occur in semi-closed communities with devastating economic consequences, *e.g.* hospitals, hotels, cruise ships, schools.

## 1.5 Key points

- This Task Force report uses the phrase *Adverse Reactions to Food* to describe a range of different types of responses to food, in particular *food intolerance* (which includes *food allergy), food aversion* and *food poisoning.* This classification of terms is consistent with current practice in the UK, although it is acknowledged that other valid classification schemes exist.

- *Food intolerance* is used here to describe a range of reproducible responses including allergic reactions, adverse reactions resulting from enzyme deficiencies, pharmacological effects and other non-defined idiosyncratic responses, each of which is manifest when the food is given without the subject's knowledge.

- Estimates suggest that no more than 5–8% of children and 1–2% of adults in the general population are affected by food intolerance. Among children, the prevalence of immunoglobulin E (IgE) mediated allergy is thought to be 1–2%, and less than 1% in adults. On the other hand, as many as 20% of people perceive themselves to be intolerant (or 'allergic') to some foods.

- Allergic reactions can either be IgE mediated and rapid (the most severe example being anaphylactic shock) or delayed and involve cell-mediated mechanisms (*e.g.* coeliac disease) or both.

- The most common intolerance linked to an enzyme insufficiency is lactose intolerance, which is widespread in some populations, although not in the UK.

- A number of food components can produce pharmacological effects, but these are usually insignificant in clinical terms.

- Dislike and subsequent avoidance of various foods (sometimes referred to as 'faddiness') is commonplace and is referred to as *food avoidance.*

- *Food aversion* (dislike and subsequent avoidance of various foods in the absence of organic disease) has been used to describe a response to a food that is associated with sickness, nausea or gastrointestinal discomfort. Sometimes the associated symptoms are similar to those resulting from true food intolerances, which can potentially lead to misdiagnosis.

- *Food poisoning* has been defined as any disease of an infectious or toxic nature caused by, or thought to be caused by, the consumption of contaminated food or water.

**Appendix A  Classification of adverse reactions to foods
(adapted from Bruijnzeel-Koomen *et al.*, 1995).**

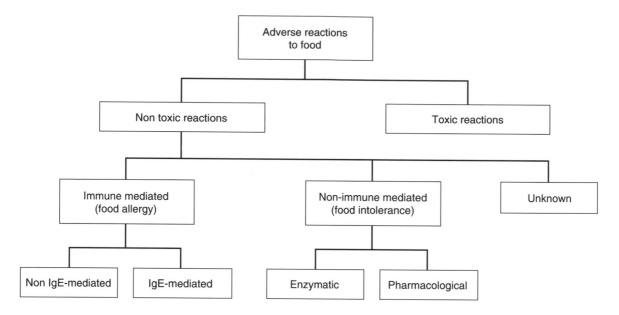

# 2
# The Immune System

## 2.1 Introduction

Many of the adverse reactions to food outlined in this publication are mediated by the immune system. These adverse reactions are more easily understood if it is realised that they are normal immunological processes, which are being inappropriately directed against food constituents to the detriment of the individual. This chapter is an attempt to outline the normal immune system and to demonstrate how these normal processes can give rise to adverse reactions to food. The chapter is not a comprehensive text, but instead is an attempt to describe the immunological processes that form the basis of several of the subsequent chapters, *e.g.* IgE-mediated food allergy (Chapter 6) and gluten sensitive enteropathy (Chapter 9). After an outline of innate (Section 2.3) and adaptive immunity (Section 2.4.1), there is a description of humoral (Section 2.4.3) and cell-mediated immunity (Section 2.4.4). The pathogenic aspects of these immune mechanisms are then detailed in the sections describing IgE and non-IgE mediated allergy (Sections 2.5.1 and 2.5.3, respectively), and finally the normal immunological responses to food are summarised (Section 2.6).

## 2.2 The immune system

We live in a microbiologically hostile world, under the constant threat of overwhelming attack by viruses, bacteria, fungi and parasites. This threat is constantly present and its nature is changing as exposure to new organisms or variants of organisms occurs. To combat this potentially devastating threat, evolution has provided humans with a highly

---

**Points to note**

- Immune responses are divided into innate and adaptive responses.
- Adaptive, but not innate immunity, is characterised by immunological memory.
- Innate immunity is considered the first line of defence, whilst the more powerful and flexible adaptive response is induced.
- Interaction between innate and adaptive immunity is essential: innate responses influence adaptive responses and adaptive immunity utilises innate mechanisms.

---

sophisticated, flexible and potent immune system. The critical protective function of the immune system becomes apparent when it fails. The inherited and acquired immunodeficiency states are characterised by increased susceptibility to all infections, including those organisms not normally considered to be pathogenic. The immune system utilises many mechanisms to combat invading microorganisms. However, the inappropriate activation of these normally beneficial mechanisms is the basis of the detrimental processes of allergy, autoimmunity and tissue rejection.

The immune response to microorganisms is divided into two general systems: innate (natural) immunity and adaptive (specific, acquired) immunity. Innate immunity is phylogenetically older with some forms present in all multicellular organisms, whereas adaptive immunity is only found in fish, amphibians, reptiles, birds and mammals.

## 2.3 Innate immunity

Innate immunity has been reviewed by Medzhitov and Janeway (1997). It comprises physical barriers, soluble factors and predominantly phagocytic cells, which internalise microbes and particulate matter. The proteins of the innate immune system that recognise microbes are either cell surface receptors (*e.g.* the CD14 lipopolysaccharide (LPS) receptor of macrophages) or soluble molecules (*e.g.* C reactive protein), both of which usually bind to microbial surface carbohydrate molecules. Innate immunity is encoded in the germline, is very similar among normal individuals and there is no memory effect, *i.e.* re-exposure to the same organism elicits the same response. Innate immunity is directed against molecular structures of microorganisms that are essential for microbial survival, such as are present in many types of microorganisms and unique to pathogenic microorganisms, *e.g.* LPS of gram negative bacteria and the teichoic acids of gram positive bacteria. The cells principally associated with innate immunity are phagocytic macrophages and neutrophils, which possess surface receptors specific for common bacterial surface molecules. Engagement of these receptors triggers phagocytosis and destruction of the microorganism. Evolutionary pressures, however, result in microorganisms that have evolved mechanisms to evade the innate immune response, *e.g.* bacterial capsules. The evolutionary response of the immune system to these evasive mechanisms is the development of a very flexible immune system that adapts to new threats (adaptive immunity). Although innate immunity is inflexible, it provides a very rapid first line of defence until the more powerful and flexible adaptive immune response takes effect. The innate and adaptive immune systems are not independent; the nature of the innate immune response probably influences the character of the adaptive immune response and the effector arm of the adaptive response harnesses innate immunity effector mechanisms (Fearon & Locksley, 1996).

## 2.4 Adaptive immunity

> ### Points to note
>
> - T lymphocytes and B lymphocytes (T cells and B cells) are the bedrock of the adaptive response.
> - Immunological surveillance of the tissues is maintained by continuous circulation of T and B cells.
> - Each T cell and B cell is specific for a single antigen.
> - Contact with a specific antigen induces rapid clonal expansion, with the antigen specificity of the numerous progeny being identical to the progenitor.

### 2.4.1 Anatomy and cells of adaptive immunity

The cells that form the mainstay of the adaptive immune system are B lymphocytes (B cells) and T lymphocytes (T cells) (for a review, see Huston, 1997). Approximately 75% of peripheral blood mononuclear leukocytes are T cells, 15% are B cells and the remaining 10% are monocytes. Lymphocytes originate in the bone marrow from a common lymphoid stem cell. B cells develop and mature further in the bone marrow, whereas T cells migrate to the thymus to undergo further development and maturation. Mature T and B cells enter the blood stream, from where they migrate into the peripheral lymphoid organs, which comprise the lymph nodes, the spleen, bronchial-associated lymphoid tissue (BALT), mucosa-associated lymphoid tissue (MALT) and gut-associated lymphoid tissues (GALT). GALT includes the tonsils, adenoids, appendix and the Peyer's patches of the small intestine. Bloodborne circulating B and T cells adhere to the capillary endothelial cells of the peripheral lymphoid organs and then migrate into the tissues. The peripheral lymphoid organs are anatomically and functionally organised to allow cellular interactions between migrating lymphocytes and antigens, which are transported from the tissues by phagocytic cells or carried passively in lymph. For the purpose of this Task Force report, an antigen is considered to be a non-self foreign substance, *e.g.* food, bacteria, virus or parasite. If the lymphocytes do not encounter antigens, they re-enter the blood stream by way of the efferent lymphatic vessels and the thoracic duct. The functional consequence of T and B cells circulating between the vascular and lymphatic systems is that all of the body tissues and mucosal surfaces are under continuous immunological surveillance for invading pathogens.

### 2.4.2 Clonal expansion of lymphocytes

Each circulating lymphocyte bears surface receptors with a single antigenic specificity, but the specificity of each individual lymphocyte is different. It has been estimated that the population of T and B cells in a human is able to recognise $10^{11}$ different antigens. This huge receptor repertoire is generated during lymphocyte development by the random rearrangement of a limited number of lymphocyte antigen receptor genes (Fanning *et al.*, 1996). Although the immune system is able to recognise a huge number of antigens, any single antigen is recognised by relatively few lymphocytes, typically 1 in 1 000 000. Therefore, when the immune system is exposed to a microorganism for the first time, initially there are not enough lymphocytes to eliminate the infection. When a lymphocyte recognises its specific antigen by way of receptor–antigen interactions, the lymphocyte stops migrating, enlarges and starts to proliferate rapidly. The resulting lymphoblasts proliferate for 3–5 days, so that a single lymphocyte gives rise to a clone of a large number of effector cells, each specific for the antigen that initiated its development. This process is known as antigen-driven clonal expansion and accounts for the characteristic delay of several days before adaptive immune responses become effective. Some of the effector cells generated by clonal expansion persist long after elimination of the microorganism and form the basis of immunological memory. Immunological memory is a characteristic of adaptive immunity and explains why re-exposure to a pathogen results in an immune response that is more rapid in onset and more effective in eliminating the microorganism. In contrast to innate immunity, the antigen specificities of adaptive immunity reflect the individual's lifetime exposure to infectious agents, and will consequently differ between individuals.

### 2.4.3 B cells, immunoglobulins and humoral immunity

> ## Points to note
>
> - Immunoglobulin secretion by B cells is the basis of humoral immunity.
> - Ig antigenic specificity is mediated by two antigen (Fab) binding sites, each with the same specificity.
> - The five immunoglobulin isotypes (IgM, IgA, IgD, IgG, IgE) possess different sets of functional properties, mediated by the Fc fragment.
> - Immunoglobulins engage effector cells of the innate response to neutralise microorganisms, *e.g.* phagocytes, complement.
> - Effective humoral responses are dependent on T cell and B cell interactions.

It is well established that protection against certain infections can be transferred by serum. This is known as humoral immunity and is mediated by circulating antibodies, also known as immunoglobulins (Ig). B cells are characterised by their production of immunoglobulins, which are the antigen-specific constituent of humoral immunity. The cell surface of B cells incorporates the membrane-bound form of immunoglobulin, which functions as an antigen-specific receptor. Upon engagement of the surface immunoglobulin, the B cell proliferates with the majority of the resulting cells transforming into plasma cells that secrete large amounts of antibody with the same specificity as the progenitor B cell. This process is illustrated in Fig. 2.1 (for a description of the function of T helper cells, see Section 2.4.6).

### (i) Structure of immunoglobulins

The general structural features of antibodies (reviewed by Huston, 1997) can be demonstrated by IgG, which has a molecular weight of approximately 150 kDa and is composed of two identical heavy chains (molecular weight of 50 kDa each) and two identical light chains (molecular weight of 25 kDa each). The two heavy chains are linked by disulphide bonds and each of the heavy chains is

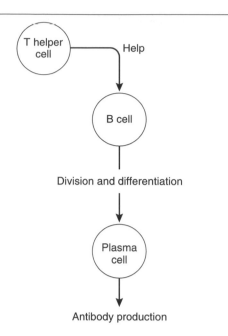

**Fig. 2.1** Schematic representation of humoral immunity. In response to a stimulus from a specific form of T cell known as a T helper cell, the B cell proliferates with the majority of the resulting cells transforming into plasma cells that secrete large amounts of antibody with the same specificity as the progenitor B cell.

linked to a light chain by disulphide bonds, giving a roughly Y shaped molecule (Fig. 2.2). The antigen binding site (Fab) of antibodies is situated at the amino end of the light and heavy chains; consequently, each immunoglobulin molecule possesses two antigen binding sites, each with the same specificity. The Fab segments of antibodies are divided into a variable (V) and a constant (C) region; it is the structural diversity of the V regions that results in the diversity of antibody specificity. There are five main types of heavy chain ($\mu$, $\delta$, $\gamma$, $\alpha$ and $\varepsilon$), which confer differing functional properties between the five major classes (isotypes) of immunoglobulin, IgM, IgD, lgG, IgA and IgE, respectively. Immunoglobulin heavy chains are encoded on chromosome 14, the light chains are encoded on chromosomes 2 and 22. The functional activity of antibodies resides at the carboxy terminal (Fc) region of the heavy chains, situated away from the antigen binding sites.

### (ii) Immunoglobulin isotypes

The antigen specificity of antibodies is mediated by the two antigen binding sites, whilst the differing Fc regions of the various Ig isotypes engage differing effector mechanisms of the humoral immune response.

Monomeric IgM and IgD are incorporated into B cell surface membranes and act as antigen-specific receptors. The C region of IgM contains an extra $C_H$ domain and an 18 amino acid 'tailpiece' allows polymerisation of IgM molecules into pentamers, the usual form of IgM in serum. The affinity of each antigen binding site tends to be low; however, a pentamer of IgM possesses 10 antigen binding sites, which gives the antibody high binding strength.

The initial humoral immune response is dominated by IgM. Later in the response IgG and IgA predominate, although during an allergic response significant quantities of IgE are secreted. This process is known as isotype switching and is the consequence of DNA rearrangements in the genes encoding for the C regions of the heavy chains; this process does not affect the V region genes (Stavnezer, 1996). The result of isotype switching is different classes of antibodies but the antigen specificity remains constant. Isotype switching is dependent on T cells and their secretion of proteins known as cytokines. These influence the behaviour of other cells. For example, the cytokine interleukin-4 (IL-4) induces B cell switching to IgE, a process that is antagonised by another cytokine, interferon-$\gamma$ (IFN-$\gamma$) (Pene *et al.*, 1988). Switching to IgA is promoted by transforming growth factor-$\beta$ (TGF-$\beta$) in combination with interleukin-l0 (IL-10) (Defrance *et al.*, 1992). More details about the effects of various cytokines can be found in Section 2.5.1, and a brief discussion of specific effects during pregnancy can be found in Chapter 5.

As the humoral immune response matures, isotype switching occurs but other changes occur in antibody structure. Point mutations take place in the genes encoding the antibody V regions. These occur in mature B cells during the immune response in the peripheral lymphoid organs. The mutant forms of the immunoglobulins are then expressed on the surface of B cells. Mutations that result in antibodies with an increased affinity for the stimulating antigen are selected, and those with reduced affinity undergo programmed cell death

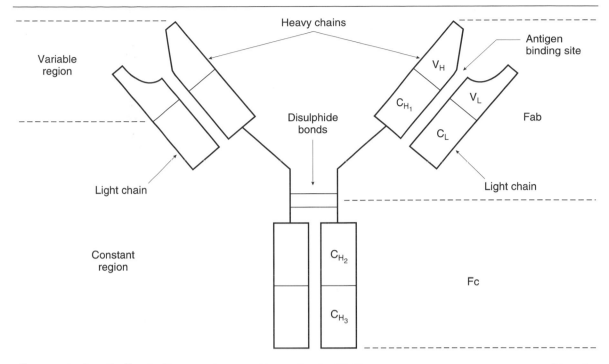

**Fig. 2.2** Schematic representation of an IgG molecule. Each IgG molecule is made up of two heavy chains (domains $V_H$, $C_{H_1}$, $C_{H_2}$, $C_{H_3}$) and two light chains (domains $V_L$, $C_L$). The antigen binding site is formed by the juxtaposition of the variable domains of the light and heavy chains ($V_H$, $V_L$). The Fab and Fc components are indicated.

(apoptosis). This process is known as affinity maturation and is T cell dependent. Consequently as the humoral immune response progresses, the affinity and specificity of the antibodies increases and the resulting memory cells provide highly effective protection against reinfection by the same microorganism (Neuberger & Milstein, 1995).

IgG antibodies are monomeric and are further subdivided into $IgG_1$, $IgG_2$, $IgG_3$ and $IgG_4$, with $IgG_1$ being found in the greatest quantities in serum. $IgG_1$ and $IgG_3$ are transferred across the placenta to the foetus. This subdivision is based upon structural differences between the heavy chains of the IgG subtypes, which confer differing biological properties between the subtypes.

IgA circulates in the blood stream but, of more functional importance, it is also secreted across mucus membranes and is found in intestinal and bronchial secretions, tears and breast milk. Circulating IgA is monomeric, whilst secreted IgA has an 18 amino acid 'tailpiece' which enables polymerisation of IgA into dimers. Polymerisation is required for transport across epithelial membranes. IgA is subdivided into $IgA_1$ (serum) and $IgA_2$ (gut).

IgE is the principal antibody isotype involved in the immune response to parasites and in allergic reactions. The ε heavy chains possess an extra $C_H$ domain and the Fc component binds with high affinity to the FcεR1 receptor found on the surface membranes of mast cells, basophils and activated eosinophils.

### (iii) Effector functions of immunoglobulins

Antibodies act in several ways to combat invading pathogens. They bind to functionally critical sites on soluble toxins and free microorganisms, preventing binding to host cell surface molecules and hence effectively neutralising the toxin or microorganism. Antibodies bound to bacteria are able to activate a series of plasma proteins, known as complement, to produce molecules that are chemotactic for phagocytes, promote phagocytosis and can also directly destroy bacteria (Lambris *et al.*, 1999).

Antibodies bind to bacteria leaving the Fc component of the antibody exposed. Phagocytic cells possess Fc receptors, which when engaged by antibody Fc segments induce phagocytosis and destruction of the coated bacterium. This process is known as opsonisation. The type of phagocyte binding to the antibody Fc segment depends on the antibody isotype; macrophages and neutrophils possess IgM-specific and IgG-specific Fc receptors, whilst eosinophils possess IgE-specific Fc receptors. Opsonising antibodies reduce the diversity that confronts phagocytic cells by transforming antigenic diversity to a couple of types by the Fc segments, which are easily recognised by phagocytes that would otherwise be unable to engage and destroy the bacteria.

Sometimes, if virally infected host cells express viral antigens on their surfaces, they become the target of antibody-dependent cell-mediated cytotoxicity. The expressed viral antigens are bound by antibodies and the exposed Fc segments are engaged by natural killer (NK) cell surface receptors, resulting in the cytotoxic destruction of the host cell by the NK cell, and effective neutralisation of the virus. NK cells are large granular lymphocytes, defined by the absence of surface Ig or T cell receptors and the presence of FcγRIII molecules and CD56 (the neutral cell adhesion molecule-1). NK cells do not undergo clonal expansion, instead they provide innate cytotoxic immune responses directed against virally infected cells. They can interact with the adaptive immune response, as outlined above, and their secretion of cytokines is attracting increasing research attention (Fearon & Locksley, 1996).

#### (iv) T cell independent stimulation of B cells

For the vast majority of antigens, the binding of antigen to B cell surface immunoglobulin, alone, is insufficient to produce activation. To elicit an effective antibody response a second signal, provided by T cells, is required. These T cell dependent responses are associated with isotype switching, affinity maturation and the efficient development of memory B cells. Certain antigens associated with

specific bacterial infections can, however, elicit a B cell response independently of T cell help (Mond *et al.*, 1995). These thymus-independent (TI) antigens tend to be components of bacterial cell walls, such as capsular polysaccharides, lipopolysaccharides and polymeric proteins. These molecules have highly repetitive epitopes, which enable extensive cross-linking of surface immunoglobulin molecules, resulting in B cell activation. Some TI antigens also possess B cell mitogenic activity, which can induce polyclonal activation of B cells.

T cell independent B cell responses are rapid and specific, and are directed against bacteria possessing antiphagocytic polysaccharide capsules, *e.g.* *Streptococcus pneumoniae.* T cell independent responses, however, do not undergo isotype switching, have limited affinity maturation and are poor inducers of memory cells, because these are all properties of a T cell assisted B cell response.

### 2.4.4 T cells and cell mediated immunity

> **Points to note**
>
> - T cell mediated immunity is directed against intracellular pathogens.
> - T cell antigen specificity is conferred by T cell receptors.
> - T cells recognise antigenic peptides in association with MHC molecules.
> - Pathogen peptides processed within the cell cytosol are presented by MHC class I molecules.
> - Phagocytosis- or endocytosis-derived pathogen peptides are presented by MHC class II molecules.
> - MHC class I associated peptides are recognised by CD8$^+$ T cells.
> - MHC class II associated peptides are recognised by CD4$^+$ T cells.

Antibodies are highly effective against extracellular pathogens but they are unable to neutralise viruses and certain bacteria that function as intracellular pathogens. T cells identify cells infected by intracellular organisms and then mount and coordinate an effective immune response.

### (i) The T cell receptor

Each T cell possesses approximately 30 000 antigen-specific T cell receptor (TCR) molecules on its surface, each with the same antigen specificity. There is structural homology between T cell receptors and immunoglobulin molecules but, unlike B cell immunoglobulin molecules, the T cell receptor is always surface bound, is not secreted and does not undergo any form of isotype switching or somatic hypermutation. The T cell receptor is composed of two transmembrane glycoprotein chains linked by a disulphide bond. The majority (90%) of T cells use a single $\alpha$ chain and a single $\beta$ chain to form the T cell receptor, with the T cell receptors of the remaining 10% of T cells comprising a single $\gamma$ chain and a single $\delta$ chain. Although differences have been identified between $\alpha\beta$ and $\gamma\delta$ T cells, the true functional significance of the T cell receptor differences are unknown. The external part of each constituent T cell receptor chain consists of a variable domain and a constant domain. The internal part of each chain consists of a short hydrophobic transmembrane region and a short 'cytoplasmic tail'. Structural comparison of T cell receptors has demonstrated that the variable region is highly polymorphic, whereas the constant region is monomorphic and provides a structural scaffold for the antigen binding variable region. Each T cell receptor has a single antigen binding site formed by the apposition of the two amino terminal variable regions. During T cell maturation, random rearrangement of gene segments encoding the T cell receptor variable $\alpha$ chain and variable $\beta$ chain regions occurs, and these determine T cell receptor antigen specificity. It has been estimated that rearrangement of the genes encoding the $\alpha\beta$ T cell receptor produces $10^{15}$ variants, each with a different antigen specificity. Similar considerations suggest even greater diversity among $\gamma\delta$ chains, with an estimated $10^{18}$ specificities.

In contrast to B cells, T cells are only able to recognise antigens that are displayed on cell surfaces. During an infection by an intracellular pathogen, corruption of the infected host cell is signalled by the surface expression of pathogen-derived peptide fragments. These peptide fragments are transported to the cell surface and expressed in conjunction with glycoproteins encoded by the major histocompatibility complex (MHC). It is the combination of the pathogen peptide fragment bound to the MHC molecule that is recognised by T cells (Fremont *et al.*, 1996).

### (ii) The major histocompatibility complex (MHC)

The major histocompatibility complex has been reviewed by Germain (1994) and Huston (1997). It is a large complex of genes that encodes the major histocompatibility glycoproteins, which are also known as human leukocyte antigens (HLA) in humans. The MHC was originally identified and characterised by its profound influence on the rejection or acceptance of transplanted organs. The MHC is the molecular basis by which T cells recognise intracellular pathogens in order to initiate or effect an immune response. MHC molecules are large cell-surface glycoproteins. There are two structural variants and they are present in some form on every nucleated cell.

An MHC class I molecule consists of a highly polymorphic 44 kDa $\alpha$ chain, which is encoded within the MHC on chromosome 6. This chain is non-covalently associated with a smaller non-polymorphic 12 kDa $\beta_2$-microglobulin chain, which is encoded by a non-MHC gene on chromosome 15. The $\alpha$ chain spans the cell membrane and forms a cleft, into which binds the pathogen-derived peptide fragment. MHC class II molecules comprise a 34 kDa $\alpha$ chain and a 29 kDa $\beta$ chain; both span the cell membrane and are MHC coded. Each chain is divided into two domains, with association of the $\alpha_1$ and $\beta_1$ domains forming an open ended peptide binding cleft, into which processed antigen peptide fragments are incorporated.

The source of the peptide, bound by the two classes of MHC molecules, differs. MHC class I molecules bind peptides that originate from pathogen proteins synthesised within the cell cytosol, typically viruses and certain bacteria. The cytosolic pathogen proteins are degraded into peptides of 8–10 amino acids by proteasomes and the generated peptides are actively transported into the endoplasmic reticulum by TAP (transporters associated with antigen processing) proteins. Within the endoplasmic reticulum, a peptide fragment is incorporated into a folding MHC class I molecule to achieve its final configuration. The MHC class I/pathogen peptide complex is very stable and is expressed on the cell surface, ready for recognition by a T cell with T cell receptors specific for the combination of peptide and MHC molecule.

The peptides that are incorporated into MHC class II molecules are derived from pathogens that have been ingested/phagocytosed by macrophages or endocytosed (ingested by invagination of its plasma membrane) by antigen-presenting cells such as macrophages, B cells and professional antigen-presenting cells (*e.g.* dendritic cells). Once internalised into vesicles, these proteins are hydrolysed by acid proteases into peptide fragments. The endosomes containing these fragments fuse with vesicles containing newly synthesised MHC class II molecules. The peptide fragments are then incorporated into the MHC class II molecule to form a very stable complex, which is expressed on the cell surface.

Antigen-specific T cell receptors recognise the MHC/pathogen peptide complex, a process known as MHC restriction. All nucleated cells constitutively express MHC class I molecules; these are recognised by T cells expressing the CD8 (a classification of cell surface proteins) antigen. The CD8 antigen is a surface molecule that acts as a co-receptor by simultaneously binding to the T cell receptor and the MHC class I $\alpha_3$ domain. The simultaneous binding of CD8 and T cell receptor to the same MHC class I/pathogen peptide complex appears to increase the sensitivity of the T cell to the presented antigen by 100-fold. MHC class II molecules are constitutively expressed by cells that can present antigens to T cells to initiate or effect an immune response, namely macrophages, B cells and professional antigen-presenting cells. MHC class II/peptide complexes are recognised by T cells expressing the CD4 antigen, which acts as a co-receptor (like CD8) by binding to the $\beta_2$ domain of the MHC class II molecules already bound by a T cell receptor. This process is illustrated in Fig. 2.3. In humans, approximately one-third of peripheral blood T cells are CD8$^+$ (*i.e.* CD8 positive), two thirds are CD4$^+$ and approximately 5–10% are CD4$^-$ CD8$^-$ (*i.e.* CD4 negative and CD8 negative), the functions of which are unclear.

The structure of the peptide binding cleft determines the peptide binding specificity of an MHC molecule, such that it binds to peptides with a broadly similar structure. There are several genetic organisational features of the MHC that result in

nucleated cells expressing a highly polymorphic set of MHC molecules, each with differing peptide binding specificities. The polymorphic nature of the MHC is the consequence of:

(1) MHC being formed by three major class I genes designated HLA-A, HLA-B and HLA-C, and three main class II genes, HLA-DP, HLA-DQ and HLA-DR;
(2) each of these loci being highly polymorphic;
(3) co-dominant expression of the antigens coded by the maternally and paternally derived loci;
(4) most individuals being heterozygous for MHC genes.

The consequence of MHC polymorphism is that each individual expresses 6 class I and 10 class II molecules, each with differing specificities. During an infection, it is highly likely that the proteins of a pathogen include peptide sequences that are incorporated into at least one MHC molecule and this can be presented to T cells. The general explanation for MHC polymorphism is that it is an evolutionary response to pathogenic diversity, enabling the immune systems of individuals to respond to a wide range of existing and evolving pathogens. The polymorphism of MHC also results in individuals with differing immunological capabilities being able to combat an individual pathogen, but on a population scale it is highly unlikely that any individual pathogen will be able to evade the immune system of every individual.

### 2.4.5 The generation of effector T cells

T cell activation is the final step in a complex process. Antigen is processed and presented in association with MHC molecules; the antigen is then transported from the site of infection to the peripheral lymphoid organs and presented to T cells. The processing, transportation and presentation of antigen is performed by antigen-presenting cells, the most important and efficient of which are dendritic cells (Fig. 2.3). Dendritic cells are mandatory for the initiation of a primary immune response against a new pathogen. However, both dendritic cells and non-professional antigen-presenting cells, such as macrophages and B cells, are able to initiate secondary (memory) responses against reinfecting organisms (for a review, see Janeway & Bottomly, 1994).

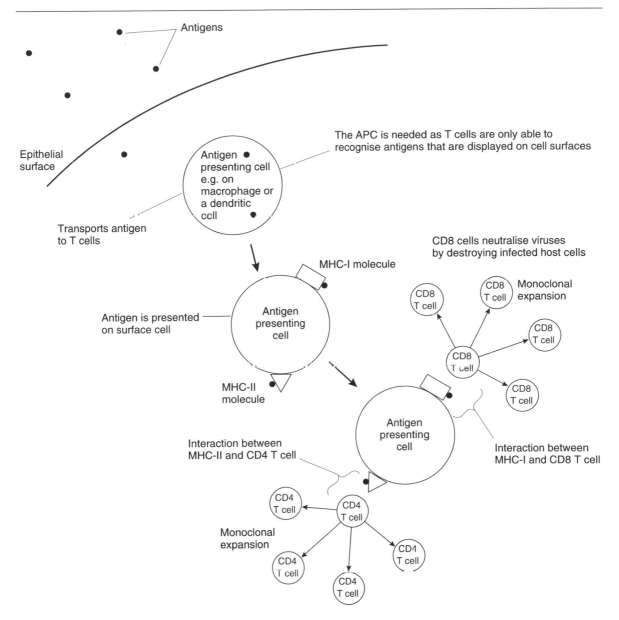

**Fig. 2.3** Interaction between antigen and T cells, and generation of effector T cells. T cells are only able to recognise antigens that are presented on cell surfaces, and so antigen presenting cells (APC), such as dendritic cells, are needed to perform this purpose. Specific molecules on the surface of the APC, known as major histocompatibility complex (MHC) I and II, bind CD8 and CD4 T cells, respectively. CD8 and CD4 are T cells that express the CD8 and CD4 cell surface proteins, respectively. This results in activation of the T cells to produce clones of themselves known as effector cells.

---

## Points to note

- Antigen-presenting cells sample tissues for antigen, then after processing migrate to local lymphoid organs to interact with T cells.
- Antigen presenting cells stimulate T cells by presentation of MHC restricted antigen and the provision of co-stimulatory signals.
- CD8$^+$ T cells neutralise viruses by destroying infected host cells (Fig. 2.4).
- CD4$^+$ Th cells neutralise intracellular bacteria, fungi and parasites by activation of phagocytic cells (Fig. 2.4).
- CD4$^+$ Th cells provide co-stimulatory signals to B cells to induce the full repertoire of the humoral response (Fig. 2.4).
- The MHC is a highly polymorphic set of cell surface antigens critical in T cell mediated immune responses.

---

### (i) Dendritic cells

Dendritic cells (reviewed by Banchereau & Steinman, 1998) are myeloid derived cells. After release from the bone marrow, they are widely distributed throughout the tissues, typically in association with epithelial surfaces. When viewed by phase contrast microscopy, dendritic cells extend long delicate motile processes in all directions. In peripheral tissues, dendritic cells are in a so-called 'immature' state and have poor T cell stimulatory activity; instead they act as sentinels, constantly sampling the surrounding tissues for pathogens. Immature dendritic cells phagocytose particulate antigens and microorganisms, and also sample the surrounding extracellular fluid for soluble antigens by macropinocytosis (a process by which cells ingest extracellular fluid). Dendritic cell surface receptors enable receptor-mediated transport across the cell membrane. These processes are so efficient that dendritic cells can initiate immune responses with pico- and nanomolar concentrations of antigens compared with the micromolar concentrations required by non-professional antigen-presenting cells such as B cells and macrophages.

Once a dendritic cell captures a pathogen-associated antigen it undergoes a series of maturational changes which reflect functional alterations. The phagocytic sampling function declines and the dendritic cell starts to process pathogenic antigens and present them in association with MHC molecules on its cell surface. Endocytosed antigens are presented in association with MHC class II molecules, whilst endogenously produced antigen, *e.g.* a virus infecting the dendritic cell, is presented in association with MHC class I molecules. Dendritic cells are able to process and present antigens in a class I restricted manner. This even includes those antigens that do not have access to the cytosolic compartment, *e.g.* viruses unable to infect dendritic cells, although the mechanism is unclear. As antigens are processed and expressed, dendritic cells upregulate surface expression of co-stimulatory molecules such as CD40 and B7, which are essential for T cell activation.

Dendritic cell maturation initiates the secretion of cytokines and chemotactic cytokines (chemokines), such as macrophage inflammatory protein 1 (MIP-1α), MIP-2, monocyte chemotactic protein 1 (MCP-1) and tumour necrosis factor α (TNF-α). These cytokines recruit macrophages, granulocytes, NK cells and more dendritic cells to counteract the invading pathogen.

In the next stage of maturation, dendritic cells bearing processed antigen migrate from the site of infection to the T cell areas of the local lymph nodes, there migration stops and dendritic cells interact with T and B cells to initiate an immune response. When localised to the local peripheral lymphoid tissue, the dendritic cells secrete cytokines, *e.g.* interleukin-12 (see Section 2.4.6), which have a profound effect on T cell function. Mature dendritic cells are extremely potent activators, with one dendritic cell being able to activate 100–3000 T cells. This potency has been attributed to the high density of MHC, and to co-stimulatory and adhesion molecules expressed on the relatively large dendritic cell surface area. Although dendritic cells are the most efficient activators of T cells, other cells are capable of presenting antigens to memory T cells.

Macrophages are phagocytic cells that play an important role in both the innate and adaptive immune responses. As part of the innate immune system they phagocytose bacteria, a process that activates and increases the ability of macrophages to present antigens and co-stimuli to T cells in a way comparable with dendritic cells.

B cells are also capable of presenting antigen. Soluble antigens bound to specific surface Ig are internalised, processed and presented on the cell surface by MHC class II molecules. In the presence of pathogenic bacteria, B cells can sometimes express the co-stimulatory B7 molecules that are essential for T cell activation.

### (ii) Interactions between dendritic cells and T cells

Naive T cells are constantly circulating between the blood stream and the peripheral lymphoid organs. During their passage throughout the peripheral lymphoid organs, they transiently adhere to antigen-presenting cells and, in the course of a day, contact is made with many thousands of dendritic cells. The transient adherence of the T cell enables the T cell receptor to 'sample' the many MHC peptide complexes on the surface of the antigen-presenting cells. Cell adhesion molecules mediate this adherence, *e.g.* lymphocyte function associated antigen-1 (LFA-1) of T cells and dendritic cell intercellular adhesion molecule-1 (ICAM-1). If the T cell receptor recognises its specific peptide/MHC molecular complex, conformational changes in the adhesion molecules are induced. These changes increase the interaction between antigen-presenting cell and T cell, and keep the T cell and its progeny in close proximity to their stimulating antigen.

Ligation or binding of a T cell receptor with a specific MHC/peptide complex, in conjunction with CD4 or CD8 co-receptors, is insufficient to trigger T cell proliferation and differentiation (Fig. 2.3). The antigen-presenting cell bearing the peptide/MHC complex must deliver a second stimulus to the T cell in order to induce the clonal expansion of the T cell. The antigen-presenting cell surface glycoproteins B7.1 (CD80) and B7.2 (CD86) provide the required co-stimulus when they are bound by their corresponding T cell surface receptor (CD28). In the induction of T cell activation, the need for simultaneous delivery of signals that are MHC restricted antigen-specific and co-stimulatory, by a single cell, means that only antigen-presenting cells can initiate T cell responses. Typically, the binding of the T cell receptor to MHC/peptide complex in the absence of co-stimulation leads to T cell anergy (unresponsiveness) or apoptosis (cell death).

### (iii) Clonal expansion and differentiation of T cells into effector cells

An antigen-specific and co-stimulatory interaction between T cell and antigen-presenting cell triggers the T cell to enter the cell cycle and proliferate (Fig. 2.3). Simultaneously, the T cell secretes the cytokine interleukin-2 (IL-2), which acts as an autocrine (stimulating secretion in local cells) protein growth factor to drive T cell proliferation and differentiation. More information about the function of cytokines can be found in Section 2.4.6. Concomitantly, the affinity of the T cell IL-2 receptors is increased by the synthesis and incorporation of the α chain of the IL-2 receptor molecule. The combination of signals from antigen-presenting cell and the autocrine secretion of IL-2 induces T cell clonal expansion, and after a few days thousands of progeny with the same antigen-specificity as the parent T cell are available to counteract the stimulating pathogen.

These effector T cells have different properties to the parent T cell. One of the most critical functional changes is that further encounters by effector T cells, with their specific antigen, result in immunological attack, with no further need for co-stimulation. The repertoire of expressed cell surface adhesion molecules also matures to enable the effector T cells to migrate out of the peripheral lymphoid organs, into the blood stream, and to adhere to vascular endothelium at sites of inflammation and/or infection. The T cells then migrate to the site of infection/inflammation to effect their immunological function. The immunological function of effector T cells is conveniently categorised by their CD4+/CD8+ status (see Fig. 2.4. for a summary of the interactions of the various components of the immune system discussed within Section 2.4).

### (iv) Effector CD8+ T cells

Effector CD8+ T cells (also known as cytotoxic T cells) are ideally suited to counteracting viral infections and are induced by MHC class I presentation of pathogen peptides to CD8+ T cells. The antiviral activity of CD8+ T cells depends on virally

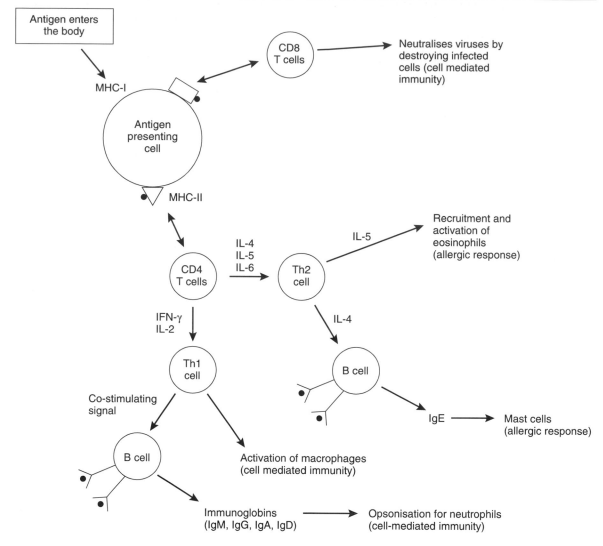

**Fig. 2.4** Simplified representation showing interactions between various components of the immune system and their roles: antigen-presenting cells, T cells and their effector cells, B cells, immunoglobulins and cytokines.

infected cells expressing viral peptide sequences in association with MHC class I molecules. The ability of effector T cells to effect immunological attack in the absence of co-stimulatory molecules is of particular relevance to effector CD8[+] T cells because most of their target cells express MHC class I restricted antigen in the absence of co-stimulatory B7 molecules. After migrating to a site of viral infection, CD8[+] T cells sample cell surfaces by transient adherence. The T cells identify virally

infected cells by the presence of cell surface MHC class I restricted viral peptides. Once a CD8[+] cell adheres to and identifies an infected cell, the corrupted cell is destroyed by directed localised secretion of cytotoxic enzymes (*e.g.* perforin and granzymes) by the CD8[+] cell; this effectively neutralises the viruses infecting the cell. Other antiviral properties of CD8[+] T cells include the secretion of the antiviral cytokine interferon-γ and expression of Fas-ligand (CD95L), which induces apoptosis in target cells bearing the Fas (CD95) receptor protein.

### 2.4.6 Effector CD4⁺ T cells

Effector CD8⁺ T cells are of major importance in the defence against viruses but they are ineffective in eliminating certain intracellular bacteria, fungi and parasites that are not neutralised by destruction of their host cell. CD4⁺ T cells are the mechanism by which the immune response neutralises these particularly resistant organisms. CD4⁺ T cells are more commonly known as T helper (Th) cells.

---

### Points to note

- T helper cells can be divided into two broad functional groups, Th1 and Th2.
- The Th1 group is defined by the secretion of interferon-γ and the Th2 group by the secretion of IL-4.
- Th1 differentiation is initiated by IL-12, secreted by macrophages and antigen-presenting cells.
- Th2 differentiation is stimulated by IL-4, the source of which is uncertain.
- Th1 cells direct coordinated IgG mediated and macrophage mediated destruction of intracellular bacteria and fungi.
- Th2 cells direct IgE mediated and eosinophil mediated destruction of helminths.
- Inappropriate Th1 responses are the basis of delayed-type hypersensitivity reactions, *e.g.* gluten sensitive enteropathy (see Chapter 9).
- Inappropriate Th2 responses are the basis of IgE mediated allergy.

---

#### (i) T helper cells and macrophages

Macrophages usually destroy phagocytosed microorganisms but certain pathogens, *e.g. Mycobacteria*, *Leishmania* and *Pneumocystis*, resist macrophage destruction, and Th cells (T helper cells) are required to increase macrophage destruction of these organisms (for a review, see Stout &

Bottomly, 1989). After directed migration of Th cells to the site of infection, Th cells sample the surface molecular repertoire of adjacent cells by transient adhesion to cell surfaces. Macrophage activation is initiated if a Th cell adheres to and recognises the particular macrophage-presented MHC class II restricted pathogen peptide, that is identical to that which induced clonal expansion of the progenitor Th cell. This interaction between macrophage and Th cell, alone, is insufficient to activate the macrophage, and two further signals are required. The first is interferon-γ, which is usually secreted locally by the engaged Th cell, but other sources of IFN-γ are also important, *e.g.* CD8⁺ T cells secrete IFN-γ. The second signal sensitises the macrophage to IFN-γ. This second signal can also be provided by Th cells that express surface CD40 ligand molecule, which interacts with macrophage surface CD40 molecules.

Clearly, Th cells are extremely potent antigen-specific macrophage activators because they provide both the IFN-γ and CD40 signals required for macrophage activation. Other signals, however, are able to sensitise macrophages to IFN-γ, amongst those identified to date are bacterial lipopolysaccharide, TNF-α and TNF-β.

Th cell induced activation greatly enhances the macrophage's antimicrobial and antigen-presenting capacity. The increased antimicrobial capacity of activated macrophages in part derives from:

(1) Increased efficiency of lysosome fusion with microbe-containing phagosomes.
(2) Increased synthesis of antimicrobial proteases and peptides, such as defensins.
(3) Release of free radicals. Induction of the respiratory burst produces extremely microbiocidal products, such as the superoxide anion $O_2^-$, singlet oxygen $^1O_2$, hydroxyl radical $OH^·$, and hydrogen peroxide $H_2O_2$.
(4) Production of the reactive nitrogen metabolite nitric oxide (NO), which is increased by activation of the enzyme, inducible NO synthase (iNOS).

Activation also increases the ability of macrophages to present antigen; the expression of MHC class I and II molecules is increased along with co-stimulatory B7 molecules. Activation increases macrophage cytokine secretion, with the cytokines

IL-12, IFN-α and TNF-α being of particular importance in the differentiation of Th cells.

Macrophage activation is associated with the release of antimicrobial mediators, which are not only toxic to microorganisms but are also extremely toxic to host cells, and these damage host tissue. Therefore, macrophage activation is tightly regulated and extremely pathogen-specific, and this control is effected by highly specialised and antigen-specific Th cells. Thus the price paid by the host, in terms of tissue damage, in order to destroy these difficult invading intracellular organisms, is minimised.

### (ii) Th cells and B cells

Th cell facilitation of B cell activation is essential for full expression of the humoral immune response, particularly isotype switching, affinity maturation and immunological memory. B cell responses to thymus-dependent antigens require activating signals from two sources; the first is the binding of B cell surface-bound IgM/IgD to the complementary microorganism surface epitope and the second is Th cell derived. After binding of antigen to B cell surface Ig, the antigen/Ig complex is internalised, degraded and peptide segments are presented on the cell surface in association with MHC class II molecules. It is these peptide/MHC class II complexes that are recognised by the Th cell. If a Th cell is to provide the appropriate B cell activating signals, it is essential that the peptide sequences recognised by the Th cell originate from the antigen recognised by the B cell via its surface Ig. This process of linked recognition means that the B cell and the Th cell respond to different epitopes but the epitopes originate from the same antigen; typically the B cell recognises a surface epitope and the Th cell possibly recognises an internal peptide sequence. For full B cell activation, the Th cell provides secreted and cell-bound signals. Effector Th cells express surface CD40 ligand and this binds to CD40 molecules present on the B cell surface. Th cell cytokine secretion is also critical in B cell activation and maturation. Once activated, B cells undergo clonal expansion and differentiation into Ig-secreting plasma cells, which secrete Ig isotypes with the same antigen specificity as the parent B cell. Cell–cell interactions are not required for plasma cells to express their anti-

microbial function because their secreted Igs are widely distributed, so plasma cells tend to localise to lymph node medullary cords and the bone marrow.

Clearly, macrophages and B cells are critically dependent on Th cells, yet clinical and experimental observations suggest that some responses mediated by CD4$^+$ Th cells are antibody-based, whilst others are macrophage based. For example, healing tuberculoid leprosy is associated with strong macrophage-mediated immunity (commonly known as delayed-type hypersensitivity [DTH] immunity) with low levels of antibodies, whilst non-healing lepromatous leprosy is associated with high levels of antibodies, weak DTH immunity and uncontrolled proliferation of microorganisms. The situation becomes even more complex when individuals experience changes in Th cell mediated immunity from lepromatous to tuberculoid leprosy. The understanding of these observations has been helped by the discovery that Th cells are functionally diverse.

### (iii) Functional diversity of Th cell

Experimental and clinical observations suggest that CD4$^+$ Th cells initiate immune responses with differing effector mechanisms (reviewed by Abbas *et al.*, 1996; Mosmann & Sad, 1996). The explanation for this came with the seminal study of Mosmann and Coffman (1989) who demonstrated that murine CD4$^+$ T cell clones could be categorised into two broad functional groups (Th1 and Th2), based on their secreted cytokines (Fig. 2.5). The Th1 cells secrete IFN-γ, IL-2 and TNF-β, whilst Th2 cells secrete IL-4, IL-5, IL-6, IL-9, IL-10 and IL-13. Both Th1 and Th2 clones secrete IL-3, TNF-α and granulocyte-macrophage colony stimulating factor (GM-CSF).

Human Th1 and Th2 cells produce similar patterns of cytokine secretion to the murine model, although the synthesis of IL-2, IL-6, IL-10 and IL-13 is not so tightly restricted to a single subset as demonstrated in mice. It has also been demonstrated in humans that individual Th cells can secrete both nominally Th1 and Th2 cytokines; these cells are commonly known as Th0. It would appear that the cytokine profiles of human Th cells form a continuum, with some extremely polarised cells typically secreting either Th1 or Th2

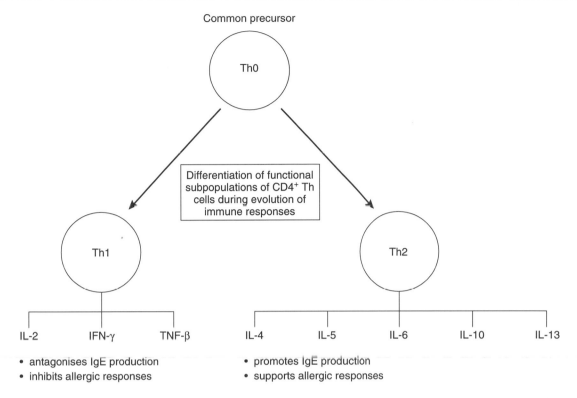

Common precursor

Th0

Differentiation of functional subpopulations of CD4$^+$ Th cells during evolution of immune responses

Th1

Th2

IL-2    IFN-γ    TNF-β

IL-4    IL-5    IL-6    IL-10    IL-13

- antagonises IgE production
- inhibits allergic responses

- promotes IgE production
- supports allergic responses

**Fig. 2.5** Functional subpopulations of T lymphocytes and allergy. T helper cells initiate immune responses with differing effector mechanisms (Th1 and Th2). In this simplified representation of the Th1/Th2 dichotomy, an undifferentiated CD4$^+$ T helper cell (Th0) is stimulated to proliferate and differentiate towards either Th1 (T helper cell 1) or Th2 (T helper cell 2) polarisation. Th1 and Th2 cells produce different sets of cytokines. The cytokines secreted determine subsequent events.

cytokines, and the majority of Th0 cells secreting a mixture of Th1 and Th2 cytokines in differing proportions (so that some are 'Th1-dominant' and others 'Th2-dominant'). The subdivision of Th cells is complicated further by the recognition that some Th2 cells predominantly secrete the suppressive regulatory cytokine, transforming growth factor-β (TGF-β), and some authorities term these cells Th3. In recent years it has become apparent that the Th1/Th2 subdivision is too simple, but the concept of the functional dichotomy of Th1/Th2 is extremely important in the understanding of the immune responses, especially allergy. In the remainder of the Chapter, Th1 refers to responses dominated by IFN-γ and Th2 refers to responses dominated by IL-4, IL-5 and IL-13, with their respective cytokine profiles being termed Th1 and Th2 cytokines.

Th1 and Th2 cytokines have important effector functions that are described below, but additionally they have important Th cell regulatory effects (Fig. 2.6). Each Th cell subset produces cytokines that function as autocrine growth factors, augmenting differentiation of Th cells in favour of that subset, *i.e.* Th1 cytokines promote differentiation towards the Th1 phenotype and Th2 cytokines toward the Th2 phenotype. Cytokines promote specific Th cell differentiation further, by inhibiting differentiation towards the reciprocal Th cell phenotype; *i.e.* Th1 cytokines inhibit differentiation towards the Th2 phenotype and Th2 cytokines antagonise the development of Th1 cells. The result of this self-amplification and mutual antagonism of the reciprocal phenotype is that once a Th cell mediated immune response deviates towards either

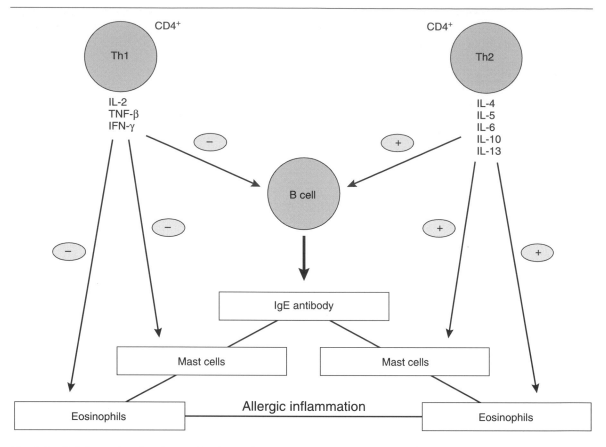

**Fig. 2.6**  Cellular and molecular mechanisms of allergy. Two main types of CD4$^+$ T helper cell are recognised and these are designated Th1 and Th2. (A similar dichotomy has also been described for CD8$^+$ T cells.) Type 1 cells produce interleukin 2 (IL-2), tumour necrosis factor $\beta$ (TNF-$\beta$) and interferon $\gamma$ (IFN-$\gamma$), whereas type 2 cell products include interleukins 4, 5, 6, 10 and 13 (IL-4, IL-5, IL-6, IL-10 and IL-13). These cytokines exert reciprocal effects on IgE antibody responses, and on the development, localisation and function of those cells (mast cells and eosinophils) that together with IgE antibody effect immediate-type hypersensitivity reactions and more chronic inflammatory responses. (Source: adapted from Department of Health, 1997.)

the Th1 or Th2 phenotype, then the Th cell response becomes increasingly polarised towards that phenotype. Not surprisingly, in humans the best evidence of Th1/Th2 functional polarisation is found in situations of chronic immune stimulation such as that present in tuberculosis, allergy and rheumatoid arthritis.

### 2.4.7 Effector mechanisms of Th1 mediated immunity

Th1 biased Th cells appear to be critical in effecting an antigen-specific phagocyte-mediated defence against microorganisms, principally bacteria, fungi and some parasites. Th1 cells are also important in type IV delayed-type hypersensitivity reactions, such as that found in coeliac disease (Chapter 9). Macrophages that have phagocytosed microorganisms normally resistant to lysosomal destruction are activated by Th1 cytokines in conjunction with surface CD40 ligand. Th1 cytokines also direct isotype switching of B cells towards IgG production. In mice, Th1 cytokines promote secretion of the opsonising antibodies IgG2a and IgG3. The influences of Th1 cytokines on human IgG secretion are not so well characterised, but extrapolation from the murine model suggests the human analogues IgG1 and IgG3 would be promoted. These opsonising antibodies bind to microorganisms and promote their phagocytosis by macrophages and neutrophils. This is the result of their affinity for phagocytes possessing Fcγ receptors (see Section 2.4.3) and their ability to activate components of complement.

Th1 cytokines also recruit phagocytic cells to sites of infection. Secretion of the haemopoetic growth factors IL-3 and GM-CSF promotes bone marrow stem cell proliferation, differentiation and the generation of large numbers of phagocytes. These are directed to the site of infection by changes in the adhesive properties of local endothelial cells, induced by the secretion of TNF-α and TNF-β by Th1 cells. Chemotaxis is promoted by the release of chemokines by the Th1 cells.

In an elegantly efficient manner, Th1 biased Th cells secrete cytokines, which not only promote Th1 differentiation and inhibit Th2 development, but also induce a complex package of biological responses directed towards the phagocytic destruction of invading microorganisms.

## 2.4.8 Effector mechanisms of Th2 mediated immunity

The Th2 cytokines are believed to be important in the immune responses against helminth infections and in the immuno-pathogenesis of allergy/type I hypersensitivity. Th2 cytokines induce the isotype switching of B cells to the synthesis of IgE; they also promote the growth, differentiation and release of mast cells and eosinophils from the bone marrow. Eosinophils are directed towards sites of helminth infection and allergy by chemokines, such as eotaxin, which are released by Th cells. Th2 cytokines also activate eosinophils. In a situation analogous to Th1-biased responses, Th2-biased Th cells induce a package of biological responses, which are characteristic of allergy and helminth infection, namely high levels of circulating IgE, mastocytosis and tissue eosinophilia (Figs 2.4 and 2.5).

It should also be mentioned that several of the cytokines characteristic of the Th2 phenotype have anti-inflammatory actions, and inhibit many pro-inflammatory macrophage functions. Some authorities have raised the possibility that Th2-biased

responses are important regulators of the immune response and principally act to limit the tissue damage associated with Th1-biased immune responses.

As mentioned in Section 2.4.6iii, the Th1/Th2 functional dichotomy is an oversimplification because there is evidence of critical involvement of Th1 cytokines in helminth infections and Th2 cytokines in responses mounted against intracellular pathogens such as leishmania. It would seem logical that CD4⁺ Th cell mediated immunity should not be as simple as outlined above, because pathogens would rapidly evolve to subvert Th1 and Th2 cytokines. Clearly, CD4⁺ Th cell responses to a microorganism should be broad, with elements of both Th1 and Th2 responses required for a healthy outcome for the host (Allen & Maizels, 1997).

### (i) Factors affecting Th1/Th2 differentiation

Unlike T cells that are predestined to mature into cytotoxic CD8⁺ T cells, Th1 and Th2 cells are not derived from distinct precommitted lineages but both subsets develop from the same CD4⁺ T cell precursor. Differentiation of naive Th cell precursors is determined by genetic and environmental factors, influential at the time of T cell antigen recognition. Several factors influencing Th1/Th2 polarisation have been proposed and demonstrated but the most potent factor is the local cytokine milieu present at the time of T cell activation. Interestingly, many of the influential cytokines are secreted by cells of the innate immune system, responding to microorganisms, and thus the nature of the innate response can influence the adaptive immune response. See Chapter 5 Section 5.2.2 for a brief discussion of the relationship between infection and allergy in early life.

The most potent cytokine stimulus for promoting development of the Th1 phenotype is IL-12 in the absence of IL-4 (Trinchieri & Gerosa, 1996). Macrophages and professional antigen-presenting cells, such as dendritic cells, secrete IL-12. This process is stimulated by bacteria (*e.g. Staphylococcus aureus*), bacterial products ( *e.g.* lipopolysaccharide) and intracellular parasites (*e.g. Toxoplasma gondil*). IL-12 is extremely potent in promoting Th1-biased differentiation by direct influences on the Th cells. Receptors for IL-12 appear to be restricted to recently activated, uncommitted Th cells and Th1 cells, and are absent from differentiated Th2 cells, although there is evidence of functional IL-12 receptors on memory Th2 cells.

The most potent Th2-promoting stimulus is IL-4 in the absence of IFN-γ. Early work suggesting that Th cell IL-4 secretion could only occur after Th2 differentiation, raised the conceptual problem of the initial source of polarising IL-4 (Ricci *et al.*, 1997). Naive Th cells can produce small amounts of IL-4 at the time of their initial activation and the local IL-4 concentration increases with increasing lymphocyte activation until IL-4 predominates locally. The stimulus to the initial secretion of IL-4 by naive Th cells is unclear, but environmental and/or genetic factors may be influential. An alternative source of Th2 polarising IL-4 is a small specialised subset of $CD4^+$ T cells, known as $CD4^+$ NK1.1 T cells, which express the NK1.1 marker normally associated with NK cells. NK1.1 cells are more fully characterised in mice, although their counterparts have been identified in humans. NK1.1 cells have been shown to account for much of the prompt IL-4 production in response to CD3 stimulation *in vivo*. The role of human NK1.1 cells in Th2 differentiation is not established, but their ability to secrete large amounts of IL-4 on primary activation is intriguing. It has also been shown that antigen presentation by B cells can stimulate Th2 differentiation (Mason, 1996). Microorganisms can induce IL-4 secretion by mast cells and basophils, but anatomical considerations rule out a major *in vivo* effect.

Although the cytokine micro-environment is the most potent determinant of Th1/Th2 polarisation, other influences have been identified. Th1/Th2 differentiation is influenced by complex interactions between antigen dose, T cell receptor and MHC antigen affinities (Murray, 1998). Influential antigenic properties include the nature of the antigen, with viruses and bacteria favouring Th1 differentiation and helminths favouring Th2. Th2 differentiation appears to be promoted by the small, highly soluble proteins characteristic of allergens. Some important allergens (house dust mite allergen, subtilisin and papain) are proteases and it is suggested that this favours Th2 differentiation because helminths secrete proteases to aid tissue penetration.

It is apparent that many factors are influential in Th1/Th2 differentiation. The cytokine milieu, type of antigen-presenting cell, co-stimulatory mole-cules, dose and antigen factors have all been shown to exert their effects. It is highly unlikely that any single criterion is the sole determinant of Th cell differentiation because this would quickly be perverted by rapidly evolving pathogens. The complex matrix of factors that eventually determine Th0, Th1 or Th2 polarisation is probably an immunological evolutionary adaptation, to reduce the scope for pathogen interference.

The human immune system has developed as a defence against pathogenic microorganisms but in a significant minority of individuals the immune system effects a response against non-pathogenic antigens. The magnitude of these inappropriate responses far outweighs any threat posed by the antigen, indeed the harmful effect of these antigens is the consequence of the maladaptive immune responses directed against them. These pathogenic immune responses are the basis of two important classes of adverse reactions to food, namely, delayed-type hypersensitivity reactions (Th1) and IgE mediated allergy (Th2) (Figs 2.4 and 2.5).

## 2.5 Allergy

### Points to note

- IgE mediated allergy is the basis of atopic asthma, atopic eczema, hayfever, IgE mediated food allergy and systemic ana-phylaxis.
- Cross-linkage of IgE on the surface of mast cells induces mast cell degranulation, releasing pro-inflammatory mediators.
- The symptoms of mast cell degranaulation are dependent on the site, dose of antigen and concentration of IgE.
- Ingested allergen may induce localised gastrointestinal symptoms, localised distant symptoms or dangerous systemic anaphy-laxis.
- Non-IgE mediated allergy/delayed-type hypersensitivity is the basis of gluten sensitive enteropathy (coeliac disease).
- Non-IgE mediated allergy/delayed-type hypersensitivity is characterised by chronic T cell mediated inflammation and tissue damage.

Allergy is derived from the Greek γγoς (allos), meaning other, and ργειν (ergein), meaning to work, and was first used in 1906 by Von Pirquet to describe altered immune reactivity. Allergy is most easily understood if it is defined as the adverse health effects derived from an immune response. In 1963, Coombs and Gell defined four classes of allergic/hypersensitivity reactions according to the underlying pathological processes. Type I hypersensitivity reactions are immediate-type reactions, mediated by IgE induced degranulation of mast cells, and are the immunopathogenic basis of IgE mediated food allergies. Type IV hypersensitivity reactions are T cell mediated and underlie gluten sensitive enteropathies (see Chapter 9) and a type of cows' milk intolerance in which the response is delayed (Chapter 7).

### 2.5.1 IgE mediated allergy

IgE mediated allergic disease occurs when a Th2 biased immune response is directed against a non-pathogenic antigen, such as food constituents, pollens, and animal or insect dander (Fig. 2.5). The IgE stimulated by the Th2 biased response is specific for the stimulating antigen and circulates in the blood stream, although most IgE is bound to tissue mast cells, which possess high affinity FcεR1 receptors on their cell surface. Exposure of IgE-coated mast cells to specific multivalent antigen induces cross-linkage of the IgE, degranulation of the mast cell and the release of pro-inflammatory mediators responsible for the clinical features of allergy (Fig. 2.7).

### (i) Mast cells and allergy

Mast cells are derived from bone marrow and, after release into the circulation in an immature form, they migrate from the vascular space into the tissues where they differentiate into recognisable mature mast cells (reviewed by Costa *et al.*, 1997; Mecheri & David, 1997). Tissue mast cells have characteristic granules that stain readily with

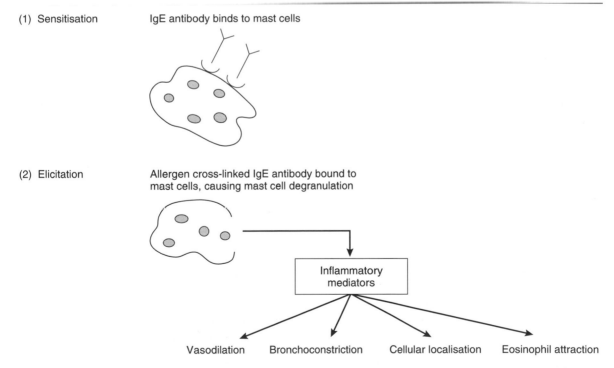

**Fig. 2.7** IgE mediated allergy. A representation of the central role of the mast cell in type I immediate type hypersensitivity. Cross-linkage of surface bound IgE induces mast cell degranulation and the release and synthesis of various inflammatory mediators.

certain basic dyes. They are widely distributed throughout connective tissue, with a tendency to lie adjacent to blood vessels, lymphatics and nerves. They are also particularly numerous in mucosal and epithelial tissues exposed to the external environment, such as those of the respiratory and gastrointestinal systems and the skin. From their distribution, mast cells appear well situated to defend against invading microorganisms. Immunocytochemical studies have shown the presence of two tissue mast cell phenotypes. The granules of $MC_T$ mast cells contain tryptase and those of the $MC_{TC}$ phenotype contain tryptase and chymase. $MC_T$ mast cells tend to be found in mucosal epithelia and appear to be involved in the immune response against pathogens; their numbers are increased at sites of Th2-biased response found in allergy and helminth infections. $MC_{TC}$ mast cells predominate in connective tissues and their numbers are increased at sites of tissue remodelling and angiogenesis; they appear not to be primarily regulated by infection, allergy or the immune system. Although there appears to be immunocytochemical heterogeneity, both $MC_T$ and $MC_{TC}$ phenotypes possess surface FcR1 receptors, can bind IgE and can degranulate.

Mast cells can be activated by a number of stimuli, the best understood of which is antigen cross-linking of surface bound IgE. The cross-linking of a few hundred IgE molecules is sufficient to induce mast cell activation, which is mediated by an influx of calcium ions into the mast cell. Mast cell expression of $Fc\varepsilon R1$ receptors is upregulated by increased circulating levels of IgE. A variety of non-specific stimuli such as bacteria, parasites, the anaphylotoxin components of complement, physical stimuli (trauma, cold) and chemical agents, such as opiates and muscle relaxants, can also activate mast cells.

Mast cell activation induces the rapid (within seconds) release of preformed and rapidly synthesised mediators. Human mast cell granules principally contain histamine, serine proteases and proteoglycans. Within the granule the proteoglycans (principally heparin and chondroitin sulphates) bind ionically with histamine and the proteases to form a crystalline structure, which is solubilised upon activation and degranulation. The biological actions of histamine include bronchoconstriction, mucus secretion, vasodilatation, nerve stimulation, increased vascular permeability and tissue oedema. The serine proteases, tryptase and chymase, have kallikrein-like activity to produce kinins, they can cleave bronchodilator peptides to produce bronchoconstriction. The proteases may also have a role in tissue remodelling because they can break down collagen and stimulate fibroblast activity. The secreted proteoglycans, heparin and chondroitin sulphate, appear to have anti-inflammatory properties, they also have anti-coagulant, anticomplement and antikallikrein activity. In addition, they are able to sequester eosinophil major basic protein and have numerous growth factor enhancing properties.

Mast cell activation also induces the liberation of membrane-derived arachidonic acid, which is metabolised to proinflammatory mediators (Fig. 2.8). Arachidonic acid is oxidised by the cyclooxygenase pathway to form prostaglandin $D_2$ ($PGD_2$) or by the 5-lipoxygenase pathway to form leukotriene $A_4$ ($LTA_4$) and the cysteinyl leukotrienes, $LTC_4$, $LTD_4$ and $LTE_4$. $PGD_2$ and the cysteinyl leukotrienes are potent bronchoconstrictors. They also promote mucus secretion, are vasodilators and increase vascular permeability and tissue oedema. $PGD_2$ is also chemotactic for human neutrophils, whilst the cysteinyl leukotrienes are eosinophil chemotactic agents.

In recent years, interest in mast cells has been rekindled by the discovery that activation induces the secretion of preformed cytokines. Activated mast cells secrete Th2 cytokines and other cytokines and chemokines, which promote Th2 differentiation and an influx of lymphocytes and eosinophils.

IgE mediated mast cell activation produces the clinical patterns associated with IgE mediated allergy because the degranulating mast cells release important inflammatory mediators that orchestrate an intense local inflammatory response (Fig. 2.9). This rapid inflammatory response is the pathophysiologic hallmark of IgE mediated allergy and is known as the immediate hypersensitivity reaction. The immediate response is rapid, intense, but short lived because of rapid degradation of the inflammatory mediators. In some individuals, the immediate response is followed 4 to 8 hours later by a slowly developing, intense and sustained response, known as the late phase reaction. The late phase response is the pathophysiologic basis for

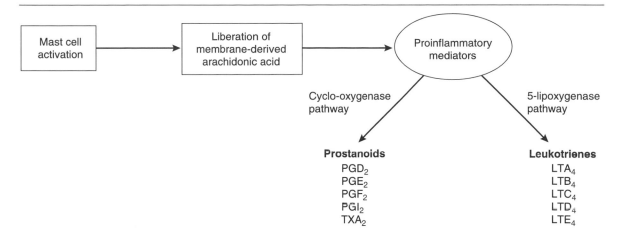

**Fig. 2.8** Proinflammatory mediators released from mast cells following stimulation by IgE. PGD$_2$, LTC$_4$, LTD$_4$ and LTE$_4$ are potent bronchoconstrictors, promote mucus secretion, are vasodilators and increase vascular permeability. PGD$_2$ attracts neutrophils and LTC$_4$, LTD$_4$ and LTE$_4$ attract eosinophils.

chronic allergic inflammatory responses such as those found in asthma (Fig. 2.9). The late phase response is initiated by the mast cell degranulation of the immediate hypersensitivity reaction, which releases leukotrienes, prostaglandins, chemokines and cytokines, which in turn recruit and activate eosinophils, neutrophils, basophils, macrophages and Th2 cells. The influx and activation of these cells releases further leukotrienes, prostaglandins, chemokines and cytokines, which induce a second phase allergic response. The recruited cells can also mobilise further inflammatory cells and this self-perpetuating response is the probable basis of chronic allergic inflammation. The process of mast cell initiation of cellular inflammation has been termed the 'mast cell leukocyte cytokine cascade'.

### (ii) Eosinophils

IgE mediated allergy and helminth infections are characterised by eosinophilia and eosinophil infiltration of tissues. Eosinophils are derived from bone marrow granulocytes, which are released into the blood stream (Costa *et al.*, 1997). Most localise to the connective tissues immediately beneath mucosal surfaces exposed to the external environment. Eosinophils have a bilobed nucleus and the cytoplasm contains distinctive granules that stain heavily with eosin. The development and differ-

entiation of eosinophils is promoted by Th2 cytokines. Eosinophils express receptors for IgG (FcγRI, FcγRII), IgA (FcαR) and, in the activated state, they express the high and low affinity IgE receptors (FcεRI, FcεRII, respectively). Eosinophils also express receptors for components of the complement cascade and Th2 cytokines.

The effector function of eosinophils is mediated by the release of their granular contents, and the secretion of lipid mediators and cytokines. Eosinophil granules contain lysosomal hydrolases and the cationic proteins, major basic protein, eosinophil cationic protein, eosinophil derived neurotoxin and eosinophil peroxidase, which are unique to eosinophils. These cationic proteins have bactericidal and antihelminthic activity, but they are also toxic to host cells and contribute to the tissue damage associated with allergy. Amongst the lipid mediators released by activated eosinophils, the products of 5-lipoxygenase oxidation of arachidonic acid predominate; principally the cysteinyl leukotrienes, the pro-inflammatory effects of which have been mentioned in Section 2.5.1*i*. The recognition that activated eosinophils secrete cytokines has focused attention on the role of eosinophils in the initiation and perpetuation of the chronic allergic inflammatory state. Activated eosinophils secrete Th2 cytokines and chemokines, which promote eosinophil differentiation, chemotaxis and

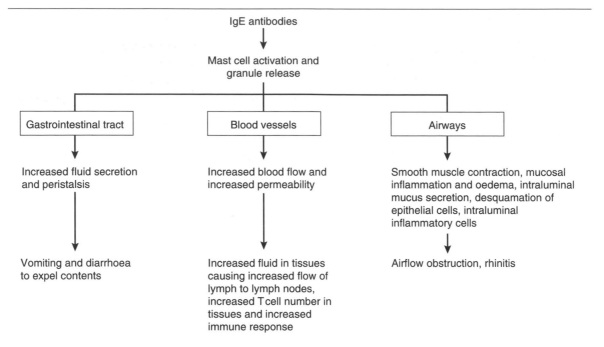

**Fig. 2.9** Effects of products of mast cells in different organs. Mast cells reside in tissues and orchestrate allergic reactions through the release of molecules, which together induce both acute and late-phase (chronic) inflammatory responses (adapted from Janeway *et al.* 1999).

activation and, unless carefully controlled, the possibility of a harmful self-perpetuating eosinophil-mediated inflammatory process can (and probably does) occur.

### (iii) Th cells

Th cells form a significant component of the cellular influx associated with the late phase response. The role of Th2-biased cells in the allergic response and their interactions with eosinophils have been mentioned in Section 2.5.1*ii*. In recent years, it has become apparent that mast cells may actively participate in the regulation of T and B cell mediated immunity. Mast cells are able to secrete preformed Th2 cytokines rapidly, with the potential to bias Th cell differentiation towards the Th2 phenotype. They are also able to orchestrate eosinophil mediated inflammation locally.

The interaction between mast cell and T cell, however, may be more direct and fundamental than traditionally thought. Mast cells are able to phagocytose bacteria and present derived antigenic

peptides in association with MHC class I and II molecules (see Section 2.4). They also express the co-stimulatory molecules B7.1 and B7.2. These findings suggest that mast cells are able to function as efficient antigen-presenting cells and may be involved in the generation of effector CD8[+] cytotoxic T cells and CD4[+] Th cells. The secreted cytokine profile of mast cells suggests that they are most likely to promote Th2 differentiation. Mast cells have also been shown to provide sufficient cell contact signals to B cells to promote the secretion of IgE; this can occur in the absence of T cells. Mast cells may also be activated by Th cells in a fashion analogous to T cell mediated activation of macrophages because they express the CD40 molecule on their surface, along with MHC-presented antigenic peptide. These are features associated with Th cell mediated activation of phagocytic cells (see Section 2.4).

The late phase response of the allergic reaction is obviously complex; the tissue damage and inflammation are the consequence of the secretion of proinflammatory mediators. The perpetuation of the inflammation into a chronic response is incompletely understood, but it is probable that continuing allergen exposure and self-perpetuating interactions between participating cells contribute to persisting allergic inflammation.

### 2.5.2 Clinical patterns of IgE mediated allergy

Sensitised individuals may be exposed to allergens by inhalation, ingestion or injection, and although the response of IgE-primed mast cells is stereotyped, the clinical expression of the allergic response is in part dependent upon the anatomic site of the allergic reaction (Fig. 2.9).

If inhaled allergens are deposited in the respiratory bronchi, acute mast cell degranulation gives rise to the symptoms of acute asthma, whereas the chronic allergic inflammatory state is associated with chronic asthma (Arm & Lee, 1992). The immediate hypersensitivity response is associated with widespread airflow obstruction resulting from bronchoconstriction, mucosal oedema and intraluminal mucus plugging. Acute and devastating bronchoconstriction usually occurs in response to exposure to allergen; fortunately, it is not common. The bronchi from most patients with asthma are chronically inflamed, with eosinophils and Th cells predominating. Chronic airflow obstruction is the consequence of bronchoconstriction, mucosal oedema and intraluminal mucus but, additionally, there is chronic remodelling of airway tissues. Growth factors released by Th cells and eosinophils may be responsible for such airway remodelling. Chronic allergic bronchial inflammation is associated with increased bronchial hyper-reactivity, which is the increased tendency of airways to bronchoconstrict in response to a stimulus. With established bronchial hyper-reactivity, bronchoconstriction can occur spontaneously or in response to non-allergic irritant stimuli such as cold air, cigarette smoke, viral infections and particulate air pollution.

Inhaled allergen may be deposited on the nasal mucosa giving rise to the symptoms associated with allergic rhinitis, namely sneezing and nasal congestion. The sneezing probably results from the stimulation of afferent nerve fibres by histamine, $PGD_2$, $LTC_4$ and kinins. Nasal congestion is induced acutely by mucosal oedema and mucus secretion; however, in the long term, chronic changes in the nasal mucosa may occur, as may nasal polyps, which are characteristically heavily infiltrated with eosinophils.

Ingestion of allergen by a sensitised subject can result in a number of different clinical manifestations depending on the dose of allergen, rapidity of absorption and the tissue distribution of the absorbed allergen (Sampson, 1997). The signs and symptoms of an immediate hypersensitivity reaction to food may occur within minutes or be delayed for up to 2 hours. If mast cell degranulation is limited to the oropharyngeal mucosa, itching or tingling of the lips, palate, tongue and pharynx may occur by neuronal stimulation. Increased vascular permeability and tissue oedema may induce life-threatening swelling of the lips, tongue and pharynx. Mast cell degranulation, limited to the gastrointestinal tract, may manifest as smooth muscle contraction and extravasation of fluid into the gut lumen, giving rise to the symptoms of vomiting, nausea, colicky abdominal pain and diarrhoea. This response to ingested allergens is analogous to the response to helminth infection, which is the natural target of IgE mediated immunity, whereby gastrointestinal tract mast cell degranulation attempts to mechanically expel the invading pathogen.

Ingested allergen may penetrate the gut mucosa and give rise to signs and symptoms in distant tissues. If the ingested allergen localises in the subcutaneous tissues of the skin, widespread wheal and flare reactions known as urticaria may occur. Wheal and flare is the term used to describe the immediate hypersensitivity response to subcutaneous allergen. Local mast cell activation results in an erythematous (vasodilatation) wheal (increased vascular permeability and oedema) surrounded by an area of vasodilatation, known as the flare induced by the stimulation of a neural reflex. The wheal and flare reaction is the basis of skin prick testing, whereby a small dose of allergen is introduced subcutaneously and a wheal and flare response is seen in the sensitised individual. Localisation of ingested allergen to the respiratory tract may induce bronchospasm and exacerbation of asthma. Localisation to the nasal mucosa may induce rhinitis, and allergic conjunctivitis may occur if the allergen localises in the conjunctiva of the eye.

Widespread dissemination of ingested allergen may induce generalised mast cell degranulation and the clinical syndrome of systemic anaphylaxis. Anaphylaxis is the consequence of the widespread release of vasoactive mediators. These induce cardiovascular shock because of vasodilatation, and extravasation of large volumes of intravascular plasma into the tissues. Anaphylaxis is also associated with acute respiratory failure, resulting from widespread bronchial airflow obstruction and compromise of the oropharyngeal airway by glossal (tongue) and pharyngeal swelling. Acute anaphylaxis may also be accompanied by urticaria, abdominal cramps, diarrhoea and vomiting. The life-threatening nature of anaphylaxis is the consequence of its rapidity and the swift compromise of the respiratory and cardiovascular systems. The rapid administration of 0.5–1 mg adrenaline intramuscularly antagonises vasodilatation, increased vascular permeability and bronchoconstriction (see Chapter 6, Section 6.6). The administration of intravenous fluids, oxygen, intravenous antihistamine and glucocorticoid may also be required. Acute anaphylaxis may also occur if an allergen is injected into the skin or vascular space. This may occur naturally with bee and wasp stings or may be iatrogenically induced if an allergen (usually an antibiotic) is administered intravenously.

### 2.5.3 Non-IgE/T cell mediated allergy

In contrast to IgE mediated allergy, delayed-type hypersensitivity (also known as type IV hypersensitivity) is mediated by antigen-specific T cells, which function in the same way when confronted by an invading pathogen. Delayed-type hypersensitivity is the immuno-pathogenic basis of gluten-sensitive enteropathy, contact hypersensitivity reactions and some reactions to insect stings. Delayed-type hypersensitivity reactions are also the basis of the tuberculin and lepromin tests used to assess exposure to *Mycobacterium tuberculosis* and *leprae*.

The tuberculin reaction demonstrates many features of delayed-type hypersensitivity. After the subcutaneous injection of tuberculin, the antigen is processed by local antigen-presenting cells and presented in an MHC class II restricted manner to circulating Th1 cells. If an individual is sensitised to the antigen, an intense Th1 cell mediated local inflammatory reaction occurs. This antigen processing and Th1 cell influx takes 24–48 hours

and is the reason for the characteristic delay in the onset of the inflammatory reaction. The Th1 cells, attracted to the site of antigen, release chemokines that attract macrophages and T cells. Th1 cells activate macrophages by cell contact and the secretion of Th1 cytokines. The visible swelling at the injection site is the consequence of cellular influx and tissue oedema, induced by pro-inflammatory cytokines that increase vascular permeability. The release of cytokines with haemopoietic activity increases the development and release of bone marrow monocytes.

In the tuberculin reaction, the dose of antigen is small and the reaction delayed but self-limiting. In coeliac disease, the antigen is ingested and the delayed-type hypersensitivity reaction occurs in the small bowel, but the reaction is not self-limiting because of further ingestion and exposure of the sensitised immune system to gliadin. This chronic cell mediated form of allergy results in the sub-villous atrophy and lymphocyte infiltrate that is so characteristic of coeliac disease. Type IV hypersensitivity reactions can also involve CD8$^+$ T cells. The delayed-type hypersensitivity response to poison ivy is a response to the hapten pentadeca-catechol, which is lipid soluble, can enter cells and can modify intracellular proteins. These modified proteins can be expressed in an MHC class I restricted manner on the cell surface to specific CD8$^+$ T cells, which will kill the cell.

## 2.6  Why do food antigens fail to produce a detrimental immune response?

> ### Points to note
> - Ingestion of food normally induces a state of immunological unresponsiveness, known as oral tolerance.
> - Oral tolerance is mediated by the generation of regulatory T cells, clonal deletion and clonal anergy.
> - Cell and IgE mediated immune responses are more easily tolerised (made unresponsive) than IgG mediated immune responses.
> - IgG responses are more difficult to tolerise and food-specific IgG antibodies are found in normal healthy people.

Clearly the human immune system is able to initiate humoral and cell mediated immune responses directed against food antigens. Clinical observation, however, is that these detrimental allergic immune responses form a significant minority rather than being the rule. These considerations raise the question as to why the human immune system does not normally induce an injurious response to food antigens (Strobel & Mowat, 1998; Faria & Weiner, 1999). The gut is exposed to a huge antigenic burden composed of ingested food, commensal bacteria and pathogenic microorganisms. This presents the immune system with a complex problem; pathogenic organisms present in ingested food must be identified and counteracted but immune responses against commensal gut organisms must be under stringent control because these organisms are essential for normal intestinal function. The proteins in our diet are intrinsically antigenic but pose no pathogenic threat to the host; indeed, they are destined to become part of the host. It is evident that exposure of the immune system to food antigens occurs because antigen can be detected in the serum within minutes of ingestion. The immune system has evolved mechanisms for preventing injurious responses to food antigens. These mechanisms appear to function at two levels:

(1) There is true immunological tolerance, with an inhibition of systemic immune responses to food antigens. This is also known as oral tolerance.

(2) There is some immunological reactivity to food antigens, which although present is not pathogenic. This can be termed immunological acceptance.

### 2.6.1 Oral tolerance/true immunological tolerance

The gastrointestinal tract has a highly structured immune network known as the gut associated lymphoid tissue (GALT), which comprises the specialised lymphoid nodules termed Peyer's patches, intra-epithelial lymphocytes, lymphocytes scattered throughout the lamina propria and the epithelial cells of the villi. Exposure of the immune system to soluble dietary antigens induces tolerance, which is highly effective and lifelong, with virtually all aspects of the immune response being susceptible to oral tolerance. Cell and IgE

mediated immunity are particularly susceptible, perhaps reflecting the potential pathological consequences of cell and IgE mediated responses to food antigens. Unfortunately, in a substantial minority (<5%), there appears to be a breakdown of oral tolerance and adverse immunological reactions occur. It is believed that a failure of oral tolerance towards food antigens is the immunopathological basis of food allergy and gluten sensitive enteropathy, and the ineffective immuno-regulation of responses against commensal organisms has been implicated in the aetiology of the inflammatory bowel conditions, Crohn's disease and ulcerative colitis.

### 2.6.2 Mechanisms of oral tolerance

The clonal deletion (elimination of immature lymphocytes upon binding self-antigen) of immature lymphocytes, able to recognise and respond to food antigens, has been demonstrated as a mechanism of oral tolerance; however, its physiological role is unclear. The oral administration of very large unphysiological doses of ovalbumin and myelin basic protein has been shown to induce clonal deletion in mice (Chen *et al.*, 1995). Other investigators have been unable to demonstrate this effect.

T cell anergy has also been proposed as a mechanism of oral tolerance, especially that induced by the ingestion of high doses of antigen. Anergy is a state of T cell unresponsiveness characterised by absence of proliferation and IL-2 production in response to antigen. It is believed that T cell anergy is the consequence of T cells recognising MHC restricted dietary antigen in the absence of co-stimulatory molecules. Once in an anergic state, T cells are refractory to activation even by antigen-presenting cells. The identity of the antigen-presenting cell responsible for anergic oral tolerance remains speculative. Conventional antigen-presenting cells, such as dendritic cells and macrophages, are abundant in the gastrointestinal tract, but it has been suggested that they are in a resting state and express low levels of co-stimulatory activity. The antigen-presenting role of the intestinal epithelial cells is under active investigation because these cells express low levels of MHC class II molecules, and ingested antigen can be detected in murine enterocytes within 5–10 minutes of feeding.

Oral tolerance to low doses of antigen is believed to be mediated by the induction of regulatory T cells, which suppress any potentially damaging immune responses by the secretion of immuno-modulatory cytokines. This form of oral tolerance can be transferred by T cells extracted from Peyer's patches, mesenteric lymph nodes and spleen, with early transfer studies suggesting that activation of $CD8^+$ suppressor T cells mediated this form of oral tolerance. $CD8^+$ T cells with the $\gamma\delta$ form of the T cell receptor are relatively abundant in the intestinal mucosa and they have also been implicated in $CD8^+$ mediated oral tolerance.

Work with knockout mice has, however, demonstrated that $CD4^+$ and not $CD8^+$ cells are essential for oral tolerance. A popular model of $CD4^+$ mediated oral tolerance proposes that Th2 biased $CD4^+$ Th cells down regulate Th1 cell mediated immunity. This model explains the relative ease with which cell mediated immune responses can be tolerised (*i.e.* made unresponsive to an antigen) by oral antigens, whereas induction of humoral tolerance is more difficult. Although Th2 cytokines are found in abundance in the intestinal mucosa, the model does not explain the observations that IgE and cell mediated immune responses are both easily tolerised, and that the oral administration of ovalbumin suppresses both Th1 and Th2 phenotypes. Furthermore, work with IL-4 and IFN-$\gamma$ knockout mice has suggested that these two cytokines are not essential for oral tolerance. The cytokine receiving most attention at present is TGF-$\beta$, which has well documented suppressive effects on many aspects of the immune response and is present at high levels in the normal intestine. TGF-$\beta$ is secreted by Th2 subsets, which have been designated Th3 and T regulatory 1(Tr1). The factors influencing Th cell differentiation towards these suppressive phenotypes are unclear, but it is assumed that the nature of the antigen, the specialised nature of gut-associated antigen-presenting cells and the cytokine milieu are important. Experimental work supports a role for TGF-$\beta$ in oral tolerance, but it remains to be seen if the enthusiasm for TGF-$\beta$ wanes as has the initial enthusiasm for IL-4 and IFN-$\gamma$.

### 2.6.3 Factors influencing oral tolerance

A number of host factors can influence the induction and maintenance of oral tolerance, these include age, genetic background, nutritional status and the intestinal microbial flora. Age seems to be particularly important, with defective induction of oral tolerance occurring in young neonates and at the time of weaning. The intestinal bacterial flora appear to modulate oral tolerance. Bacterial lipo-polysaccharide (LPS) appears to facilitate the induction of oral tolerance and may bias intestinal Th cell differentiation towards the Th2 (and possibly also the Th3) phenotype. The prescription of antibiotics to infants has been shown to be associated with IgE mediated allergy, with the implication that the adverse effects of antibiotics on the gut commensal flora may interfere with the normal development of oral tolerance and the development of allergy (Farooqi & Hopkin, 1998). Antigen-associated influences include the dose and the nature of the antigen. In general, high antigen doses induce anergic tolerance, while low doses or continuous exposure to low dosing tend to generate the regulatory form of tolerance. The nature of the antigen is also influential, with soluble antigens being the most effective inducers of oral tolerance. Particulate or replicating antigens tend to activate antigen-presenting cells and induce a defensive immune response rather than tolerance.

Oral tolerance is, therefore, a highly effective mechanism that has evolved to prevent the damaging, sensitising immune responses directed against food antigens. Although not fully understood, it is probable that several mechanisms are involved and it is unlikely that any one mechanism predominates. Furthermore, it is likely that differing mechanisms are implicated under different circumstances. As mentioned above, IgG mediated immune responses to food are not as easily tolerised as cell- and IgE mediated responses. It is becoming increasingly obvious that IgG mediated responses against food antigens occur, but that the individual is able to live with this situation. This phenomenon has been termed immunological acceptance (reviewed by Barnes, 1995) (see Section 2.6.4).

### 2.6.4 Immunological acceptance

Several studies have demonstrated that children and adults have circulating IgG specific for food antigens (Barnes, 1995). These antibodies appear as early as 3 months of age and increase during the first 5 years of life. It is also of interest that food-specific IgE antibodies decline during the same time period. IgG1 and IgG4 isotypes, specific for egg, wheat and cows' milk proteins, have been detected in normal healthy individuals and in individuals with food allergies. Reviews of the literature have demonstrated that the determination of food-specific IgG has no predictive value for dietary manipulation or management of patients with classical food allergy. These findings suggest that the production of IgG antibodies to dietary antigens is a normal immunological response to food. The circulating IgG binds to the absorbed dietary antigen and is increased in circumstances that allow increased absorption of partially digested food proteins and peptides, *e.g.* mucosal damage. This has led to the concept that IgG antibodies to food proteins may represent a normal mechanism for clearing inadvertently absorbed protein or peptides.

Clearly the response of the immune system to food is complex and incompletely understood. Suppression of cell- and IgE mediated immune responses to food is clearly important as witnessed by their failure.

Complete suppression of all immune responses to food does not occur because the body appears to be able to function completely normally despite the presence of IgG generating immune responses.

## 2.7 Conclusion

Many of the common adverse reactions to food described in this report are immunologically mediated and the various processes involved are summarised in Fig. 2.10. The immune system is broadly divided into humoral (antibody) and cell mediated immunity, which interact with each other to generate the optimal mechanisms to eliminate invading microorganisms. The immune responses directed against food constituents are no different to those directed against invading microorganisms, it is just that they are directed against the 'wrong' target. Whereas the elimination of invading microorganisms by the immune system is beneficial to the host, the same immune responses directed against food constituents result in tissue damage and disease.

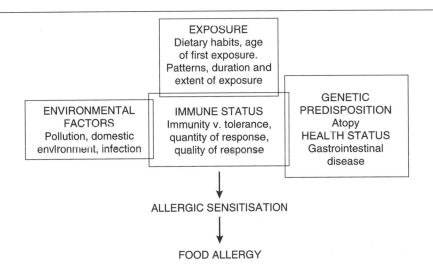

**Fig. 2.10** Interaction of factors that lead to the development of allergy. The ability of a protein antigen to induce allergic sensitisation is determined by a number of factors. The exposed individual must be susceptible. Such inherent susceptibility is governed by both heritable factors and by environmental factors which influence the characteristics of the immune system. Perhaps the most important is atopy, this being a predisposition to mount IgE antibody responses. It is likely also that general health status and in particular pre-existing gastrointestinal disease will affect the induction of allergic sensitisation and/or the elicitation of food allergic reactions. (Source: Food Standards Agency, 2000.)

# 3
# Nutrition and the Immune System

## 3.1 Introduction

Associations between famine and epidemics of infectious disease have been noted throughout history, and Hippocrates recognised that poorly nourished people are more susceptible to infectious disease. Generally undernutrition impairs the immune system, suppressing immune functions that are fundamental to host protection against pathogenic organisms. The detailed evidence for all aspects of this subject has been referred to elsewhere (for further reading, see Scrimshaw & SanGiovanni, 1997; Calder & Jackson, 2000). Undernutrition leading to impairment of immune function can be due to insufficient intake of energy and macronutrients and/or due to deficiencies in specific micronutrients (vitamins and minerals). Often these occur in combination such that protein-energy malnutrition and deficiencies in micronutrients such as vitamin A, iron, zinc and iodine can occur together.

Clearly the impact of undernutrition is greatest in developing countries, but it can also be important in developed countries especially amongst the elderly, individuals with eating disorders, alcoholics, patients with certain diseases and premature and small-for-gestational age babies. Many studies have been performed in animals and these have often compared the effects of diets containing insufficient or deficient, sufficient and, in some cases, excess amounts of an individual nutrient under study. Such studies are valuable because they allow the effect of the nutrient to be studied in a highly controlled setting, and because the immune system of experimental animals is more accessible than that of humans. In humans, studies of the immunological impact of nutrient deficiencies have been imposed by nature either through famines, natural disasters or habitual consumption of diets deficient in one or more nutrients, or, by diseases that result in inability to absorb or transport nutrients. These studies have made it clear that there are some nutrients whose availability at an appropriate level is essential if the immune response to bacteria, viruses, fungi and parasites is to operate efficiently. However, in considering the effects of various nutrients on the human immune system, it is important to emphasise that nutrient deficiencies are unlikely to occur in healthy people consuming a mixed diet, and that overconsumption of some nutrients can in fact be harmful.

## 3.2 Impact of infection on nutrient status

While undernutrition decreases immune defences against invading pathogens and makes the individual more susceptible to infections (see below), certain pathogens can diminish nutritional status (see Scrimshaw & SanGiovanni, 1997; Calder & Jackson, 2000 for reviews). Thus, there is a bidirectional interaction between nutrition, infection and immunity. The changes in nutrient status caused by infection are mediated by changes in dietary intake, nutrient absorption and nutrient requirements and losses of endogenous nutrients (Fig. 3.1). Growth of the individual can be impaired due to the combination of poor nutrition, malabsorption and the host response to infection. Infection also alters behaviour which can affect feeding practices.

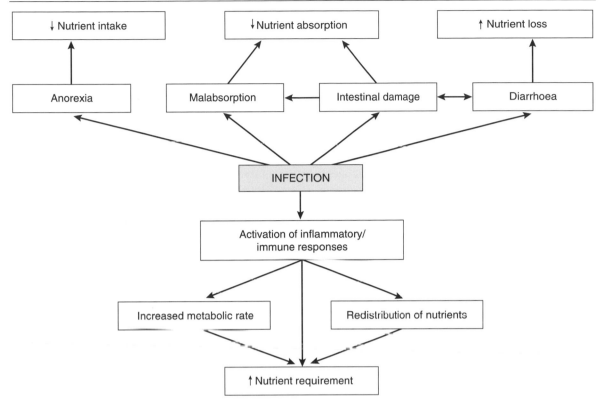

**Fig. 3.1** Mechanisms by which infection can affect nutrient status.

### 3.2.1 Infection is characterised by anorexia

Clearly, a reduction in food intake (anorexia) will result in reduced intake of all macro- and micro-nutrients. This could lead to nutrient deficiencies even if the host was not already deficient and it could make apparent existing borderline deficiencies.

### 3.2.2 Infection is characterised by nutrient malabsorption and loss

Markedly decreased absorption of total energy, nitrogen, fat, carbohydrate, fat-soluble vitamins, water-soluble vitamins and iron has been reported during a wide range of infections and there may also be nutrient loss caused by diarrhoea, vomiting or damage to the intestinal wall caused by some infective agents (see Calder & Jackson, 2000).

### 3.2.3 Infection is characterised by increased resting energy expenditure

Infection increases the basal metabolic rate: there is a 13% increase for each 1°C increase in body temperature. During a period of high fever, metabolism may increase by nearly one third, so increasing the requirement for energy-yielding nutrients and the co-factors that participate in their metabolism. This places a significant demand on body pools of nutrients, particularly when coupled with anorexia, diarrhoea and other nutrient losses (*e.g.* in urine and sweat).

### 3.2.4 Infection is characterised by altered metabolism and redistribution of nutrients

The acute phase response is the name given to the metabolic response to infections and it includes the onset of fever and anorexia, the production of specific 'acute-phase reactants' and the activation and proliferation of immune cells. Such a catabolic response occurs with all infections even when they are subclinical and may occur in response to immunisation. This response serves to cause redistribution of nutrients away from skeletal muscle and adipose tissue and towards the host immune response. This redistribution is mediated by production of pro-inflammatory cytokines (by leukocytes) and associated endocrine changes. These lead to mobilisation of amino acids, primarily from skeletal muscle, which are used as gluconeogenic substrates in the liver with the nitrogen released being lost in the urine. Some of the amino acids are used by the liver for the synthesis of the so-called acute phase proteins and by leukocytes and other cells for synthesis of immunoglobulins (Ig) and cytokines. The average loss of protein over a range of infections has been estimated to be 0.6 to 1.2 g per kg body weight per day, with severe infections inducing the greatest loss. The metabolic response to infection also results in increased oxidant stress, which can potentially deplete reserves of cellular and plasma antioxidant vitamins.

## 3.3 Protein-energy malnutrition and immune function

A large number of studies in animals have demonstrated the adverse effects of protein deficiency on immunity and these effects have been confirmed in various human settings (*e.g.* Chandra, 1975, 1979, 1983; Chandra *et al.*, 1982, 1984; Rivera *et al.*, 1986). It is not surprising that protein deficiency diminishes immune responses and increases susceptibility to infection because immune defences are dependent upon cell replication and the production of proteins with biological activities (*e.g.* Ig, cytokines, acute phase proteins). It is, however, important to note that protein-energy malnutrition is often characterised not simply by insufficient intake of total energy and macronutrients but by micronutrient deficiencies as well.

Practically all forms of immunity may be affected by protein-energy malnutrition but non-specific defences and cell mediated immunity are more severely affected than humoral (antibody) responses (see Gross & Newberne, 1980; Kuvibidila *et al.*, 1993; Woodward, 2001 for reviews). Protein-energy malnutrition causes atrophy of the thymus, spleen, lymph nodes and tonsils in laboratory animals and humans. The circulating white blood cell count can be increased but this is due to increased numbers of neutrophils; the absolute and relative numbers of monocytes, lymphocytes, $CD4^+$ cells and $CD8^+$ cells are decreased, as is the CD4/CD8 ratio. The extent of the decline in lymphocyte numbers is proportional to the extent of malnutrition (Rivera *et al.*, 1986). The proliferative responses of T lymphocytes to mitogens and antigens and the synthesis of IL-2 and IFN-$\gamma$ are decreased by malnutrition. Natural killer cell activity is decreased in malnutrition, as is the production of tumour necrosis factor alpha (TNF-$\alpha$), IL-1 and IL-6 by stimulated monocytes (see Woodward, 1998 for references). The skin response to antigens is decreased by malnutrition and the extent of the decrease is related to the degree of malnutrition (Rivera *et al.*, 1986). Bactericidal activity and respiratory burst of neutrophils are decreased by malnutrition, but the phagocytic capacity of neutrophils and monocytes appears to be unaffected. B cell numbers and circulating Ig levels are not affected or may even be increased by malnutrition (see Kuvibidila *et al.*, 1993; Woodward 2001), although differences in findings might reflect the level of underlying infection. Although the level of secretory IgA in tears, saliva and intestinal washings is decreased by malnutrition, this may relate to decreased expression of the polymeric Ig receptor, which is responsible for transepithelial transport of IgA, rather than to reduced IgA synthesis (see Woodward, 1998 for references). Protein-energy malnutrition renders the host more susceptible to infection with bacteria, viruses, fungi and parasites.

## 3.4 The influence of individual micronutrients on immune function

### 3.4.1 Vitamin A

Humans consuming diets containing suboptimal amounts of vitamin A show a range of immune impairments, including atrophy of the lymphoid organs, decreased numbers of circulating T and B lymphocytes, a reduced CD4/CD8 ratio, a decreased antibody response and a lowered concentration of sIgA in tears and saliva, decreased phagocytosis and respiratory burst by neutrophils, decreased natural killer activity, cytotoxic T lymphocyte (effector CD8[+] T cells, see Chapter 2, Section 2.4.5*iv*) activity and lymphocyte proliferation, and a decreased delayed-type hypersensitivity response (see Friedman & Sklan 1993; Semba, 1998, 1999 for reviews). Information on the functioning of the immune system and the implications of these changes can be found in Chapter 2. Vitamin A is essential for maintaining epidermal and mucosal integrity, and vitamin A deficient mice have histopathological changes in the gut mucosa consistent with a breakdown in gut barrier integrity and impaired mucous secretion. Vitamin A regulates keratinocyte differentiation and vitamin A deficiency induces changes in skin keratinisation which may explain the observed increased incidence of skin infections (see Semba, 1998).

While vitamin A deficiency is endemic in some underprivileged communities, especially in South East Asia and India, sporadic cases are occasionally seen in malnourished children elsewhere, precipitated in most cases by infectious diseases. It in turn predisposes to respiratory infections, diarrhoea and severe measles (see Scrimshaw & San-Giovanni, 1997; Semba 1999; Calder & Jackson, 2000 for references).

Replenishment of vitamin A in depleted or deficient subjects leads to restoration of lymphoid organ development, circulating immune cell populations, immune cell functions and delayed-type hypersensitivity response and improved resistance to infection (see Friedman & Sklan, 1993; Semba 1998). Although there are suggestions that high levels of vitamin A in the diet might enhance immune responsiveness above 'normal', excess intakes of vitamin A can cause immunological defects identical to those induced by vitamin A deficiency and can decrease resistance to infection (see Friedman & Sklan, 1993).

### 3.4.2 Carotenoids

The results of studies of β-carotene supplementation on immune function in humans have been inconsistent, with some studies showing effects and others not (see Roe & Fuller, 1993; Hughes, 1999 for a review). Thus, whether β-carotene influences human immune function is uncertain at this point in time.

### 3.4.3 Vitamin B$_6$

The estimated average requirement for vitamin B$_6$ in the adult population in the UK is 1.2 mg/day for males and 1.0 mg/day for females (Department of Health, 1991). Feeding healthy elderly humans a vitamin B$_6$ deficient diet (3 µg/kg body weight or about 0.17 and 0.1 mg/day for men and women, respectively) for 21 days resulted in a decreased percentage and total number of circulating lymphocytes, decreased T and B cell proliferation in response to mitogens and decreased IL-2 production (Meydani *et al.*, 1991). Repletion studies over a 21 day period suggested that the optimum to return the immune functions to starting values was achieved by 33.75 µg/kg body weight per day (about 1.9 and 1.1 mg/day for men and women, respectively). These data indicate that vitamin B$_6$ deficiency impairs human immune function and that this impairment is reversible by repletion. Lymphocyte functions were not enhanced at levels of vitamin B$_6$ above those recommended.

### 3.4.4 Vitamin C

Vitamin C is a water soluble antioxidant found in high concentrations within circulating leukocytes. The estimated average requirement for vitamin C in the adult population in the UK is 25 mg/day (Department of Health, 1991). Although Jacob *et al.* (1991) claim that increased intake of vitamin C can improve immune function, studies on the immunological impact of vitamin C in humans provide conflicting results. Most studies report that vitamin C is ineffective in reducing the incidence of the common cold, although it may reduce the severity of symptoms (see Siegel, 1993 for references).

### 3.4.5 Vitamin E

Vitamin E is the major lipid-soluble antioxidant in the body and is required for protection of membrane lipids from peroxidation. Since free radicals and lipid peroxidation can damage cells, it has been claimed that vitamin E should optimise or enhance the immune response (see Bendich, 1993; Meydani & Beharka, 1998; Han & Meydani, 1999 for reviews). Habitual intakes of vitamin E among adults in the UK are between 3.5 and 19.5 mg α-tocopherol/day for males and 2.5 to 15.2 mg α-tocopherol/day for females (Department of Health, 1991). Except in premature infants and some elderly subjects, clinical vitamin E deficiency, defined by existing criteria, is rare in humans, but cigarette smokers have been reported to have low levels of lung and serum vitamin E, increased numbers of neutrophils and macrophages in the lung, increased reactive oxygen species production by phagocytes and depressed immune responses (see Bendich, 1993; Tappia *et al.*, 1995).

The only case that has been made for the use of vitamin E supplements is in premature infants and the elderly. Chavance *et al.* (1989) found a positive association between plasma vitamin E levels and delayed-type hypersensitivity responses and a negative association between plasma vitamin E levels and incidence of infections in healthy adults aged over 60. Administration of vitamin E to premature infants enhanced neutrophil phagocytosis

but decreased the ability of neutrophils to kill bacteria. Because premature infants are often deficient in vitamin E, preterm infant formulas now contain vitamin E at adequate levels. The case for supplementing the diet of elderly subjects is less clear. Although a vitamin E intake of no more than 20 mg daily seems to be compatible with normal health in the population at large, Meydani and colleagues (1990, 1997) have claimed that vitamin E supplements of 60 to 200 mg daily in elderly subjects increase the antibody response to hepatitis B vaccination. Although a higher dose (800 mg/day) did not (Fig. 3.2), this dose was capable of enhancing delayed hypersensitivity reactions. Since other parameters of immune function were unaffected it remains unclear if there are any clinical benefits to be obtained by adding vitamin E to the diet at levels beyond those normally consumed.

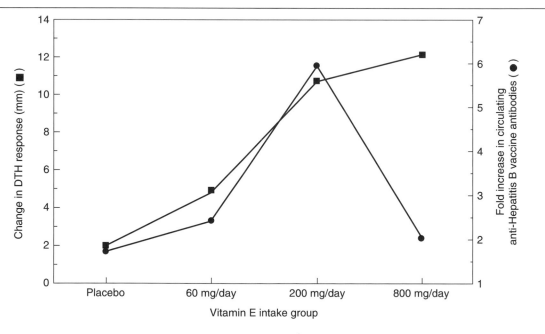

**Fig. 3.2** Vitamin E and human immune function. Healthy elderly subjects supplemented their habitual diet with a placebo or with vitamin E at levels of 60, 200 or 800 mg/day. The delayed-type hypersensitivity (DTH) response to seven recall antigens was assessed at baseline and after 4 months. Total delayed-type hypersensitivity induration response at baseline was approximately 20 mm in each group. Subjects were then vaccinated against hepatitis B (with subsequent boosters); antibodies to the vaccine were measured prior to vaccination and 3 months later. Plasma vitamin E concentrations (μmol/L) after 4 months' supplementation were 23 (placebo), 38 (60 mg/day), 51 (200 mg/day) and 71 (800 mg/day). Data are taken from Meydani *et al.* (1997).

### 3.4.6 Zinc

The mean habitual intakes of zinc among adults in the UK are 11.4 and 8.4 mg/day for men and women, respectively (Department of Health, 1991). In Indian infants – who may also have other nutritional problems – low plasma zinc levels predicted the subsequent development of lower respiratory tract infections and diarrhoea. Indeed, diarrhoea is considered a symptom of zinc deficiency. There are a number of studies showing that zinc supplementation decreases the incidence of childhood diarrhoea and respiratory illness (see Scrimshaw & SanGiovanni, 1997; Shankar & Prasad, 1998; Calder & Jackson, 2000 for references), although some studies fail to show benefit of zinc supplementation in respiratory disease (see Calder & Jackson, 2000 for references). As well as decreasing the risk of young infants developing diarrhoea, zinc supplementation reduces diarrhoea-induced growth faltering (see Calder & Jackson, 2000). Zinc administration to preterm low body weight infants

(1 mg/kg per day for 30 days) increased the number of circulating T lymphocytes and lymphocyte proliferation (Chandra, 1991). Providing 5 mg zinc/day to low birth weight, small-for-gestational-age infants for 6 months increased measures of cell mediated immune function and decreased the incidence of gastrointestinal and upper respiratory tract infections (Lira *et al.*, 1998); a zinc dose of 1 mg/day was without effect.

Other studies have shown considerable disturbances of immune function in zinc-deficient subjects, but without clarifying their clinical significance, *e.g.* in patients with zinc deficiency related to sickle cell disease and with acrodermatitis enteropathica, and also in experimental zinc deficiency in man (induced by consumption of <3.5 mg zinc/day), which could be returned to normal by zinc supplementation (Beck *et al.*, 1997; Shankar & Prasad, 1998). The clinical significance of these effects on the immune system is not clear but these data suggest that zinc deficiency impairs Th1 but not Th2 responses and alters the balance

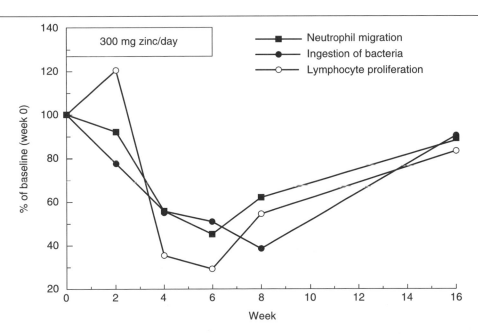

**Fig. 3.3** Suppression of human immune function by excess zinc intake. Healthy adult males consumed 150 mg zinc twice daily for 6 weeks and then ceased zinc supplementation and were followed for a further 10 weeks. Neutrophil migration (■), phagocytic ingestion of bacteria by neutrophils (●) and lymphocyte proliferation (▲) are expressed as % of values at entry to the study. Data are from Chandra (1984).

between CD4+ and CD8+ cells and within CD4+ subsets.

Excessive zinc intakes impair immune responses. For example, giving 300 mg zinc/day for 6 weeks to young adult humans decreased lymphocyte and phagocyte function (Fig. 3.3) (Chandra, 1984). High zinc intakes can result in copper depletion, and copper deficiency impairs immune function (see below).

### 3.4.7 Copper

Overt copper deficiency is believed to be rare in humans. Zinc and iron impair copper uptake so that taking high doses of these might induce mild copper deficiency. Copper deficiency has been described in premature infants and in patients receiving total parenteral nutrition. The classic example of copper deficiency is Menkes syndrome, a rare congenital disease which results in the complete absence of ceruloplasmin, the copper-carrying protein in the blood. Children with Menkes syndrome have increased bacterial infections, diarrhoea and pneumonia. Some workers have reported impaired blood T lymphocyte responses in patients with Menkes syndrome, but these have not been confirmed by others (see Prohaska & Failla, 1993 for references). The average intake of copper among adults in the UK is estimated to be about 1.5 mg/day (Department of Health, 1991). Putting human volunteers on a low copper diet (0.38 mg/day for 42 days) resulted in decreased lymphocyte proliferation but did not affect neutrophil phagocytosis or the proportions of different immune cells in the bloodstream (Kelley *et al.*, 1995). As with some other micronutrients, excess copper can impair immune responses (Pocino *et al.*, 1991).

### 3.4.8 Iron

The Department of Health (1991) comments that iron deficiency is common among some segments of the UK population, but also that the degree to which physiological requirements for iron vary from person to person is not known precisely. Iron deficiency causes multiple effects on immune function in humans, including atrophy of the thymus, decreased numbers of circulating T lymphocytes, a reduced CD4/CD8 ratio, decreased respiratory burst by neutrophils, decreased natural

killer activity, cytotoxic T lymphocyte activity and lymphocyte proliferation, decreased IL-1, IL-2 and IFN-γ production and a decreased delayed-type hypersensitivity response (see Sherman & Spear, 1993 for a review). Iron deficient individuals have normal phagocytic function but there is impaired ability to kill bacteria by neutrophils, probably as a result of an alteration in respiratory burst. Iron deficiency is associated with gastrointestinal and respiratory infections.

Despite the suppressive effects of iron deficiency on immune responses, iron overload and excessive iron supplementation are associated with increased risk of infection. For example, if iron-deficient individuals who have compromised resistance to infection are given large doses of iron parenterally or orally, an exacerbation of infection and death can occur. Parenteral iron administration to low birth weight babies increased the incidence of septicaemia, while supplemental iron has been observed to increase the incidence of infections among Somali nomads, the incidence of diarrhoea among Chilean children and the duration of diarrhoea among Bangladeshi children (see Calder & Jackson, 2000 for references). These effects of iron administration might in part be because micro-organisms require iron and so providing it may favour the pathogen. Excess iron has also been shown to impair immune responses. Iron overload decreases the number of T lymphocytes and CD4+ cells, the CD4/CD8 ratio, lymphocyte proliferation and IL-2 production, cytotoxic T cell and natural killer cell activities, and phagocytic activity of neutrophils (see Sherman & Spear, 1993). It is not clear what the mechanism of the effect of iron overload is but it might relate to deposition of iron in lymphoid tissues affecting cell movement and function or to increased peroxidative damage which is favoured by increased levels of free iron.

### 3.4.9 Micronutrient combinations and resistance to infection

Elderly humans given a multi-nutrient mix containing the US recommended amounts of vitamins A, B$_6$, B$_{12}$, D, thiamin, riboflavin, niacin, folate, and minerals iron, zinc, copper, selenium, iodine, calcium and magnesium and higher than the US recommended amounts of vitamin C (80 mg/day), vitamin E (44 mg/day) and β-carotene (16 mg/day) for 12 months had a higher antibody response to influenza vaccine and less infection-related illness than the placebo group (Chandra 1992). Girodon *et al.* (1996) reported fewer infections in elderly subjects supplemented with minerals (20 mg zinc plus 100 mg selenium per day for 2 years) alone or in combination with vitamins (120 mg vitamin C, 6 mg β-carotene, 15 mg vitamin E per day for 2 years) than in those who were supplemented with vitamins alone.

### 3.4.10 Micronutrients and HIV infection

Many individuals with HIV infection consume less than the recommended amounts of a range of micronutrients (see Semba & Tang, 1999 for references). Nutrient intake by patients with HIV infection may be decreased as a result of loss of appetite, aversion to food and throat infections, while vomiting, diarrhoea and malabsorption may also contribute to deficiencies (see Semba & Tang, 1999 for a discussion). The prevalence of micronutrient deficiencies (based largely upon concentrations measured in the plasma or serum) varies widely depending upon the population and the stage of the disease; Semba and Tang (1999) conclude that low plasma or serum levels of vitamins A, $B_6$, $B_{12}$, C, D and E, β-carotene, selenium and zinc are common.

Micronutrient deficiencies may increase oxidative stress and compromise host immunity, so contributing to HIV disease progression. Low plasma or serum vitamin A levels are associated with accelerated HIV progression, increased mortality, higher rates of transmission of HIV from mother to baby, child growth failure and increased HIV load in breast milk and the birth canal (see Semba & Tang, 1999 for references). Low serum or plasma concentrations of vitamins $B_{12}$ or E or of zinc increase the risk of progression to AIDS (see Semba & Tang, 1999 for references).

Various supplementation studies have been reported. Vitamin A supplementation resulted in a significant reduction in mortality and morbidity among HIV infected children (Coutsoudis *et al.*, 1995). However, maternal vitamin A supplementation throughout the third trimester of pregnancy and at delivery did not alter the rate of mother-to-child HIV transmission up to 3 months of age of the infants (Coutsoudis *et al.*, 1999).

Multivitamins (vitamins $B_6$, $B_{12}$, C and E, folate, thiamin, riboflavin, niacin) decreased foetal death (miscarriage and still birth), lowered the incidence of low birth weight, lowered severe preterm birth and decreased the number of small-for-gestational-age infants; however vitamin A alone was without effect (Fawzi *et al.*, 1998). Likewise, multivitamins, but not vitamin A, increased the number of T, $CD4^+$ and $CD8^+$ lymphocytes in the bloodstream (Fawzi *et al.*, 1998).

### 3.4.11 Micronutrients and asthma

Respiratory diseases, such as asthma, impose oxidant stress on the individual as a result of inappropriate production of reactive oxygen species (*e.g.* superoxide and hydroxyl radicals, hydrogen peroxide, hypochlorous acid) (see Rahman *et al.*, 1996; Repine *et al.*, 1999 for reviews). These reactive species damage host tissues, upregulate the production of inflammatory cytokines and adhesion molecules thereby amplifying the inflammation, induce bronchoconstriction, elevate mucous secretion and cause microvascular leakage (see Repine *et al.*, 1999). Oxidant stress can deplete cells and tissues of antioxidants, if these are not replenished sufficiently through the diet. Furthermore, a low dietary intake of antioxidants may exacerbate the problem by allowing generation of reactive species to proceed unchecked. Among the important antioxidants to consider are vitamins C and E (vitamin C is the major antioxidant present in the airway surface of the lung), glutathione, the glutathione recycling enzyme glutathione peroxidase and the enzymes which remove superoxide and hydrogen peroxide (superoxide dismutase and catalase, respectively); glutathione peroxidase, superoxide dismutase and catalase contain selenium, copper and zinc, and iron, respectively.

Fogarty and Britton (2000) have recently reviewed the evidence for associations between intakes of various micronutrients and asthma; they have surveyed cross-sectional, case-control, prospective and intervention studies. Epidemiological studies have suggested an association between increased asthma risk and low dietary intakes of selenium, vitamin C and vitamin E (see Schwartz & Weiss, 1994a; Greene, 1995; Troisi *et al.*, 1995; Dow *et al.*, 1996; Soutar *et al.*, 1997). Trials using vitamin C in asthma have provided mixed results, with some showing benefit and others not (see Bielory & Gandhi, 1994; Hatch, 1995 for reviews). These contradictions most likely relate to the dose and duration of vitamin C used, the types of patients studied and the outcomes measured. However, the lack of consistency suggests that the impact of vitamin C in asthma is probably small. Selenium supplementation in asthmatics (100 µg/day for 4 weeks) did not significantly change lung function or airway hyper-responsiveness (Hasselmark *et al.*, 1993). Vitamin $B_6$ (300 mg/day for 9 weeks) did not improve symptoms or skin test reactivity in steroid-requiring asthmatics (Sur *et al.*, 1993).

## 3.5 Dietary fat and immune function

### 3.5.1 Fatty acids in the human diet

The types and amounts of fat in the human diet have been described in detail elsewhere (British Nutrition Foundation, 1992). By far the most important component of dietary fat in quantitative terms is triacylglycerol, which in the UK diet constitutes >95% of dietary fat. Each triacylglycerol molecule is composed of three fatty acids esterified to a glycerol backbone, and so fatty acids are a major constituent of dietary fat. Because of the range of foodstuffs consumed, the human diet contains a variety of fatty acids (British Nutrition Foundation, 1992). Detailed information on the structure, intakes and metabolic relationships among the different fatty acids may be obtained elsewhere (British Nutrition Foundation, 1992, 1999). Fatty acids have systematic names but most also have common names and are described by a shorthand nomenclature (*e.g.* 18:2*n*-6 for linoleic acid; see British Nutrition Foundation, 1992). This nomenclature indicates the number of carbon atoms in the chain, the number of double bonds in the chain and the position of the first double bond from the methyl terminus of the chain. Mammals cannot synthesise linoleic acid (18:2*n*-6) or α-linolenic acid (18:3*n*-3), and so these two fatty acids are termed essential fatty acids. Plant tissues and plant oils tend to be rich sources of linoleic and α-linolenic acids.

Once consumed in the diet, linoleic acid can be converted via γ-linolenic (18:3*n*-6) and dihomo-γ-linolenic (DGLA; 20:3*n*-6) acids to arachidonic acid (20:4*n*-6) by the pathway outlined in Fig. 3.4.

Using the same pathway (Fig. 3.4) dietary α-linolenic acid can be converted into eicosapentaenoic acid (EPA; 20:5*n*-3) and docosahexaenoic acid (DHA; 22:6*n*-3). Intake of longer chain polyunsaturated fatty acids is low in the UK. EPA and DHA are found in relatively high proportions in the tissues of so-called 'oily fish' (*e.g.* herring, mackerel, fresh [*i.e.* not tinned] tuna, sardines) and in the commercial products called 'fish oils' which are a preparation of the body oils of oily fish or the liver oils of other species of fish (*e.g.* cod). EPA and DHA comprise 20–30% of the fatty acids in a typical preparation of fish oil, which means that a one gram fish oil capsule provides 200 to 300 mg of these fatty acids. In the absence of significant consumption of oily fish, α-linolenic acid is the major dietary *n*-3 fatty acid.

### 3.5.2 Amount of dietary fat and immune function

A reduction in total dietary fat intake by healthy male subjects (from 40% to 25% of total energy) resulted in greatly enhanced human blood lymphocyte proliferation in response to mitogens (Kelley *et al.*, 1989, 1992). Human natural killer cell activity was significantly increased by a reduction in fat intake to <30% energy (Barone *et al.*, 1989). IL-1 production by lipopolysaccharide-stimulated monocytes from elderly subjects was increased when fat intake was reduced from 36% to 27% of energy (Meydani *et al.*, 1993). Taken together these data suggest that a high fat diet suppresses the activity of cellular components of both natural and cell mediated immunity in humans.

### 3.5.3 Eicosanoids: a link between fatty acids and the immune system

The key link between fatty acids and immune function is that a group of mediators termed eicosanoids are synthesised from fatty acids, in particular DGLA, arachidonic acid and EPA (Fig. 3.5). Because the membranes of most cells contain large amounts of arachidonic acid, compared with DGLA and EPA, arachidonic acid is usually the principal precursor for eicosanoid synthesis. Arachidonic acid can act as a substrate for cyclooxygenase (COX), forming 2-series prostaglandins (PG) and related compounds, or for one of the lipoxygenase (LOX) enzymes (Fig. 3.5). There are

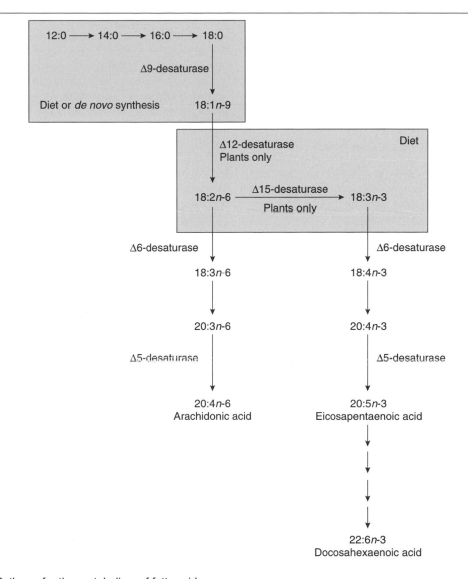

**Fig. 3.4** Pathway for the metabolism of fatty acids.

at least 16 different 2-series prostaglandins and these are formed in a cell-specific manner. For example, monocytes and macrophages produce large amounts of $PGE_2$ and $PGF_2$, neutrophils produce moderate amounts of $PGE_2$ and mast cells produce $PGD_2$. The LOX enzymes have different tissue distributions with 5-LOX being found mainly in mast cells, monocytes, macrophages and granulocytes and 12- and 15-LOX being found mainly in epithelial cells. Metabolism of arachidonic acid by the 5-LOX pathway gives rise to hydroxy and hydroperoxy derivatives (5-HETE and 5-HPETE, respectively), and the 4-series leukotrienes (LT), $LTA_4$, $LTB_4$, $LTC_4$, $LTD_4$ and $LTE_4$ (Fig. 3.5). Prostaglandins and leukotrienes have a number of physiological roles, but of relevance to this report they are involved in modulating the intensity and duration of inflammatory and immune responses and in regulating immune cell function. However, PG and LT often have opposing effects so that the

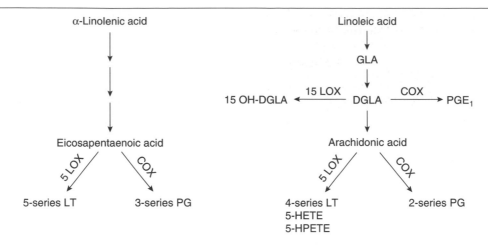

**Fig. 3.5**  Eicosanoid synthesis from *n*-6 and *n*-3 polyunsaturated fatty acids.

overall physiological effect will be governed by the concentrations of these mediators, the timing of their production and the sensitivities of target cells to their effects.

### 3.5.4 Linoleic acid and immune function

The average intake of linoleic acid in the adult UK population is approximately 10 g/day (approximately 5% of energy) (British Nutrition Foundation, 1999), although habitual intakes among healthy adults vary from less than 5 to greater than 15 g/day and have increased over the last 30 years. Surprisingly, few human studies have investigated the immunological impact of linoleic acid. The most detailed are those of Kelley *et al.* (1989, 1992), which involved providing volunteers with low fat diets (25% energy as fat) that were rich in linoleic acid (12.9% of energy) or poor in linoleic acid (3.5% of energy). No differences were observed in the responses of lymphocytes to various T cell mitogens, in circulating IgM, IgG, IgE or IgA levels, or in the delayed-type hypersensitivity response to seven recall antigens. Similarly, 5.5 g linoleic acid/day for 12 weeks (provided as a 9 g daily supplement of encapsulated sunflower oil) had no effect on lymphocyte proliferation, natural killer cell activity or production of TNF-α, IL-1α, IL-1β, IL-2, IFN-γ by mononuclear cells (Yaqoob *et al.*, 2000). These studies suggest limited impact of

linoleic acid (at a level of 3.5% dietary energy and above) upon human immune function.

### 3.5.5 α-Linolenic acid and immune function

The average intake of α-linolenic acid in the adult UK population is approximately 1.5 g/day (approximately 0.7% of energy) (British Nutrition Foundation, 1999), although habitual intakes among healthy adults vary from less than 0.5 to greater than 2 g/day. Two studies have reported the effects of large amounts of α-linolenic acid on some immune responses in healthy humans (Kelley *et al.*, 1991; Caughey *et al.*, 1996). A high dose of α-linolenic acid (approximately 14 g/day for 4 weeks) decreased IL-1 and TNF production by lipopolysaccharide-stimulated human monocytes (Caughey *et al.*, 1996). Adding linseed oil (providing about 18 g α-linolenic acid/day) to a low fat diet (total fat provided 29% energy) resulted in a significant decrease in human blood lymphocyte proliferation and in the delayed-type hypersensitivity response to seven recall antigens after 6 weeks, but circulating antibody levels were unaffected (Kelley *et al.*, 1991). In contrast to these effects, there was no effect of daily supplements of linseed oil (providing 2 g α-linolenic acid/day) in healthy subjects aged 55 to 75 years on natural killer cell activity (Thies *et al.*, 2001), or of supplements of oil (providing 4.1 g α-linolenic acid/day) on neutrophil respiratory burst in healthy males aged < 40 years (Healy *et al.*, 2000). These studies suggest that a moderate increase in α-linolenic acid intake by healthy adults does not affect immunity, but that a marked increase in α-linolenic acid intake (*e.g.* 7- to 15-fold) can induce effects. It is not clear whether these are exerted by α-linolenic acid itself or by EPA, a product of α-linolenic acid metabolism.

### 3.5.6 Fish oil and immune function

The average intake of long chain *n*-3 poly-unsaturated fatty acids in the adult UK population is probably less than 0.25 g per day (British Nutrition Foundation, 1999), although habitual intakes among healthy adults can vary greatly and will differ substantially between those who eat oily fish regularly and those who do not. Feeding humans increased amounts of fish oil results in a decrease in the amount of arachidonic acid in the membranes of most cells in the body, including those involved in inflammation and immunity (Gibney & Hunter, 1993). This means that there is less substrate available for synthesis of eicosanoids from arachidonic acid. Furthermore, EPA competitively inhibits the oxygenation of arachidonic acid by COX. Thus, fish oil feeding results in a decreased capacity of immune cells to synthesise eicosanoids from arachidonic acid. In addition, EPA is able to act as a substrate for both COX and 5-LOX (Fig. 3.5), giving rise to derivatives which have a different structure from those produced from arachidonic acid (*i.e.* 3-series prostaglandins and thromboxanes, and 5-series LT). Thus, the EPA induced suppression in the production of arachidonic-acid derived eicosanoids is mirrored by an elevation in the production of EPA derived eicosanoids. The eicosanoids produced from EPA are often less biologically potent than the analogues synthesised from arachidonic acid, although the full range of biological activities of these compounds has not been investigated. The reduction in generation of arachidonic acid-derived mediators, which accompanies fish oil consumption, has led to the idea that fish oil is anti-inflammatory and might modulate immune function. Since dietary fish oil leads to decreased $PGE_2$ production, it is often stated that it should reverse the effects of $PGE_2$. However, the situation is likely to be more complex than this because $PGE_2$ is not the sole mediator produced

from arachidonic acid and the range of mediators produced have varying, sometimes opposite, actions. Furthermore, EPA will give rise to mediators with varying actions. Thus, the overall effect of fish oil feeding cannot be predicted solely on the basis of an abrogation of $PGE_2$ mediated effects.

Some studies report that supplementation of the diet of healthy humans with EPA plus DHA (2.4 to 14 g/day) results in decreased lymphocyte proliferation, decreased monocyte and neutrophil chemotaxis, decreased production of IL-1, IL-2, IFN-γ, IL-6 and TNF, and decreased expression of MHC-II and adhesion molecules on monocytes (see Calder, 1997, 1998a,b,c for references). These levels of long chain *n*-3 polyunsaturated fatty acids would require the consumption of at least 6 standard one gram fish oil capsules per day (this would provide approximately 2 g EPA plus DHA). Several studies in healthy humans indicate that low to moderate intake of EPA plus DHA has little impact on immune function, at least in the short term (see Calder 1997, 1998a,b,c for references). There are no detailed human studies that seek to determine the dose dependence of fish oil on a range of immune parameters. There is some evidence, especially from animal studies, of interaction between *n*-3 polyunsaturated fatty acids and vitamin E with respect to immune function. However, the relationship between dietary, plasma and immune cell vitamin E levels is a complex one. It seems important to examine the relationship between the levels of polyunsaturated fatty acids and vitamin E in the diet, plasma and immune cell vitamin E status, and immune cell function in man.

### 3.5.7 Dietary fat and Th1 skewed immunological diseases

Chronic inflammatory diseases are characterised by a dysregulated Th1-type response (see Chapter 2) and often by an inappropriate production of arachidonic acid-derived eicosanoids, especially $PGE_2$ and $LTB_4$. The effects of fish oil suggest that it might have a role in prevention and therapy of chronic inflammatory diseases. A number of clinical trials have assessed the therapeutic benefits of dietary supplementation with fish oils in several inflammatory diseases in humans, including rheumatoid arthritis (see Volker & Garg, 1996; James & Cleland, 1997; Geusens, 1998 for reviews), Crohn's

Disease (see Belluzzi & Miglio, 1998 for a review), ulcerative colitis (see Rodgers, 1998 for a review) and psoriasis (see Ziboh, 1998 for a review). Many of the placebo-controlled, double-blind trials of fish oil in chronic inflammatory diseases reveal benefit, including decreased disease activity and a lowered use of anti-inflammatory drugs; the evidence for a beneficial effect of fish oil supplements is strongest in rheumatoid arthritis. Most trials of fish oil supplementation in systemic lupus erythematosus and multiple sclerosis have failed to show clinical improvement.

### 3.5.8 Fatty acids and Th2 skewed immunological diseases

$PGD_2$, $LTC_4$, $LTD_4$ and $LTE_4$ are produced by the cells that mediate pulmonary inflammation in asthma, such as mast cells, and are believed to be the major mediators of asthmatic bronchoconstriction. Although its action as a precursor for leukotrienes has highlighted the significance of

arachidonic acid in the aetiology of asthma, a second link concerns the ability of $PGE_2$ (for which it is also a precursor) to regulate the activities of macrophages and lymphocytes. Of particular relevance in the context of asthma and allergic diseases is the ability of $PGE_2$ to inhibit the production of the Th1-type cytokines IL-2 and IFN-$\gamma$, without affecting the production of the Th2-type cytokines IL-4 and IL-5, and to stimulate B cells to produce IgE. These observations suggest that $PGE_2$ regulates the development of these diseases (Fig. 3.6). As a result of this, there has been speculation that the increased intake of linoleic acid, the precursor of arachidonic acid, which has occurred since the mid-1960s, is causally linked to the increased incidence of asthma and allergic diseases over this period (Black & Sharpe, 1997; Hodge *et al.*, 1994). However, the idea that increased intake of linoleic acid is associated with allergic disease is opposed by the frequently reported lowered proportions of $\gamma$-linolenic acid, DGLA and/or arachidonic acids in the blood, cells and milk of allergic mothers and/or

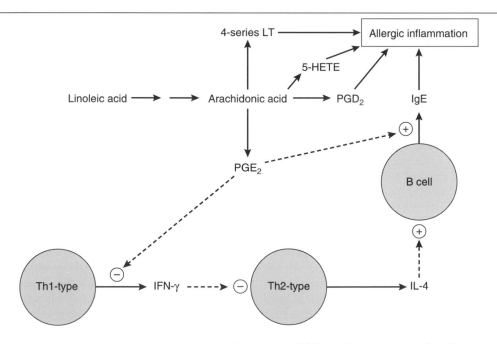

**Fig. 3.6**   Putative roles of arachidonic acid in allergic inflammation. $PGE_2$ inhibits production of the Th1-type cytokine, IFN-$\gamma$, so allowing the production of Th2-type cytokines (*e.g.* IL-4) to proceed without inhibition. IL-4 promotes Ig class switching in B cells to produce IgE; $PGE_2$ also directly promotes IgE production by B cells. Thus, $PGE_2$ acts to promote the Th2-type response and IgE production. The 4-series LT (and some 2-series PG, such as $PGD_2$) are the direct mediators of allergic inflammation.

their offspring (see Calder & Miles, 2000 for references). There are also abnormalities in the proportions of the long chain *n*-3 polyunsaturated fatty acids in these types of disease (see Calder & Miles, 2000), and a case has been made for increasing the consumption of these fatty acids by patients with allergic diseases (Black & Sharpe, 1997; Hodge *et al.*, 1994). Although there is some epidemiological evidence to support a protective role of long chain *n*-3 polyunsaturated fatty acids in asthma (Schwartz & Weiss, 1990, 1994b; Hodge *et al.*, 1996), several studies of fish oil supplementation in asthma reveal limited clinical impact (see Calder & Miles, 2000 for references), despite significant biochemical changes. In contrast, some studies have shown significant clinical improvements in some patient groups and suggest that this type of approach may be useful in conjunction with other drug- and diet-based therapies (see Calder & Miles, 2000). A careful study by Broughton *et al.* (1997) found that increased *n*-3 fatty acid ingestion improved lung function in response to methacholine challenge in more than 40% of the 26 adult asthmatics studied. However, some patients did not respond to the high *n*-3 fatty acid intake, which in some cases probably worsened respiratory function. This study suggests that there are subjects who respond positively to fish oil intervention and subjects who do not respond and who might even be worsened by such intervention; therapies should be approached cautiously until more is understood about the interaction between fatty acid consumption and disease activity.

## 3.6 Dictary amino acids and related compounds and immune function

### 3.6.1 Sulphur amino acids and glutathione

Sulphur amino acids are essential in humans. Deficiency in methionine and cysteine results in atrophy of the thymus, spleen and lymph nodes, and prevents recovery from protein-energy malnutrition (see Gross & Newberne, 1980 for references). When combined with a deficiency of isoleucine and valine (also essential amino acids), sulphur amino acid deficiency results in severe depletion of gut lymphoid tissue, which is very similar to the effect of protein deprivation (see Gross & Newberne, 1980).

Glutathione is an antioxidant tripeptide which consists of glycine, cysteine and glutamate. Glutathione concentrations in the liver, lung, small intestine and immune cells fall in response to inflammatory stimuli, and this fall can be prevented in some organs by provision of cysteine in the diet. Glutathione can enhance the activity of human cytotoxic T (effector $CD8^+$ cells) cells and depletion of intracellular glutathione diminishes lymphocyte proliferation and the generation of cytotoxic T cells. Cell culture studies indicate that glutathione can alter the Th1/Th2 balance in favour of a Th1 response (Peterson *et al.*, 1998).

### 3.6.2 Arginine

Arginine is a non-essential amino acid in humans. It is involved in protein, urea and nucleotide synthesis and ATP generation (see Redmond & Daly, 1993). It is the precursor of nitric oxide, a potent immunoregulatory mediator which is cytotoxic to tumour cells and to some microorganisms. Arginine is also the precursor for synthesis of polyamines, which have a key role in DNA replication, regulation of the cell cycle and cell division. In healthy human subjects, arginine supplementation (30 g/day; a typical Western diet provides about 4 g/day) has been shown to increase blood lymphocyte proliferation in response to mitogens, to decrease $CD8^+$ cell numbers while not affecting total lymphocyte or $CD4^+$ cell numbers and to promote wound healing (Barbul *et al.*, 1981, 1990). There are very few other studies of the effect of arginine on immune function in healthy humans. In patients, following surgery, arginine provision (25 g/day enterally for 7 days) increased circulating $CD4^+$ cell numbers and enhanced lymphocyte proliferation to mitogens (Daly *et al.*, 1988). These observations have led to the development of enteral formulas containing arginine for use in trauma patients. A number of studies have investigated the immunological and clinical effects of such formulas, which typically also contain other potentially immunomodulatory substances such as *n*-3 fatty acids and nucleotides, in surgery, trauma and burns patients. These studies show a lower number and reduced severity of infectious complications and decreased hospital stay (see Evoy *et al.*, 1998 for references), but it is very difficult to attribute these benefits to any one of the constituents of the formulas used.

### 3.6.3 Glutamine

Glutamine is the most abundant amino acid in the blood and in the free amino acid pool in the body (Elia & Lunn, 1997), with skeletal muscle being the most important site of production. Important users of glutamine include the kidney, liver, small intestine and cells of the immune system. In healthy subjects, plasma glutamine concentrations show little variation ($600\,\mu M$), but levels are lowered by up to 50% by sepsis, injury and burns and following surgery (see Wilmore & Shabert, 1998; Calder & Yaqoob, 1999 for references). Furthermore, the concentration in skeletal muscle is lowered by more than 50% in at least some of these situations (see Calder & Yaqoob, 1999), indicating that a significant depletion of the skeletal muscle glutamine pool is characteristic of trauma. The lowered plasma glutamine concentrations which occur are most likely the result of demand for glutamine (by the liver, kidney, gut and immune system) exceeding the supply, and it is proposed that glutamine be considered a conditionally essential amino acid during catabolic stress (Lacey & Wilmore, 1990).

It has been suggested that the lowered plasma glutamine contributes, at least in part, to the impaired immune function which accompanies such situations, and that restoring plasma glutamine concentrations should restore immune function (Newsholme & Calder, 1997). Although animal studies support this idea (see Calder & Yaqoob, 1999 for references), there are relatively few human studies of the influence of dietary glutamine on immune function, and there have been no studies of glutamine and immune function in healthy free-living humans, not undergoing some form of stress. However, the potential application of glutamine in trauma patients is now widely recognised and formulas containing glutamine or its precursors for use in such patients have been developed. Glutamine has been shown to decrease infection rates, mortality and hospital stay in various patient groups in intensive care (see Calder & Yaqoob, 1999 for references); but most of these studies have not measured immune function and so the benefit of glutamine cannot be attributed to improved host defence. In addition to a direct immunological effect, glutamine, even when provided parenterally, improves gut barrier function in patients at risk of infection (van der Hulst et al., 1993).

## 3.7 Probiotics, immune function and allergy

### 3.7.1 The theoretical basis for the use of probiotics

Indigenous bacteria are believed to contribute to the immunological protection of the host by creating a barrier against colonisation by pathogenic bacteria. This barrier can be disrupted by disease and by use of antibiotics, so allowing pathogens easier access to host tissues once they are in the gut. It is postulated by some that this barrier can be maintained by providing supplements containing live 'desirable' bacteria: such supplements are called probiotics (see Goldin, 1998; Naidu et al., 1999 for extensive reviews). Probiotic organisms are found in fermented foods, including traditionally cultured dairy products and newer kinds of fermented milks. The organisms included in commercial probiotics include lactic acid bacteria (e.g. Lactobacillus acidophilus, Lactobacillus casei, Enterococcus faecium) and Bifidobacteria. These organisms only colonise the gut temporarily, making their regular consumption necessary. In addition to creating a barrier effect, some of the metabolic products of probiotic bacteria (e.g. lactic acid and a class of antibiotic proteins termed bacteriocins produced by some bacteria) may inhibit growth of pathogenic organisms, compete for nutrients with the pathogens, or perhaps enhance the gut immune response against pathogenic bacteria (Fig. 3.7) (see Naidu et al., 1999 for a review).

### 3.7.2 Probiotics and immune function

Studies in animals reveal that lactic acid bacteria administered orally increase the numbers and functions of various immune cell populations, including those in the intestinal mucosa, and protect against challenges with pathogenic bacteria, reverse some of the immunosuppressive effects of malnutrition and cause the symptoms of enterocolitis to be less severe (see Naidu et al., 1999). Despite extensive animal studies, the effects of probiotic bacteria on human immune function and host defence remain unproven although some positive studies have emerged (see Naidu et al., 1999).

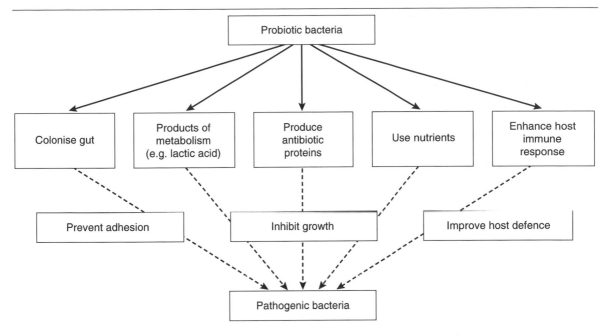

**Fig. 3.7** Potential roles of probiotic bacteria in the human intestinal tract. Probiotic bacteria may act in a variety of ways to prevent the growth and colonisation of pathogenic bacteria.

### 3.7.3 Probiotics and allergy

Gut microflora play a role in the development of the gut immune system. Recent studies suggest a link between gut microflora and allergic sensitisation, although this is far from proven. Animal studies indicate that 'desirable' intestinal microorganisms could downregulate allergic inflammation by counterbalancing Th2-type lymphocyte responses and by enhancing the IgA response. Infants with atopic eczema and cows' milk allergy showed significantly improved clinical scores and significantly decreased faecal concentrations of TNF-α and α-1-antitrypsin after inclusion of *Lactobacillus* in hydrolysed whey formula for one month (Majamaa & Isolauri, 1997); this study is difficult to interpret, however, because the addition of *Lactobacillus* to the diet was concurrent with the elimination of cows' milk. A recent double-blind, cross-over study investigated the effects of *Lactobacillus* on milk challenge in milk-hypersensitive and healthy adults (Pelto *et al.*, 1998). This study found different effects of *Lactobacillus* between the milk-sensitive and healthy subjects: *Lactobacillus* had an immunostimulatory effect in healthy subjects, but appeared to downregulate some aspects of inflammation in milk-hypersensitive subjects (see Pelto *et al.*, 1999 for a discussion of these findings).

## 3.8 Breast feeding and immune function

### 3.8.1 The composition of breast milk

Breast milk is the best example of a foodstuff with immune-enhancing properties. It contains a wide range of immunologically-active components including cells (macrophages, T and B lymphocytes, neutrophils), immunoglobulins (IgG, IgM, IgD, sIgA), lysozyme (which has direct antibacterial action), lactoferrin (which binds iron, so preventing its uptake by bacteria), cytokines (IL-1, IL-6, IL-10, IFN-γ, TNF-α, TGF-β), growth factors (epidermal growth factor, insulin-like growth factor), hormones (thyroxin), fat-soluble vitamins (vitamins A, D, E), amino acids (taurine, glutamine), fatty acids, amino sugars and nucleotides (see Emmett & Rogers, 1997; Bernt & Walker, 1999 for reviews). Breast milk contains factors which prevent adhesion of certain microorganisms to the gastrointestinal tract and so prevents bacterial colonisation. Human breast milk contains factors which promote the growth of useful bacteria (*e.g. Bifidobacteria*) in the gut; this factor is absent from milks of all other species. The content of many factors varies among milks of different species, and is different between human breast milk and many infant formulas. Human milk is rich in Ig, in the antimicrobial proteins lactoferrin and lysozyme, in vitamins A, D and E, in polyunsaturated fatty acids, in free amino acids and in nucleotides; in contrast, cows' milk either lacks or contains much lower amounts of many of these factors (Jackson & Golden, 1978). Jackson and Golden (1978) speculate that the role of cows' milk is to aid development of the rumen in the calf; thus the composition of cows' milk should be one which will promote growth of certain types of bacteria in the gastrointestinal tract. Clearly, this may be undesirable in the new born human infant and could have disastrous consequences, particularly when combined with exposure to microorganisms. The factors in human milk (*e.g.* the sIgA antibody to P6, the Bifidus factor, lactoferrin) seem designed to promote growth of *Bifidobacteria* and *Lactobacilli* and to prevent growth of potentially pathogenic gram-negative bacteria (see Levy 1998, for a discussion).

### 3.8.2 Breast feeding, immune function and infection

Mata *et al.* (1977) provided elegant data which suggest that breast feeding reduces the incidence of infections in children in developing countries. Other studies support the notion that breast feeding has a key role in the prevention of infectious disease: the risk of diarrhoea, respiratory infections and mortality was lowest in exclusively breast-fed Peruvian infants and highest in those who were not breast fed (Brown *et al.*, 1989). In the absence of diarrhoea, linear growth of exclusively breast-fed infants was three times higher than those who were not breast fed. A study in Scotland found that babies who were breast fed for 13 or more weeks had significantly less gastrointestinal illness than those who were bottle fed from birth (Howie *et al.*, 1990); the protective effect of breast feeding was maintained beyond the breast feeding period and resulted in a decreased rate of hospital admissions.

Breast feeding for less than 13 weeks was not protective (Howie *et al.*, 1990). Golding *et al.* (1997a,b,c) have reviewed the impact of breast feeding and conclude that during the first 4 to 6 months of life it protects against gastroenteritis and diarrhoea in both the developed and developing world, and that it may be protective against lower, but probably not against upper, respiratory tract infections. In addition to preventing infectious disease, breast feeding enhances the antibody responses to vaccination, and there may be stronger T cell responses as well (see Hanson *et al.*, 1997 for references). The proposed benefits of breast feeding in atopic infants are discussed in Chapter 5.

## 3.9  General comments

Deficiencies of total energy or of one or more essential nutrients, including vitamins A, $B_6$, $B_{12}$, C, E, folic acid, zinc, iron, copper, selenium, essential amino acids and essential fatty acids, impair immune function and increase susceptibility to infectious pathogens. This is most likely because these nutrients are involved in the molecular and cellular responses to challenge of the immune system. Providing these nutrients to deficient individuals restores immune function and improves resistance to infection. For some nutrients the dietary intakes which result in greatest enhancement of immune function are above currently recommended intakes. However, excess intake of some nutrients also impairs immune responses. Thus, four potential general relationships between the intake of a nutrient and immune function appear to exist (Fig. 3.8).

These different types of relationship might in part reflect interactions between nutrients, such that an excess of one nutrient negatively affects the status of a second nutrient (*e.g.* zinc and copper). There appear to be interactions between similar classes of nutrients (*e.g. n*-6 and *n*-3 polyunsaturated fatty acids) which have yet to be fully unravelled, and there are most likely interactions between nutrients that contribute to oxidative stress (*e.g.* polyunsaturated fatty acids) and those which protect against it (*e.g.* vitamin E). It is often assumed, when defining the relationship between nutrient intake and immune function, that all components of the immune system will respond in the same dose-dependent fashion to a given

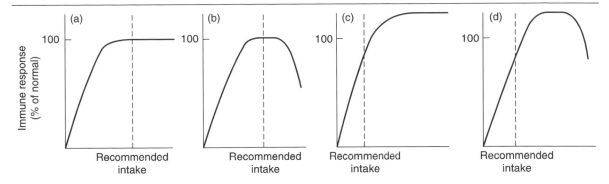

**Fig. 3.8** Potential patterns of relationship between nutrient status and immune function. All patterns assume that a deficiency of the nutrient impairs the immune response. In pattern (a) the immune response is maximal, in terms of relationship to the intake of the nutrient under study, at the recommended level of intake and intakes somewhat above the recommended intake do not impair immune function. In pattern (b) the immune response is maximal, in terms of relationship to the intake of the nutrient under study, at the recommended level of intake and intakes somewhat above the recommended intake impair immune function. In pattern (c) the immune response is submaximal, in terms of relationship to the intake of the nutrient under study, at the recommended level of intake and intakes somewhat above the recommended intake do not impair immune function. In pattern (d) the immune response is submaximal, in terms of relationship to the intake of the nutrient under study, at the recommended level of intake and intakes somewhat above the recommended intake impair immune function.

nutrient. This is not correct, at least as far as some nutrients are concerned, and it appears likely that different components of the immune system show an individual dose–response relationship to the availability of a given nutrient.

One aspect not touched upon in this overview is the role of hormones in regulating immune function. An inadequate supply of nutrients to the body may cause physiological stress, leading to elevations in the circulating concentrations of glucocorticoids and catecholamines. Both these classes of hormones have an inhibitory effect on immune function, and so may be important factors when considering the relationship between nutrient supply and immunological outcome.

An early point of contact between nutrients and the immune system occurs within the intestinal tract. There is relatively little work relating nutrient status to function of the gut-associated immune system. This is of particular relevance when considering adverse reactions to foods: the role of immunoregulatory nutrients in responses to food components and in sensitisation to food/borne allergens is largely unknown. An understanding of the interaction between nutrients, the types of

bacteria which inhabit the gut, and gut-associated and systemic immune responses is beginning to emerge.

Some consider that the immune system does not respond optimally to challenge in apparently healthy, free-living humans even if they are not overtly deficient in any single nutrient. Individuals may be marginally deficient in one or more nutrients, or may be consuming some nutrients in excess. There is now much interest in optimising the immune response in such individuals, not simply by correcting marginal deficiencies but by increasing the intake of certain micronutrients, amino acids and probiotics. At this stage, the immuno-enhancing effect of such supplementation is unproved and, as far as micronutrients are concerned, might even be dangerous. An extension to this idea is that diseases involving immune dysregulation might be subject to control by nutrient supplementation or dietary modification. However, more needs to be known about the relationship between nutrients and immune responses in these disease conditions before such approaches can be considered.

## 3.10 Key points

- Deficiencies of a wide variety of essential nutrients may impair immune function and increase susceptibility to infectious pathogens. Particular examples of those at most risk include premature infants and in malnutrition, especially in childhood, in old age and in the presence of infections, especially HIV.
- While immune function can be improved when deficient nutrients are replaced, as in institutionalised elderly people, an overcorrection of deficiencies, *e.g.* from zinc or iron, can damage the immune response.
- For some nutrients, the dietary intakes that result in the greatest measurable enhancement of immune function are above currently recommended intakes, but this should not be taken to mean that supplementation is the answer as excess intake of some nutrients can also impair immune function. There is no convincing evidence that the immune systems of non-deficient healthy people on a normal mixed diet benefit from vitamin or other dietary supplements.
- A high fat diet can damage the immune response. Fatty acids are, however, an important substrate for the production of eicosanoids, and fish oils may have beneficial effects which are the subject of on-going investigation.
- A number of nutrients can be shown to influence different components of the immune system in a dose–response fashion. The outcomes of these effects can also interact with one another and also with other substances, such as hormones.
- Relatively little is known about the relationship between nutrient status and function of the gut-associated immune system.
- Despite growing interest in the potential of nutrient supply to influence outcome in diseases involving immune dysregulation, the available evidence is insufficient to support recommendations.

# 4
# Epidemiology of Food Intolerance and Food Allergy

## 4.1 Introduction

Food intolerance and allergy are emerging as major consumer and public health concerns. However, the actual magnitude of the problem remains unknown because of a paucity of quality information regarding the prevalence (established cases per unit time) and incidence (new cases per unit time) of these conditions. The absence of scientifically authoritative studies is surprising given the media and public interest in the subject. This chapter aims to outline the epidemiology of food intolerance with particular attention to IgE mediated food allergy. The epidemiology of non-IgE mediated food allergy is discussed briefly, followed by a description of the epidemiology of IgE mediated allergy in children and adults. Possible time trends are mentioned and IgE mediated food allergy, in the context of general IgE mediated allergy, is also discussed.

## 4.2 The adequacy of currently available epidemiological data for food intolerance

The epidemiology of food intolerance is poorly characterised and a number of factors have probably contributed to this. The traditional epidemiological tool of the postal or interviewer-administered symptom questionnaire is an unreliable method for identifying food intolerance because of positive response bias, and the prevalence of suggestive but not diagnostic symptoms greatly and variably exceeds the true prevalence of food intolerance. Even in the clinical setting, the identification and confirmation of food intolerance is difficult, time consuming and expensive in terms of patient and medical time and commitment. The clinical protocols of elimination diets, open food challenges and double-blind placebo-controlled food challenges (DBPCFC) to identify food intolerance are not easily applied to large scale epidemiological studies because of difficulties with subject compliance as well as logistic and economic considerations (see Chapter 11). There are no simple tests that reliably identify food intolerance. Skin prick tests and food specific serum IgE, although commonly used in epidemiological studies, merely reflect IgE sensitisation. Many individuals possess these antibodies but apparently do not display symptoms when they eat the food, *i.e.* they are clinically asymptomatic.

Review of the studies that have investigated the epidemiology of food intolerance and food allergy reveals several limitations. Many studies have described the prevalence of food intolerance and allergy in groups that are not representative of the general population; for example, patients referred to allergy clinics and the children of atopic parents. Very few of the general population studies have corrected for non-response bias. In one study that did adjust for this phenomenon, the prevalence of symptoms in the responders to a postal survey was considerably greater than the prevalence rate in a sample of non-responders (7.4% vs 1.1%), (Young *et al.*, 1987). Therefore, the prevalences of food intolerance and allergy, derived from the several large general population studies reliant on postal screening questionnaires, are probably over-estimates. The working definitions of adverse reactions, food intolerance and food allergy are not consistent between studies, with the term food allergy sometimes being loosely applied to all adverse reactions and with many studies failing to report the individual prevalences of IgE and non-IgE mediated food allergy.

### 4.2.1 Non-IgE mediated allergy

In this chapter, discussion of non-IgE mediated food allergy is limited to gluten sensitive entero-pathy (coeliac disease) and the epidemiology of this condition will be discussed briefly here; for a more detailed description refer to Chapter 9, in particular Sections 9.5 and 9.10.

When compared with non-allergic food intoler-ance and IgE mediated food allergy, the epide-miological features of gluten sensitive enteropathy are well characterised. This is largely the con-sequence of the readily available, sensitive and specific antigliadin and IgA antiendomysial anti-body assays (see Chapter 9, Section 9.7.2), which have enabled screening of sections of the general population and have led to the identification of unrecognised clinical cases and additional sub-clinical/latent cases.

The prevalence of clinical cases of biopsy-proven coeliac disease in adults has been calculated as between 1 in 1000 and 2.7 in 1000 people (Hallert *et al.*, 1983; Midhagen *et al.*, 1988; Collin *et al.*, 1997; Sjoberg & Eriksson, 1999), but the prevalence of coeliac disease in general populations screened for the condition is inevitably greater.

Using these new techniques, the consensus for the prevalence of gluten sensitive enteropathy in Europe is typically 3 to 4 cases per 1000 people (Catassi *et al.*, 1994; Rostami *et al.*, 1999), although some studies, for example in Belfast and Sweden, have suggested a higher prevalence in some popu-lations (Johnston *et al.*, 1998; Ivarsson *et al.*, 1999). Ivarsson *et al.* (1999) screened 1894 Swedish adults and noted that the prevalence of biopsy-proven coeliac disease was 5.3 per 1000, with 80% of identified cases being previously undiagnosed. There was a 7:3 female to male dominance in this Swedish population. For a more detailed discus-sion, see Chapter 9.

Several studies have identified time trends (at least among those cases that have been confirmed) and also evidence of geographical variation. Collin *et al.* (1997) reported a ten-fold increase in the prevalence of proven coeliac disease between 1975 and 1994. In addition to geographic variation, George *et al.* (1997) reported an increase in the cumulative incidence rates of proven coeliac dis-ease in children from 0.1 per 1000 to 0.54 per 1000 live births between 1976 and 1993/4.

As is discussed in more detail in Chapter 9, the apparent increase in prevalence is likely to be mainly due to improved identification of cases, as a result of increasing awareness, changes in diag-nostic practice and the easy access to diagnostic serology and endoscopy. However, changes in dietary patterns, particularly in early life (*e.g.* infant feeding and weaning practices), over the past half century may also have contributed to some extent (see Chapter 9, Section 9.10).

## 4.3 Infants and children

The prevalence of food intolerance and of allergy is undoubtedly influenced by a number of factors, namely age, gender, genetic constitution, dietary habits, the allergenicity of dietary components and perhaps by as yet unidentified environmental fac-tors. The prevalence of food intolerance and allergy is greater in infants and children than in adults and will be considered first.

Most of the studies (summarised in Table 4.1) that have characterised the prevalence of food intolerance and allergy in the general paediatric population have focused on individual dietary components such as milk, eggs and peanuts. How-ever, an insufficient number of relatively small studies have measured the overall prevalence of food intolerance and allergy in the paediatric population. Bock (1987) recruited a cohort of 480 neonates and studied them prospectively for 3 years, with any symptoms suggestive of food intol-erance and allergy being investigated by elimina-tion diets, open challenge and DBPCFC. Suspected food-related symptoms were reported by the par-ents of 28% of the infants, with 80% of these being reported in the first year, 16% in the second and 4% in the third year of life. Food intolerance or allergy (see Chapter 1 for definitions) was con-firmed in only 8% of the total group, with nearly all of the reproducible reactions being independent of

**Table 4.1**  Summary of the epidemiological studies of food intolerances and allergy in children.

| Author | Age group (years) | Study size and Country | Prevalence of reported symptoms | Foods responsible | Prevalence of food intolerance/allergy |
|---|---|---|---|---|---|
| Bock (1987) | 0–3 | 480 USA | 28% (+16% fruit and juices) | Milk, soya, eggs, peanuts (fruit and juices) | Intolerance 8% (+12% fruit and juices) |
| Douwes *et al.* (1988) | 0–0.5 | 1004 Netherlands | 5.3% | Milk, soya, eggs, peanuts | Intolerance 1.7% |
| Høst & Halken (1990) | 0–1 | 1749 Denmark | 6.7% | Cows' milk | Intolerance 2.2% IgE allergy 1.2% |
| Schrander *et al.* (1993) | 0–1 | 1158 Netherlands | 18% | Cows' milk | Intolerance 2.8% |
| Bock (1987) | 0–3 | 480 USA | 15% | Cows' milk | Intolerance 5.2% |
| Sampson (1999) | 0–3 | 1314 Germany | | Hens' eggs | IgE allergy 1.3% |
| Tariq *et al.* (1996) | 4 | 1218 UK | | Peanuts | IgE allergy 0.5% |
| Sicherer *et al.* (1999) | <18 | 2998 USA | | Peanuts, treenuts | Peanut intolerance 0.4% Treenut intolerance 0.2% |
| Young *et al.* (1987) | 0–9 | 2255 UK | 15% | Food additives | Not given |
| Fuglsang *et al.* (1993) | 5–16 | 4274 Denmark | 6% | Food additives | Intolerance 1–2% |

IgE dependent mechanisms, *i.e.* either non-allergic reactions or non-IgE mediated allergy. The foods responsible were milk, soya, peanut and egg, but a further 16% of the children were reported to have reactions to fruits and fruit juices. Reproducible reactions, including skin rashes and/or diarrhoea, to fruit and fruit juices were confirmed in 12% of the total group. This intolerance developed later than those to milk, soya, egg and peanuts. Douwes *et al.* (1988) followed a random population of 1004 Dutch infants, from birth until the age of 6 months. Of these children, 5.3% showed symptoms that were suggestive of food intolerance/allergy and this diagnosis was confirmed by positive results (elimination and challenge protocol) in 1.7% of the sample. From a review of the literature, Chandra (1997a) has stated that the true prevalence of incontrovertible food allergy in the general population of young children is about 1.4% (0.5–3.8%).

In general, the prognosis of childhood food intolerance is good, with most non-allergic intol-erance being outgrown in the first few years of life. Similarly, most IgE mediated allergies to milk, eggs and soya resolve with age, although in some children they may remain severe. Unfortunately, children with IgE mediated food allergy to peanuts, nuts, fish and shellfish are unlikely to grow out of their allergy and should, therefore, be suitably advised.

### 4.3.1  Cows' milk intolerance and allergy

The prevalence of cows' milk intolerance and allergy has been studied more extensively. In a study of 1749 randomly selected neonates, Høst and Halken (1990) reported that 6.7% developed symptoms suggestive of cows' milk intolerance (see Chapter 6 for information on clinical features). Use of a strict elimination and challenge protocol (see Chapter 11 for details) confirmed cows' milk intolerance to be present in 2.2% of the sample during the first year. Further investigation of these indicated that an IgE mediated mechanism was present in just over half (54%), giving a prevalence of IgE mediated cows' milk allergy of 1.2% in the first year. The prognosis for recovery from cows' milk intolerance was good, with 56% able to consume cows' milk by their first birthday, 77% by their second and 87% by the age of 3 years. Cows' milk intolerance was associated with intolerance to other foods in 54% of cases, mainly to eggs, citrus fruit and tomatoes. In a similar study of 1158 randomly selected infants, the prevalence of symptoms suggestive of cows' milk intolerance during the first year was 18%; however, subsequent detailed investigation suggested that the prevalence of proven cows' milk intolerance in the first year of life was 2.8% (Schrander *et al.*, 1993). In the study of Bock (1987), 15% of the 480 children followed for 3 years developed symptoms of cows' milk intolerance, with the prevalence of proven intolerance being 5.2%. Virtually all of the cases of cows' milk intolerance developed in the first year of life (5%) and the remainder (0.2%) in the second year. The prognosis for cows' milk intolerance is usually good (especially if not mediated by IgE); most cases occur during the first year of life and the child usually 'grows out' of the condition. In a study of 100 children with proven cows' milk allergy (Bishop *et al.*, 1990), 28% developed tolerance by the age of 2 and, by the age of 6, 78% had developed tolerance and had been re-established on milk-containing diets. In this study, cows' milk allergy was defined by either an elevated specific IgE (25% of cases) or *in vitro* evidence of sensitisation, as manifested by cytokine secretion in response to milk protein. The authors also demonstrated that cows' milk allergy was associated with reports (from parents) of adverse reactions to other foods, such as egg (58%), soya milk (47%) and peanuts (34%).

### 4.3.2 Allergy to egg

It is difficult to ascertain the prevalence of childhood hens' eggs allergy from the published literature. Sampson (1999) states that the prevalence of hens' eggs hypersensitivity in young children is about 1.3%. This figure is based on the study of Nickel *et al.* (1997), which reported the prevalence of egg-specific IgE in 1314 randomly identified infants followed from birth to 3 years. However, it is not immediately apparent from the data of Nickel

*et al.* (1997) how Sampson (1999) has derived the prevalence rate of 1.3%.

### 4.3.3 Peanut allergy

The recent emergence of peanut allergy as the most frequent cause of food-associated anaphylaxis in Europe and North America has stimulated epidemiological research. Bock and Dorion (1992) identified all cases of food-related anaphylaxis presenting at all the emergency rooms serving the 3.3 million population of Colorado and calculated the annual incidence of food-induced anaphylaxis as 1 person per 234 000 people, with peanuts being responsible for one third of these cases. Bresser *et al.* (1995) reported a higher rate of food-related anaphylaxis, at 1 in 90 900 people per year, this being derived from a population of 1.5 million centred on Munich, Germany.

The allergens found in peanuts (a legume) and in nuts (sometimes referred to as tree nuts) appear to be the major causes of food-related episodes of anaphylaxis. In a study of 13 cases of fatal and near fatal anaphylaxis in children and adolescents, Sampson *et al.* (1992a) reported that peanuts were responsible for 4 out of 13 and nuts for 6 out of 13 cases, with egg being responsible for 1 in 13 and milk 2 in 13. Similarly, Yunginger *et al.* (1988) reported that peanuts were responsible for 4 out of 7 fatal food-related anaphylactic episodes in children and adults, pecan nuts were responsible for 1 in 7, crab 1 in 7 and fish 1 in 7. A random telephone survey of 12 032 individuals in the USA revealed that, after adjustment for response bias, the prevalence of symptoms strongly suggestive of peanut allergy in children aged under 18 years was 0.4% and for tree nuts, 0.2% (Sicherer *et al.*, 1999). It should be noted that the definition of food allergy used by Sicherer *et al.* (1999) differs from that used in this report, with the 'food allergies' reported by Sicherer *et al.* being more correctly described as food intolerances because the very nature of a telephone survey excludes comment on the allergic/non-allergic status of any adverse reactions. Tariq *et al.* (1996) reported on a year cohort of 981 4-year-old children from the Isle of Wight, UK, and demonstrated that the prevalence of IgE mediated peanut allergy was 0.5% and that one-third of these children had suffered episodes of peanut-related anaphylaxis. In contrast to allergy to cows' milk, egg and soya, the remission rate for childhood peanut allergy is low. (For further discussion, see Chapter 6, Section 6.5.2.)

### 4.3.4 Intolerance to food additives

The prevalence of intolerance to food additives in 4274 children aged 5–16 years has been estimated by Fuglsang *et al.* (1993) to be 1–2%, using open challenges and DBPCFC. This represents a 3- to 6-fold reduction compared with the 6% of children in the sample who had reported symptoms consistent with intolerance to food additives (synthetic colourings and citric acid). In a large general population survey, Young *et al.* (1987) reported that the parents of 15% of 0–9-year-old children believed that their children were intolerant of food additives. Unfortunately it is not clear from the paper how many of these childhood cases were confirmed using challenge protocols (see Table 4.2 for overall figure). Further information on food additives can be found in Appendix 1.

## 4.4 Adults

Given the generally good prognosis associated with childhood food intolerance and food allergy, it would seem logical for the prevalence of these conditions in adults to be lower than in children, and indeed this appears to be so. The prevalence of food intolerance and food allergy in adults (summarised in Table 4.2) has been measured in several studies, although direct comparisons between stu-dies are difficult because of differences in study populations, methodology and working definitions. Niestijil Jansen *et al.* (1994) studied a random sample of 1483 adults, of whom 12.4% reported symptoms of food intolerance/allergy during a postal survey. Subsequent detailed investigation of these subjects, including DBPCFC, suggested that the prevalence of food intolerance in this popula-tion was 2.2% and that the prevalence of IgE mediated food allergy was 0.2%. The authors also reported a sex difference in symptom reporting and in the prevalence of food intolerance/allergy, with 15% of women and 9% of men reporting symp-toms. The prevalence of food intolerance/allergy was 2.9% in women and 1.8% in men. Cohen *et al.* (1985) investigated 2385 adult US blood donors, among whom 4.9% reported adverse reactions to food. After detailed investigation, including DBPCFC, the prevalence of proven food intoler-ance was reported as 1% and the prevalence of food allergy was about 0.5%. The low prevalence of symptoms reported in this study has been attributed to the questionnaire that was used, but it should be noted that healthy blood donors are a highly selected healthy group of individuals and may not be representative of the general adult population. Young *et al.* (1994) reported that the prevalence of food intolerance in a general population setting, after detailed investigation including DBPCFC, was 1.4–1.8% depending on the criteria used. The prevalence of self-reported symptoms of food intolerance was again high at about 20%. Chandra (1997a), in his review of food allergy, states that the prevalence of incontrovertible food allergy in the adult population is 0.3% (range 0.1–1.0%).

**Table 4.2** Summary of the epidemiological studies of food intolerance and allergy in adults.

| Author | Study size and country | Prevalence of reported symptoms | Foods responsible | Prevalence of food intolerance/allergy |
|---|---|---|---|---|
| Young *et al.* (1994) | 18 880 UK | 20% | 8 foods | Intolerance 1.4–1.8% |
| Niestijil Jansen *et al.* (1994) | 1483 Netherlands | 12.4% | | Intolerance 2.2% IgE allergy 0.2% |
| Sicherer *et al.* (1999) | 12 032 USA | | Nuts | Peanut intolerance 0.7% Tree nut intolerance 0.7% |
| Young *et al.* (1987) | 18 582 UK | Food 15.6% Food additives 7.4% | | Intolerance to food additives 0.01–0.23% |

### 4.4.1 Peanut allergy in adults

The prevalence of adult intolerance to peanuts has been addressed in the study of Sicherer *et al.* (1999). A random telephone survey of 12 032 individuals in the USA revealed, after adjustment for response bias, that the prevalence of symptoms strongly suggestive of peanut allergy in adults aged over 18 years was 0.7% and for tree nuts 0.7%. In this study, the prevalence of peanut allergy was greater in adults than children, which is the reverse of the observations for other food allergies, such as cows' milk and hens' eggs, probably reflecting the persistence of peanut allergy in children as they grow up, giving a greater cumulative adult prevalence. However, the age distribution of peanut allergy may alter in the coming decades as there is some evidence that the age of onset of peanut allergy is decreasing with successive generations (Hourihane *et al.*, 1996).

### 4.4.2 Intolerance to food additives in adults

The prevalence of intolerance in adulthood to food additives was addressed by Young *et al.* (1987), who reported that 15.6% of adults reported adverse reactions to food and 7.4% reported adverse reactions to food additives. The prevalence of these self- (or parentally-) reported reactions was greater in women than in men, and adult prevalence was less than in children. Following a detailed assessment protocol, the prevalence of proven intolerance to food additives was 0.01–0.23%. The reported prevalence rate is for the additives tartrazine E102, quinolone yellow E104, sunset yellow El10, carmoisine E122, amaranth E123, indigo carmine E132, green S E142, annatto E160(b), benzoates E210-E219, butylated hydroxyanisole E320 and butylated hydroxytoluene E321. It is likely to be an underestimate because, in spite of the known ability of sodium metabisulphite (see Appendix 1) to provoke asthma attacks (Schwartz 1997), intolerance to this substance was not assessed.

## 4.5 Time trends and geographic differences

Most European and North American paediatricians would agree with the generally held view that the prevalence of food intolerance and food allergy has increased in the past 30 years. Published medical literature cannot support or refute these clinical observations because there have been virtually no repeated cross-sectional or longitudinal studies specifically designed to investigate time trends in food intolerance and allergy. There is some evidence suggesting that episodes of food-related anaphylaxis have increased in recent years. In his review of peanut allergy, Hourihane *et al.* (1996) summarises the history of publications on peanut allergy and suggests that the first scientific reports of peanut allergy started in the late 1970s, with reports of peanut-related anaphylaxis starting in the mid 1980s. Peanut-related anaphylaxis is a dramatic condition and it is highly unlikely to have been previously missed or misdiagnosed. Moneret-Vautrin and Kanny (1995) have provided more direct evidence demonstrating that, in France, episodes of food-related anaphylaxis increased five-fold over a 10-year period. The most likely explanation for the increase in food-related anaphylaxis is a general increase in the prevalence of IgE mediated food allergy, with the cases of anaphylaxis representing those most severely affected by IgE allergy.

It is highly likely that the prevalence of IgE mediated food allergy in prosperous/developed countries has increased in the last 30 years and, unfortunately, probably continues to do so. This increase is consistent with clinical anecdote, the increase in food-related anaphylaxis and the well documented increases in the prevalence of the other IgE mediated allergic diseases of atopic asthma, atopic eczema and allergic rhinitis (hayfever) (see Section 4.7). Despite the clinical impression that the prevalence of non-IgE mediated food allergy is increasing, it is not possible to make an authoritative comment because of the lack of data. Given the recent increases in the prevalence of diseases mediated by non-IgE immune mechanisms, *e.g.* juvenile onset diabetes mellitus, rheumatoid arthritis and inflammatory bowel disease, it is not inconceivable that the prevalence of non-IgE mediated food allergy may also be increasing. There is an urgent need for studies to determine whether or not food allergy (and food intolerance) is on the increase, as extrapolation from time trend data for non-food allergic conditions cannot be relied upon.

Discussion about geographic differences in the prevalence of food intolerance and allergy is limited by a similar paucity of quality published data. The study of Gislason *et al.* (1999) investigated the prevalence of IgE sensitisation to food allergens in adults living in Iceland and Sweden. It should be emphasised that the presence of food-specific IgE is not always associated with symptoms. Gislason *et al.* reported that the prevalence of food-specific IgE to peanuts, wheat and soya beans was higher in Sweden, along with IgE specific for timothy grass, cat, birch and cladosporium. The general impression is that there is indeed geographic variation in the prevalence of these conditions with, for example, fish allergy being common in children who live in countries with a high fish consumption and peanut allergy being very rare in countries with a low consumption of peanuts. Feeding practices do not, however, fully explain anecdotal geographical differences. For example, the consumption of peanuts is high in Indonesia (Ewan, 1998) yet the anecdotal prevalence of peanut allergy in this country is either very low or unheard of. The same applies to parts of Africa where peanuts are a staple part of the diet. Of course, this may be the result of a failure to diagnose cases of peanut allergy; it has been described in black people (from Africa and the Caribbean) living in Britain. There is a growing consensus in the field of allergy research that IgE mediated allergy is more prevalent in affluent westernised countries and that the allergens to which children become sensitised reflect early exposure to the local commonly ingested and inhaled allergens.

## 4.6 The relationship between IgE mediated food allergy and other IgE mediated allergies

Atopy is the inherited tendency to generate immune responses, dominated by IgE, in response to environmental antigens and is by far the most influential risk factor known that predisposes to asthma, eczema and hayfever. Atopy can be objectively quantified by the measurement of total serum IgE, allergen specific IgE and by skin prick tests. Several lines of evidence strongly suggest that IgE mediated food allergy, especially in young children, should be considered as one component of an atopic quadrad (Sampson, 1996a).

The prevalence of the atopic conditions (asthma, eczema and hayfever) is much greater in children and adults with IgE mediated food allergies than in subjects who do not have food allergies (Bishop *et al.*, 1990; Høst & Halken, 1990; Hill *et al.*, 1994; Niestijil Jansen *et al.*, 1994). This association is particularly strong in children with peanut allergy; Tariq *et al.* (1996) demonstrated that all children in their study with peanut allergy had other atopic diseases. In particular, the prevalence of asthma, eczema and allergic rhinitis was 46%, 62% and 31%, respectively, in the children with peanut allergy, compared with prevalences of 14.5%, 11.4% and 5.1%, respectively, in the control group of children (which comprised non-allergic children and children with non-peanut allergies). Studies in cows' milk allergic children (Høst & Halken, 1990; Hill *et al.* 1994) have demonstrated that the prevalence of atopic disorders is greatest in those who remain intolerant and that, even in children who grow out of their allergy, the prevalence of atopic disorders is greater than in the general population.

It has been suggested that IgE mediated food allergy tends to occur in those children who are highly atopic (Hill *et al.*, 1994; Zimmerman *et al.*, 1989). When compared with subjects who are not food allergic, the prevalence of IgE sensitisation to inhalant and ingested allergens is greater in those with food allergy (Høst & Halken, 1990; Hill *et al.*, 1994; Tariq *et al.*, 1996). Bjornsson *et al.* (1996) noted that IgE sensitisation to food allergens was uncommon in adults who were IgE sensitised to less than two inhalant allergens.

In common with other atopic conditions, food allergy is associated with a positive family history of atopic conditions including food allergy. Høst and Halken (1990) reported a positive family history of atopy in 55% of their children with cows' milk allergy. Tariq *et al.* (1996) reported a positive family history in 93% of their subjects with peanut allergy compared with 58% of children without peanut allergy. By characterising the history of IgE mediated allergy in the relatives of children with peanut allergy, Hourihane *et al.* (1996) demonstrated that the prevalence of peanut allergy in the siblings of probands (cases identified independently of their relatives) with the allergy was 7%. Furthermore, the authors also demonstrated an increase in all forms of atopic disease in the relatives of proband children, and interestingly they also demonstrated that atopy was becoming increasingly prevalent in successive generations, as was the prevalence of peanut allergy.

Thus it would appear that IgE mediated food allergy, especially in young children, should be considered as one component of the atopic spectrum. Given this association and the lack of data related to food allergy, it is reasonable to describe briefly the epidemiology of the other atopic diseases. Although this may shed light on the epidemiology of IgE mediated food allergy, it is no substitute for data from studies specifically designed to characterise the epidemiology of food intolerance and food allergy.

## 4.7 General epidemiology of IgE mediated allergy

The prevalence of the IgE mediated diseases of atopic asthma, atopic eczema and allergic rhinitis (hayfever) is greater in children than in adults, and this is consistent with the observed prevalence rates of food intolerance and food allergy. It is also fairly well established that atopic conditions in children are more prevalent in boys, whereas in adults there is a female excess (Dodge & Burrows, 1980; Clough, 1993; Sears *et al.*, 1993; Peat, 1996); again the available data on food intolerance and allergy are consistent with these observations. There is increasing evidence that atopic diseases are associated with the affluent 'westernised' lifestyle. In the rural areas of developing countries, the prevalence of atopic conditions is extremely low when compared with affluent urban areas (Godfrey, 1975; Cookson, 1987; Hijazi *et al.*, 1998). The very low anecdotal prevalence of peanut allergy in rural West Africa and Indonesia (where peanut consumption is high) is consistent with this. In westernised countries, this urban rural difference is not present (Devereux *et al.*, 1996). The rapid increase in the prevalence of atopy in Pacific islanders who had migrated from the relatively underdeveloped island of Tokelau to New Zealand emphasises the adverse influence of westernisation on atopy and probably food allergy (Brown & Gadjusek, 1978). The collapse of the communist systems in Eastern Europe has enabled the comparison of populations of similar genetic constitution who have lived under markedly different environmental, social and political conditions.

Comparison of the former West Germany with the former state of East Germany revealed that the prevalence of asthma, eczema, hayfever and IgE sensitisation was significantly lower in East Germany (Von Mutius *et al.*, 1992, 1994; Nicolai *et al.*, 1997). Furthermore, as the former East Germany has become more affluent and westernised, the prevalence of allergic rhinitis and IgE sensitisation appears to be on the increase (Von Mutius *et al.*, 1998). This population base could provide the ideal opportunity to quantify changes in food intolerance and food allergy with increasing affluence.

The prevalence of atopic diseases has increased dramatically in the past 30 years (Fleming & Crombie, 1987; Burr *et al.*, 1989; Aberg, 1989) and this is consistent with the clinical impression of an increase in food allergy in the same time period. For example, repeated cross-sectional studies of 8–13-year-old Aberdonian school children in 1964, 1989 and 1994 have revealed that the prevalence of hayfever has increased from 3.2% to 11.9% to 12.7%, respectively, that the prevalence of atopic eczema has increased from 5.3% to 12% to 17.7% and that the prevalence of asthma has increased from 4.1% to 10.2% to 19.6% (Ninan & Russell, 1992; Omran & Russell, 1996). Undoubtedly atopy has a strong genetic predisposition and the molecular basis of this is becoming clearer (Borish, 1999). However, the recent rapid increases in the prevalence of atopy (and presumably food allergy) cannot be attributed to alterations in the candidate genetic loci; instead, changes in environment and/or lifestyle must be increasing the expression of this genetic susceptibility. The recognition that environmental factors must be driving the recent increases in atopy has led to the realisation that if the factors can be identified, then public health measures should be effective in reversing the observed increase (Haby *et al.*, 2001). Consideration of geographic and longitudinal changes in atopy has led to two potential environmental/lifestyle factors being proposed as the factors responsible for the recent increases in IgE mediated allergy, namely exposure to infectious disease and change in dietary habits, and these are presently being investigated.

Children in affluent westernised societies are exposed to relatively few infectious diseases and when they are exposed they receive antibiotics. It has been proposed that this lack of infection-driven immunological stimulation promotes the maintenance or the development of Th2 biased immune development and IgE based allergy (Shaheen, 1997) (see Chapters 2 and 5, and Chapter 3, Section 3.5.8).

There have been various changes in the diets of westernised countries in recent decades; for example, there has been a change in the fatty acid composition of the diet, with a shift towards a greater intake of *n*-6 (ω-6) fatty acids, which are abundant in vegetable oils such as sunflower and corn oils (British Nutrition Foundation, 1999), and a relative decline in consumption of the long chain *n*-3 fatty acids found in oil-rich fish, consumption of which has fallen markedly over the past 50 years, although there has been a partial reversal of this trend recently, as shown by National Food Survey data (Ministry of Agriculture, Fisheries and Food, 2000). Fatty acids in these two series are essential precursors for the synthesis of eicosanoids, which in turn influence cytokine secretion (see Chapter 2, Section 2.4.3 and Chapter 3, Section 3.5 for details). These fatty acids, being unsaturated, are vulnerable to peroxidation and the body has devised a multi-tiered defence against such damage, which involves a whole host of antioxidants, many of which are provided by the diet, *e.g.* vitamin E, vitamin C and carotenoids. There is currently considerable interest in the potential of a range of plant food constituents to benefit health,

for example through antioxidant mechanisms, and this is the subject of another British Nutrition Foundation Task Force, due to report in 2002. This interest is fuelled by concern that vegetable consumption has fallen progressively in recent decades and although fruit consumption has risen recently, the content of antioxidant substances such as flavonoids and carotenoids is not usually a primary driver in modern plant breeding selection processes. Consequently, consumption of the wide range of potentially advantageous substances may well be declining.

Such epidemiological data, when considered in conjunction with immunological data (see Chapter 3, Section 3.5.8), has led to the proposal that the current diet of affluent societies promotes the differentiation of T helper cells towards the Th2 phenotype and IgE mediated allergy (Seaton *et al.*, 1994; Black & Sharpe, 1997). It has even been suggested that such a diet, when consumed by a pregnant woman, promotes the development of the Th2 phenotype and IgE mediated allergy in her unborn child (see Chapter 5 for background information, particularly Section 5.2.2). It should, however, be emphasised that these proposals are merely working hypotheses and are included for general interest, and until evidence is produced to support these proposals, no recommendations can or should be made.

## 4.8 Key points

- The epidemiology of gluten sensitive enteropathy (coeliac disease) is fairly well characterised, with a prevalence of clinically proven disease being 1 to 3 cases per 1000 people. However, screening of the general population suggests there may be a significant number of latent/subclinical cases. The European consensus for the prevalence of all cases of coeliac disease is 3 to 4 cases per 1000 people. Superficially there appears to have been an increase in the prevalence of coeliac disease, but increased awareness and new serological tests probably account for most, if not all, of the increase.

- However, in general, it is very difficult to make meaningful comments on the prevalence of food intolerance and allergy to individual foods, and without further research it is virtually impossible to identify time trends and geographical variation. This is mainly due to the paucity of studies and the lack of consensus regarding standard working definitions, which has resulted in different studies using non-comparable methodologies.

- The limited data available suggest that a significant proportion of people (up to 30% of children and adults) believe they are intolerant of one or more foods. However, estimates suggest that in fact the prevalence of proven food intolerance in children is of the order of 5–8% and in adults 1–2%.

- The prevalence of proven IgE mediated food allergy in children is about 1–2% and in adults less than 1% (typically 0.2–0.5%).

- In children, the prevalence of intolerance to individual foods ranges between 0.5% and 5%, with peanut allergy being present in up to 0.5%. In adults, the prevalence of peanut allergy is between 0.5% and 1%, depending on the study population.

- The most potent risk factor predisposing to food allergy is a personal or family history of atopy.

- In common with other forms of atopic allergy (*e.g.* atopic asthma), it is highly likely that IgE mediated food allergy has increased in the last 30 years and will probably continue to do so in the foreseeable future. No reliable data on these time trends are yet available.

- Both genetic and environmental factors influence susceptibility. Recent research has demonstrated associations between certain genetic loci and IgE mediated allergy. The relevance of these associations and the potential impact on them of environmental factors, such as changes in the patterns of childhood infection and consumption of dietary constituents, is under active investigation.

# 5
# Pre- and Postnatal Sensitisation to Foods

## 5.1 Introduction and definition of terms

This chapter considers the factors that may influence sensitisation to food in the pre- and neonatal period and during infancy. Allergy to foods that are introduced into the diet for the first time occurs more frequently in the first year of life than at any other time. This is likely to be because the baby is the recipient of a wealth of new exposures during this period, but also because susceptibility may be greater early in life. In most (80–90%) cases, food allergy in infants resolves naturally with time (see Chapter 4, Section 4.3.1).

### 5.1.1 IgE mediated allergy

Most food allergies are mediated by IgE antibody dependent mechanisms (see Chapter 2). IgE antibodies bind, via specific receptors, to the membranes of mast cells and basophils. Following subsequent exposure, the inducing allergen binds to and cross-links membrane-bound IgE and this results in degranulation of mast cells and the release of both pre-formed and newly-synthesised inflammatory mediators. Thus, IgE triggered reactions can have profound and lasting effects exemplified in babies by eczema, the onset of which may be delayed for many hours, or even days, after the food was eaten. Other symptoms, which occur in allergic people of all ages, include vomiting, diarrhoea and the oral allergy syndrome (Amlot *et al.*, 1987). For a detailed description of the various immunological mechanisms see Chapter 2, and for a discussion of food allergy see Chapter 6.

Childhood food allergy can also be T cell mediated (*i.e.* non-IgE), the most common examples being coeliac disease (see Chapter 9) and a form of intolerance to cows' milk (see Chapter 6).

## 5.2 Factors that influence neonatal sensitisation to food

### 5.2.1 Genetic background

Genetic predisposition plays an important role in determining susceptibility to allergic disease in general, particularly the development of childhood allergy (Rowntree *et al.*, 1985). If one parent has an allergy to grass pollen, dust mite or cat/dog dander then the offspring is more likely to become allergic to foods (during the first few months of life) and to inhaled antigens in childhood or early adult life (Burr *et al.*, 1989). However, allergy to a particular inhalant allergen in a parent does not predict that an offspring will also react to the same antigen. In other words, the capacity to mount vigorous IgE responses may be inherited, but the specific protein against which an allergic response is directed appears not to be genetically programmed. Other factors, including infection and pollution, may influence the nature of immune responses (Hide & Warner, 1997; Howarth 1998). For a review see Geha (2000).

Of all the factors that govern sensitisation to foods in early life, the inherited susceptibility to allergic disease is usually the most powerful. Studies have suggested that allergy is more likely to be inherited from the mother than the father, though atopy in both parents dramatically increases the likelihood of atopy in their child (Ruiz *et al.*, 1992).

A number of other factors are also important in determining whether a food, or more specifically a protein, is allergenic (Astwood *et al.*, 1996). These include the size and stability of the protein, its glycosylation status, the food matrix in which the protein is present and the immunogenicity of the protein.

### 5.2.2 Prenatal exposure

The environment experienced by the developing foetus is an extremely complex balance between factors that prevent the rejection of the developing baby (which is genetically different from the surrounding maternal tissue due to inherited traits from the father) and those which promote its growth and development.

Trophoblasts, cells derived from the developing embryo, carry antigens from both parents. During pregnancy, the mother's immune response is downregulated so as to prevent fetal rejection (Warner *et al.*, 1997). This is thought to be brought about by switching from the normal Th1-type response by T lymphocytes to a Th2 response (see Chapter 2 and Fig. 2.5). Different series of cytokines are associated with these two responses. Knowledge is growing about the positive and negative roles of individual cytokines in the various stages of pregnancy (Warner *et al.*, 1997).

Warner and colleagues (1997) speculate that the interactions between Th1 and Th2 cytokines (see Chapter 2) during pregnancy are influential in determining the type of antigenic response that develops in the foetus following maternal exposure and that in infants who do not become atopic, intrauterine antigen exposure is most likely involved in the generation of immune tolerance, rather than sensitisation. However, in those in whom the bias towards a Th2-type response (which predominates during pregnancy) persists unduly after birth, antigen exposure *in utero* may have established a primary sensitisation that is then sustained by the infant's own antigen exposure following birth. They also speculate that, against the background of a critical Th1/Th2 cytokine balance to preserve the materno–fetal relationship, it is possible that a fetus with a particular genetic predisposition (*e.g.* a deficient IFN-γ response at the time that T cell responses are initiated) will develop a Th2-type reaction to the antigen (and associated IgE production) rather that the normal Th1 response (see Fig. 2.5 in Chapter 2). The drive

towards the Th2 response is strong in early pregnancy, but declines in late pregnancy as placental function decreases (Howarth, 1998).

The whole question of *in utero* sensitisation remains very speculative; nevertheless, the factors that have been suggested as potential influences on sensitisation include:

- The nature and characteristics of the developing immune system of the fetus and neonate (see below).
- The exposure of the mother, during pregnancy and breastfeeding, to allergens and the characteristics of her immune responses to these allergens. It has been speculated that mothers with a predominantly IgG response to a given antigen may clear circulating antigen more effectively than mothers with a predominantly IgE response, or little or no response, and hence process the antigen before it is allowed to induce sensitivity in the baby (Warner *et al.*, 1997).
- Exposure to allergens in infancy.

Early infection (particularly viral infection) has been found to have a negative association with the development of atopy (*i.e.* reduce the likelihood of it happening), perhaps through promotion of a Th1 response (Howarth, 1998). This hypothesis is supported by work in countries that still have a high prevalence of infant infection (see Howarth, 1998 for references). On this basis, it is suggested that the decrease in the occurrence of infection in the very young (and during pregnancy) as a consequence of improved social conditions and modern health care may explain, at least in part, the observed increases in the rates of atopy and some allergic conditions (see Chapter 4). If this is the case, it is important to understand the events that cause the persistence of the Th2 type response. Further consideration of Th1 and Th2 responses can be found in Chapter 2.

Collateral evidence for the sterile/aseptic environment hypothesis (sometimes referred to as the hygiene hypothesis), described above, exists in so much as epidemiological studies have identified that the risk of atopic disease is more common in first-born children than in subsequent children within a family (Von Mutius *et al.*, 1994). Here, the hypothesis is that subsequent children are exposed early to infection from their older siblings and this promotes a Th1 response and downregulates any tendency to allergic disorders (Warner *et al.*, 1997). Other hypotheses should not be ruled out though, for example that in subsequent pregnancies changes in placental function or maternal nutrition may also be relevant. It has also been suggested that birth weight of the child is a factor. Low birth weight was found to be a highly significant risk factor for the development of allergic disorders (not just food allergy) in 2-year-old children participating in a study conducted on the Isle of Wight (Arshad *et al.*, 1992).

It has been speculated that fetal T cells might be primed against common antigens during the second trimester of pregnancy (Warner *et al.*, 1997). In this context it is of interest that most studies involving maternal avoidance of allergen-containing foods have taken place during the third trimester, *i.e.* potentially too late to be expected to be influential in high risk infants (see Section 5.7). It should be noted, however, that this and related concepts are speculative and regarded by some as controversial.

There is currently no evidence concerning the ability of antigens or antigen fragments to cross the placenta from mother to fetus (Warner *et al.*, 1997), but it is known that IgG crosses the placenta (to provide passive immunity to the developing fetal system), albeit by highly specific mechanisms, and the potential for antibody/antigen immune complexes to travel the same path has been speculated by these authors.

It is for this reason that COT (the Committee on Toxicity of Chemicals in Food, Consumer Products and the Environment) made recommendations on the consumption of peanuts by pregnant women with a family history of allergic disease. Although it is acknowledged that the evidence that peanut allergy can result from exposure *in utero* is inconclusive, the COT report (Department of Health, 1997) on peanut allergy recommended that

'pregnant women who are atopic, or for whom the father or any sibling of the unborn child has an atopic disease, may wish to avoid eating peanuts and peanut products during pregnancy.'

The main reason for the recommendation was that many peanut-sensitive children react on first known exposure, suggesting that sensitisation has already occurred. The report also noted that there is no

justification for avoidance of peanuts in the absence of atopy in parents or siblings.

### 5.2.3 Antibody responses

During pregnancy, the human placenta develops a specific transport mechanism for IgG (see above). This is not equally efficient for all four subclasses of IgG, and IgG1 is transferred preferentially while the slowest transfer is seen with IgG2 (Malek *et al.*, 1996). Furthermore, other factors may play a part in influencing the effectiveness of transport. There is evidence, for example, for the exclusion of specific IgG4 but not IgG1 antibody to ovalbumin and casein (Kemeny *et al.*, 1986; Devey *et al.*, 1993), and that these antibodies differ in affinity. The exclusion of high affinity antibody could be explained by the inability of complexes to cross the placenta, as the exclusion of IgG4 was antigen specific. However, this explanation is only a possibility.

The infant's immune system is immature at birth. IgA is not produced until birth and the presence of IgA in cord blood is indicative of contamination with maternal blood. There is no clear evidence that babies mount an IgE, IgG or IgA antibody response to foods *in utero*. Normally, it typically takes 3–6 months for babies to make their own IgE or IgG response to food antigens (Kemeny *et al.*, 1986).

## 5.3 Assessment of abnormal immune response

The development of most types of food allergy is dependent upon the generation of IgE antibody responses. The type of antibody that is generated during immune responses is to a large extent dependent upon the local cytokine microenvironment and, in particular, the relative availability of type 1 and type 2 cytokines secreted by functional subpopulations of T lymphocytes. The generation of IgE antibody is favoured by type 2 cytokines, such as IL-4, and antagonised by type 1 cytokines such as IFN-γ. In addition to regulating IgE antibody responses, type 1 and type 2 cytokines also influence isotype distribution of IgG antibody. Thus, for instance, IL-4 is known in humans to favour the production of IgG4. The balance between IgG and IgE antibodies may impact on allergic responses.

### 5.3.1 Cord blood or term IgE concentration

While the positive association between an elevated cord blood IgE level and the development of allergy has been shown in many studies (Croner *et al.*, 1982; Magnusson & Masson, 1985), it is now clear that cord blood IgE only identifies a fraction of those who later become allergic (Ruiz *et al.*, 1990, 1991; Croner & Kjellman, 1992). In addition, elevated cord blood IgE is not usually at a very high level when one takes into account the average amount of IgE that can be made by a plasma cell (0.5 ng/week *in vitro*) (Dhanjal *et al.*, 1992) and it is therefore unlikely that the amounts detected necessarily represent a significant immune response. Caution needs to be taken in interpretation of results as maternal blood may contaminate that of the infant during birth. If the mother makes a large amount of IgE, this could lead to a falsely high cord blood IgE level.

### 5.3.2 CD4$^+$ T cell responses to allergens in cord blood

There has been intensive investigation of cord blood T lymphocyte responses. Cord blood T cells secrete reduced amounts of IFN-γ compared with adult T cells (Warner *et al.*, 1994) and it is reported that levels of soluble IL-2 receptor (CD25) are elevated in infancy (Jones *et al.*, 1994), suggesting immune activation. Indeed, pregnancy is normally associated with a Th2 bias (see Section 5.2.2), which may explain why Th1 inflammatory diseases, such as rheumatoid arthritis, may improve during pregnancy. However, it has been proposed that IL-13 (another Th2 cytokine) is produced at a lower level by cord blood T cells of babies who subsequently become allergic by 3 years of age (Williams *et al.*, 2000).

Cord blood T cell responses to specific food allergens, and interestingly to inhalant allergens, have been reported by a number of groups (Holt *et al.*, 1995; Szepfalusi *et al.*, 1997). However, antigen-specific T cell responses have not been followed postnatally to determine whether these cells are part of a coherent immune response. It has been suggested that cord blood T cells that proliferate in response to food allergens play an important part in the development of allergy. But it is presently uncertain whether these responses are 'real'.

One way of assessing an immune response is to follow the frequency of antigen-specific T cells in the circulation. Because of the small amounts of infant blood available, T cell responses have only been measured at a single time point, *i.e.* at birth. This makes it difficult to assess time trends in response. Furthermore, as the baby's own IgG1 antibody response to milk and egg proteins is thought not to be triggered until 3 to 6 months of age (Kemeny *et al.*, 1986), there is a discrepancy between T and B cell priming, which needs to be explained. There is also a discrepancy with reports of associations between development of cows' milk allergy and exposure to cows' milk in the first few days of life (Høst *et al.*, 1988) (see also Section 5.7.2).

### 5.3.3 CD4$^+$ T cell responses and IgG antibodies to constituents of foods

Ongoing research is addressing several relevant questions. Is it likely that substantial T cell responses to food antigens occur *in utero*? IgG, IgA and IgE antibody responses require T cell help (see Chapter 2, Section 2.4.3). How does the T cell response to ovalbumin in cord blood match with the IgG antibody response in cord serum? First, there is clear evidence that the transport of IgG across the placenta is an active process. No such mechanism has been identified for ovalbumin or any other food allergen. Secondly, studies of specific IgG1 and IgG4 antibody responses to ovalbumin in neonates have shown that there is, as in adult life, a transition from IgG1 to IgG4 (Aalberse *et al.*, 1983; Urbanek *et al.*, 1986; Kemeny *et al.*, 1986). As in adults, this is associated with a rise and then a fall in the affinity of IgG1 antibodies and the generation of a high affinity IgG4 response (Devey *et al.*, 1993). This has been interpreted to mean that the first significant immune response of the neonate to ovalbumin occurs when it is introduced into the diet, typically at around 4–6 months of age.

## 5.4 Trigger foods

The most common triggers of food allergy in the first 2 years of life will in part depend on the foods to which the child is exposed, which in turn will depend on where the child lives and also the food culture of the country. For example, allergy to fish is less common in UK infants but more common in Scandinavia where fish is more prominent in the diet. Other foods, for example egg, are widely introduced early in infant feeding and hence are common triggers. In many cases detailed information about the prevalence of allergy to these foods in early life, or indeed later in life, is absent (a summary of the available information can be found in Chapter 4).

## 5.5 Dietary factors in the development of atopy in infants

The major factor determining development of food allergy in infants is genetic inheritance. Non-genetic factors, not linked to diet or exposure, such as infection can also play a part in a genetically susceptible child. A number of dietary factors have also been implicated, including:

- the possibility of intrauterine sensitisation to food allergens;
- the protective effect of breast milk on allergen sensitisation;
- the sensitising potential of food allergens in breast milk;
- the protective effect of protein hydrolysate formula;
- the early introduction of solid food (*i.e.* before 4 months of age).

A number of dietary intervention studies have explored the role of each of these dietary factors in the prevention of food allergy but the results are conflicting and inconclusive.

## 5.6 Maternal diet during pregnancy

There is little published evidence to support any associated benefit of dietary intervention during pregnancy and the development of allergic disease in the genetically susceptible child. In a Cochrane review, Kramer (2000) concludes that prescription of an antigen avoidance diet to a high-risk woman during pregnancy is unlikely to reduce substantially the risk of giving birth to an atopic child. Moreover, such a diet may have an adverse effect on maternal and/or fetal nutrition.

It is still uncertain whether or not sensitisation occurs *in utero* and, if so, whether this occurrence is restricted to specific stages of gestation. So far, the majority of studies have focused on modifying diet during the third trimester of pregnancy (see comment in Section 5.2.2). Two of the earlier randomised studies investigating the impact of diet during the third trimester reported no advantages. Falth-Magnusson *et al.* (1987) compared the effect of a third trimester milk- and egg-free diet with a normal diet. Infants in both study groups were given either breast milk or a casein hydrolysate formula until 3 months of age. No differences were found between study group infants with respect to cord blood IgE concentrations; incidence of food sensitisation or development of atopic diseases at 18 months of age (Falth-Magnusson *et al.*, 1988), and 5 years of age (Falth-Magnusson & Kjellman, 1992). In addition, Lilja *et al.* (1988) failed to detect any effect of a third trimester diet that was either high or low in cows' milk and egg on the development of specific egg or cows' milk IgE antibody in paired cord sera from any infant with IgE specific to milk formula or egg at 4 months of age.

Other studies have claimed a protective role of diet during pregnancy, but these studies have advocated dietary change during both pregnancy and lactation (Chandra *et al.*, 1986; Zeiger *et al.*, 1989), or have studied diet retrospectively (Frank *et al.*, 1999). Chandra *et al.* (1986) found that exclusion of cows' milk, egg, peanut, fish and beef throughout both pregnancy and lactation, coupled with breast feeding, and delayed introduction of solid food for the first 6 months of life reduced the incidence of eczema in high risk infants. However, no evidence was provided for a reduction in skin prick sensitivity or RAST in the intervention group. A similar approach (excluding cows' milk, egg and peanut) during the last trimester of pregnancy and lactation, together with the use of casein hydrolysate infant formula and delayed introduction and use of low allergenic weaning foods, reduced food associated atopic dermatitis, urticaria and gastrointestinal disease at 12 months (Zeiger *et al.*, 1989). By 7 years of age, however, in this study there were no differences in the prevalence of food allergy or other atopic disease (Zeiger & Heller, 1995) (see also Section 5.8).

Manipulating maternal diet during pregnancy is potentially hazardous (Zeiger *et al.*, 1989; Falth-Magnusson *et al.*, 1987). Requirements for many nutrients, *e.g.* energy, protein and folic acid, increase during pregnancy (Department of Health, 1991), and maternal third trimester dietary restrictions have been associated with a substantial reduction in maternal weight gain and a small decrease in term birth weight (Zeiger *et al.*, 1989). In addition, mothers find compliance with dietary modification particularly difficult (Zeiger *et al.*, 1989) and dietary restriction of eggs during pregnancy has even been associated with more persistent egg intolerance in the offspring (Falth-Magnusson & Kjellman, 1992), suggesting that such a strategy might be counterproductive.

Therefore, there is little support for any dietary restrictions during pregnancy as a means of preventing food allergy. Nevertheless, because of the severity of reactions experienced, COT decided to advise against the consumption of peanuts during pregnancy where there is a family history of atopy, as a safeguard. The basis for this is the speculation that the increasing prevalence of peanut allergy is due to increased consumption of peanuts by pregnant women and breast feeding mothers (Hourihane *et al.*, 1996; Frank *et al.*, 1999), and because children react on first known exposure, suggesting that sensitisation has already occurred (see Section 5.2.2).

## 5.7 Breast feeding

There is long standing controversy regarding the degree to which breast feeding prevents, reduces, delays or even increases the development of allergic disease. Breast milk has a number of nutritional, physiological and immunological advantages and has been strongly recommended for the infant at risk of developing atopy (Department of Health, 1994). The components in human milk with immunological properties comprise three overlapping groups of bioactive agents. These are direct-acting antimicrobial agents (*e.g.* lysozyme, secretory IgA), anti-inflammatory factors (modulators of leucocytes) and immuno-modulating components (*e.g.* TNF-α) (Lo, 1997). The protective effects of breast milk have been attributed to the enhancement of the postnatal growth of intestinal epithelial cells and maturation of mucosal functions in several experimental models (Høst *et al.*, 1999). Although the protection by breast milk against infectious gastrointestinal disease is well established, particularly in developing countries

(Hanson *et al.*, 1985), there is a lack of objective data to suggest it can prevent atopic disease.

It is 65 years since Grulee and Sandford (1936) first reported that breast feeding protected against 'infantile eczema'. They found eczema to be seven times more common in formula-fed infants. Almost 40 years later, Matthew *et al.* (1977) reported less eczema at 6 and 12 months of age in a prospective study of infants who where breast fed in combination with other prophylactic measures. More recently, Wilson *et al.* (1998) reported reduced respiratory mortality lasting until at least 7 years of age, in an industrialised setting, if exclusive breast feeding continued until the age of 15 weeks. Although some subsequent studies have supported these early findings, others have shown no benefit and some have even suggested that breast-fed infants may be at increased risk.

### 5.7.1 Evidence supporting the protective effect of breast milk

The bulk of published papers support the benefit of breast feeding in reducing allergic disease (Table 5.1). In a retrospective study of 1749 Danish infants, Høst *et al.* (1988) demonstrated that the 39 infants who developed cows' milk allergy had all been exposed to cows' milk either purposely or inadvertently during the first 3 days of life. In contrast, none of the 210 exclusively breast-fed infants had cows' milk allergy. Exclusive breast feeding in high-risk infants with a family history of atopy has been associated with less atopic disease at 5 years (Chandra, 1997b) and at 17 years of age (Saarinen & Kajosaari, 1995). However, the methodology of many of these studies has been widely criticised (Kramer, 1988; Zeiger, 1997) and the main problem in interpreting the results is the lack of random assignment to early diet. Clearly, random assignment to breast feeding or formula feeding is considered unethical in healthy infants, but the social and demographic differences normally found between breast-fed and formula-fed infants confound comparative analysis (Lucas *et al.*, 1990). Other common design criticisms include lack of blinding, *e.g.* of the investigator, the means of confirmation of immune response, failure to document compliance, inadequate sample size, brief duration of breast feeding and different control

**Table 5.1**  Studies supporting breast feeding in the prevention of atopy.

| Authors | Subject number | Maternal diet restrictions during lactation | Infant diet | Outcome |
|---|---|---|---|---|
| Lucas *et al.* (1990) | 75 preterm | None | BM vs preterm formula | Reduced atopic dermatitis at 1.5 years in BM group in high risk infants |
| Host *et al.* (1995), reported in Halken *et al.* (1995) | 88 | None | BM and/or extensive hydrolysed formula vs cows milk formula for 6 months | At 5 years: 5.7% cumulative prevalence of cows' milk allergy in BM group; 20% in control group |
| Saarinen & Kajosaari (1995) | 236 | None | Group 1: BM > 6 months Group 2: BM 1–6 months Group 3: BM < 1 months | Age 17 years, % substantial atopy: Group 1: 8% Group 2: 23% Group 3: 54% |
| Chandra (1997b) | 216 | None | BM (4 months) or partial hydrolysate formula (6 months) or soya formula (6 months) or cows' milk (6 months) | Prevelence of eczema and asthma lowest in BM and partial hydrolysate formula at 5 years |

BM – breast milk

measures in the various treatment groups (Kramer, 1988; Zeiger, 1997).

There is one published prospective, randomised study, which compared the effect of banked or donor breast milk with a cows' milk preterm formula on the development of atopy in a preterm infant cohort (Lucas *et al.*, 1990). There was no difference in the incidence of allergic reactions between the two groups. However, in the subgroup of infants with a family risk of atopy, those who received a preterm formula based on cows' milk had a significantly greater risk of developing one or more allergic reactions, particularly eczema, by 18 months of age.

The optimal duration of breast feeding is unclear. Variations in the duration of exclusive breast feeding confound the interpretation and comparison of studies. However, it has been shown that prolonged breast feeding over 6 months was associated with less eczema at 1 and 3 years of age compared with breast feeding for intermediate periods (1–6 months) and short periods (< 1 month) (Saarinen & Kajosaari, 1995).

It has been suggested that the IgA concentration in breast milk may be important in determining whether allergy subsequently develops in geneti-

cally predisposed children. Among genetically high-risk infants and their mothers in Helsinki, who were followed to 1 year of age, breast milk IgA was significantly lower in mothers of those babies who later developed allergy to cows' milk (Jarvinen *et al.*, 2000). An IgA concentration of less than 0.25 g/l at between 6 days and 4 weeks postpartum increased the risk by 15 fold. The authors suggest that breast milk IgA may limit ingress of food allergens through the intestine and possibly also limit the amount of allergen available to the infant through breast milk (Jarvinen *et al.*, 2000).

### 5.7.2  Evidence against breast feeding

Several studies have not demonstrated any protective effect of breast feeding against atopic disease (Hide & Guyer, 1985; Gustafsson *et al.*, 1992; Savilahti *et al.*, 1987; Lindfors & Enocksson, 1988; de Jong *et al.* 1998; Saarinen & Savilahti, 2000). Long term follow up at 7, 11 and 14 years of age of a group of 736 healthy full-term infants, who received either breast milk or a combination of breast milk and cows' milk formula on the maternity ward, found no differences in the incidence of atopic disease (Saarinen & Kajosaari, 1995). In a carefully designed, double-blind intervention trial, de Jong *et al.* (1998) concluded that early and brief exposure to cows' milk in breast-fed infants did not increase the risk of atopic disease in the first 2 years of age. In this study, a group of 1533 healthy breast-fed neonates were randomised to receive either cows' milk protein or a placebo (a mixture of maltodextrin, glucose and mineral solution emulsified with vegetable fats). The intervention feeding was given at least three times during the first 3 days of life, supplementary to or instead of a breast feed (a median volume of 120 ml was taken). Mothers were encouraged to breast feed for at least 6 weeks. In the first year, atopic disease was 10% in the cows' milk group and 9.3% in the placebo group. In the second year, atopic disease was 9.6% and 10.2%, respectively.

In contrast, others have found that use of cows' milk formula is associated with a lower incidence of atopy. Lindfors and Enocksson (1988) found a reduced incidence of allergic symptoms at 18 months and 5 years of age in 216 small-for-gestational age children who received cows' milk formula before breast feeding.

Savilahti *et al.* (1987) found prolonged breast feeding to be associated with a higher incidence of atopy. In a further study, investigating a cohort of 6209 unselected healthy infants fed either breast milk or infant formula, the chief factors associated with the development of cows' milk allergy were exclusive breast feeding or breast feeding combined with infrequent exposure to cows' milk during the first 2 months of life (Saarinen & Savilahti, 2000).

In addition, the potential presence of various dietary allergens in breast milk and the possible atopic disposition of some mothers who breast feed add to confusion in this area. Therefore, there is a lack of agreement and objective validation regarding the effect of breast feeding on the development of allergic disease.

## 5.8 Maternal diet during lactation

It is well recognised that drugs, other chemicals, toxins and components of foods are passed to an infant via breast milk. Food allergens in breast milk have been implicated in the development of food allergy in high-risk infants who have been exclusively breast fed. It was as early as 1923 that Stuart identified the presence of egg white protein in breast milk (Stuart, 1923). Three bovine milk antigens ($\beta$-lactoglobulin, casein and $\gamma$-globulin), hens' egg ovalbumin and gliadin (from wheat) have been detected in minute quantities in most samples of breast milk provided by mothers within 2–6 hours of consuming these foods (Zeiger, 1997). Molecular size analysis suggests that these food antigens, presented in this way, maintain their potential for infant sensitisation (Cavagni *et al.*, 1988). However, it is not entirely clear whether it is these particular food antigens and route of delivery or other sources of allergens, such as inhaled food proteins or even hands contaminated with such proteins, that play a role in sensitisation (Høst *et al.*, 1999). Even so, infants with cows' milk allergy, whose lactating mothers were already on cows'-milk-free diets, have reacted when challenged with cows' milk through their mother's own breast milk (Jarvinen *et al.*, 1999). It has been shown also that consumption of whey hydrolysate formula by the lactating mother reduces the transfer of $\beta$-lactoglobulin into human milk (Fukushima *et al.*, 1997), although the extent of secretion of this immunoglobin into breast milk varies widely after cows' milk ingestion among lactating women (Sorva *et al.*, 1994).

There have been a few studies that have evaluated the efficacy of maternal exclusion diets during lactation (Chandra *et al.*, 1989; Sigurs *et al.*, 1992; Arshad *et al.*, 1992). In a randomised controlled trial, in a group of 97 high-risk infants, lactating mothers followed either a diet free from milk, egg, fish, soya and peanut or a normal diet. Eczema was significantly less common in a group of breast-fed infants whose mothers were on a restricted diet (Chandra *et al.*, 1989). Sigurs *et al.* (1992) reported that an exclusion diet, free of cows' milk, eggs and fish, during the first 3 months of lactation, resulted in a lower cumulative prevalence of atopic dermatitis at 4 years but not at 10 years of age (Hattevig *et al.*, 1996). In a further study, on the Isle of Wight (Arshad *et al.*, 1992), high-risk infants were randomly allocated to either a control group or to an intervention group with three characteristics. The mothers all breast fed and excluded from their own diets milk, eggs and fish; low-allergen foods were used at weaning and the infants received reduced exposure to environmental irritants and allergens such as smoking and housedust mite, respectively. The prevalence of allergic disorders, particularly eczema and asthma, was less at 12 months (Arshad *et al.*, 1992) and food and/or aeroallergen sensitisation was less at 2 years (Hide *et al.*, 1994).

In the context of the mechanisms being proposed by Warner and colleagues (1997), which remain speculative, there are a number of possible and overlapping interpretations of these findings. Firstly, there may be no benefit in excluding foods from the diet if the mother's IgG response is sufficiently strong to 'mop up' allergen. On the other hand, a full and total exclusion of allergens from the maternal diet might be expected to be effective in preventing allergic disease, but this assumes that the presence of allergen in the maternal diet is not necessary to induce tolerance in the baby. Also, it has to be recognised that total exclusions will usually fail because they are so difficult to achieve.

It has been suggested by a COMA Working Group (Department of Health, 1994) that where there is a family history of atopy, in addition to exclusive breast feeding for 4–6 months, breast-feeding mothers should exclude common food allergens from their diets to help prevent food allergy. However, this latter approach should be applied with caution. During lactation, maternal nutritional requirements are increased and there is no information reporting the effect of maternal exclusion diets on maternal anthropometric and biochemical nutritional status. If the decision is made to adopt this approach, maternal exclusion diets should always be started prenatally to ensure food allergen elimination from the maternal circulation *before* breast feeding is started (Wolfe, 1995).

## 5.9 Use of protein hydrolysate formula

Not all mothers of high-risk infants can or wish to breast feed. Many studies have used protein hydrolysate formulas for such infants, as an alternative to standard formulas, in an attempt to prevent atopic symptoms in infants whose mothers choose not to breast feed. Protein hydrolysates are derived from several sources, including hydrolysed cows' milk casein, cows' milk whey, bovine or porcine collagen, soya or a combination of these. Protein hydrolysates are generally categorised by the degree of hydrolysis, *i.e.* extensive or partial protein hydrolysates. In the extensively hydrolysed casein formulas, the peptides have a molecular

weight below 1200 daltons, whereas in the partially hydrolysed whey formulas, a significant proportion of peptides have a molecular weight between 800 and 4000 daltons (Halken *et al.*, 1995). The practical advantages, *i.e.* taste, cost and low osmolarity, of partial protein hydrolysates are discussed in Chapter 11, Section 11.6.1ii.

There have been a number of prospective intervention studies that have successfully used extensively hydrolysed formulas, as an alternative (*i.e.* for women who choose not to breast feed) or in combination with breast milk, together with low allergen weaning foods (not before 4 months) for the first 6 months of life, to reduce the cumulative prevalence of atopic dermatitis in early life (Zeiger *et al.*, 1989; Hattevig *et al.*, 1989; Chandra *et al.*, 1989). Equally, Marini *et al.* (1996) reported a reduced incidence of various allergic manifestations, particularly atopic dermatitis at 1, 2 and 3 years of age, compared with normal cows' milk formula, when exclusive partial hydrolysate was given to high-risk infants during the first 5 to 6 months of life (in combination with a low allergen weaning diet from 5 months to 12 months of age). There is also evidence from some studies that the cumulative incidence of atopy and cows' milk allergy is significantly reduced at 5 and 7 years of age following use of both extensive and partial protein hydrolysates (rather than normal formula) for the first 6 months of life (Kerner, 1997; Vandenplas *et al.* 1995; Chandra, 1997b). However, not all studies have been consistent (Zeiger, 1997).

In a 5-year follow up of high-risk infants with a family history of allergy (Chandra & Hamed, 1991; Chandra 1997b), exclusive feeding of a partial whey hydrolysate for 6 months was associated with a significant lowering of the cumulative incidence of atopic disease, compared with a standard cows' milk formula. Exclusive breast feeding for at least 6 months had a similar effect to the partial hydrolysate. Soy formula was not effective in reducing atopic disease. DBPCFC in the partial hydrolysate group showed a lower prevalence of food allergy at 5 years compared with the other formula-fed groups.

Two recent studies comparing extensive and partial protein hydrolysate formulas have demonstrated the superiority of extensive protein hydrolysate formula in allergy prevention, at least in the short term. In an allergy-prevention intervention study, 155 infants with a family history of allergy were allocated randomly to either an extensive or partial protein hydrolysate or to normal formula until the age of 9 months, following a period of breast feeding. The cumulative incidence of atopic symptoms was 51%, 64% and 84%, respectively, in the extensively hydrolysed, partially hydrolysed and normal infant formula groups (Oldaeus *et al.,* 1997). Halken *et al.* (2000) compared two extensively hydrolysed formulas with a partial hydrolysate formula in a group of over 500 infants at risk of developing allergy. The formulas were used to replace normal formula or to complement or replace breast milk until the age of 4 months. The cumulative incidence of confirmed cows' milk allergy at 18 months was 0.6% (1 in 161) in infants fed extensively hydrolysed formula, 4.7% (4 in 85) in infants fed partially hydrolysed formula and 1.3% (3 in 232) in exclusively breast-fed infants. The authors note that these results should be interpreted with caution because of the small number of cases.

## 5.10  Introduction of solids

There is some evidence from a New Zealand birth cohort followed for 10 years that early introduction of solids before 4 months of age may predispose high-risk infants to eczema (Fergusson *et al.,* 1990). The rate of eczema increased in almost direct proportion to the number of different types of solid food given to the infant in the first 4 months of life. Children given four or more different solid foods before 4 months of age had over twice the risk of recurrent or chronic eczema when compared with children given no solid food during this period. Kajosaari and Saarinen (1983) also demonstrated that early introduction of solid foods (by 3 months of age) was associated with a higher prevalence of atopic dermatitis in high-risk infants, compared with introduction of solids at 6 months of age. It is generally recommended that early weaning is avoided and, in high-risk infants the advice is preferably that solids are not introduced before 5 to 6 months of age, although delayed weaning after this age is likely to be associated with inadequate nutrition. There is little consensus on the first type of weaning foods to introduce, but it is probably advisable to introduce low allergen foods such as potatoes, baby rice, fruit and vegetables. The COT report on peanut allergy (Department of Health, 1997) recommends that high-risk infants should not be given peanuts and peanut products until they are at least 3 years of age.

---

### 5.11  Key points

- There is little published evidence to support any benefit of dietary intervention during pregnancy regarding the development of allergic disease in the genetically susceptible child.

- It is generally agreed that exclusive breast feeding should be encouraged for all infants for 3 to 4 months (for a range of reasons, many of which are unrelated to atopy). Exclusive breast feeding for 4 to 6 months may be particularly important for infants at high risk of atopic disease, although benefits beyond 6 months of age are unclear.

- Early introduction of solids (before 4 months) may predispose high-risk infants (*i.e.* those with a family history) to atopic disease, *e.g.* eczema.

- Protein constituents of foods may be identified in breast milk but there is no consensus that this is harmful, even in infants at high risk of atopic disease.

- There is some evidence to support the exclusive use until 5 to 6 months of hydrolysed infant formulas in bottle-fed infants at high risk of developing atopic diseases. In some studies, the benefit has been similar to that reported with exclusive breast feeding.

- If dietary restriction is advised to reduce the risk of allergy developing in a high risk child, there is little consensus regarding the ideal dietary plan. Prevention programmes are costly and demanding for both families and health professionals.

# 6
# Common Food Allergies

## 6.1 Introduction

It has been estimated that the intestinal tract of an average person will process 100 tonnes of food in a lifetime. It is therefore vital for the body to be able to process that food into digests and then to absorb nutrients through the intestinal wall selectively, discarding other materials as waste. Perhaps not surprisingly, the protective mechanisms which discriminate between useful substances and those which could be harmful are not infallible.

An important function of the immune system is to distinguish self from non-self (Chapter 2). The processes that lead to recognition are particularly active at the body surfaces, including the surfaces of the intestinal tract. Once recognised, the system is able to mount a specific immune response to non-self, which can promote the rejection or localisation of foreign substances. When a food component is treated as non-self, an immune response may be elicited and a number of health problems can arise. Allergy describes the changes which occur when a specific immune response is itself the cause of adverse health effects, producing symptoms which may occur within minutes of a new contact with the allergenic substance. In this context, allergy can appear to be 'immunity gone wrong'. In some 'atopic' people, this allergic tendency can be inherited.

Allergies such as hay fever affect one in six of the population, but the medical care of allergic conditions generally, especially food allergy, has been slow to receive serious attention. It is now accepted that food reactions are not uncommon (Chapter 4), that they can be serious or even life threatening, and that they are particularly common in infancy and childhood. Fortunately, many childhood reactions subside as the child – and the child's immune system – matures. Peanut allergy is an exception and is frequently life-long (Bock & Atkins, 1989) (see Section 6.5.2).

Not all food intolerance is allergic (Table 6.1; Chapters 1 and 7), and symptoms can be caused by a number of other non-immunological mechanisms, for example by a failure of the enzymatic digestion of sugars (Chapter 8) or fats. Food allergy is certainly not the most common type of adverse reaction to food, but it is one of the most dramatic.

## 6.2 Allergens involved

Apart from the genetic make-up of the individual, the circumstances in which food allergic reactions occur depend on the integrity of the intestinal wall barrier and on the nature of the food itself. The allergens that are involved are largely proteins or glycoproteins and many, though not all, have a molecular weight between 10000 and 40000 daltons, and ability to resist digestion (Astwood et al., 1997). Heat, by denaturing proteins, usually has the opposite effect and can reduce or abolish allergenicity (see Chapter 5, Section 5.2.1).

Many protein allergens have now been identified and characterised. For example, in codfish, a single parvalbumin (allergen M) appears to have the most important but not the only role (Food Standards Agency, 2000). In contrast, the allergenicity of peanuts depends on several heat-stable proteins. In hens' eggs, ovalbumin, ovomucoid and conalbumin are all important allergens. Of these only ovomucoid is heat stable, but undenatured ovalbumin and conalbumin may also be present in home-made

**Table 6.1**   Main causes of food intolerance.

| Mechanisms | Examples of causes |
|---|---|
| *Immunological* Allergy (usually IgE antibody-mediated) | Skin reactions to egg Intestinal reactions to cows' milk Severe (anaphylactic) reactions to peanuts |
| Delayed hypersensitivity (T lymphocyte mediated) | Coeliac disease, some (delayed) reactions to cows' milk (typically skin reactions) |
| *Non-immunological* Enzyme defects | Inability to digest milk lactose (hypolactasia) Inability to tolerate alcohol (alcohol dehydrogenase deficiency) |
| Pharmacological (drug effects) | Caffeinism (and caffeine withdrawal symptoms) Histamine effects (*e.g.* from badly stored mackerel) |
| Irritant and multi-factorial | Asthma attacks caused by metabisulphite preservatives (see Appendix 1) Fatty diarrhoea in liver and gall bladder disease |

mayonnaise. Most cows' milk allergic individuals are sensitised to more than one milk protein, the most prominent being casein and β-lactoglobulin.

When allergy has developed cross-reactions can occur. For instance, the pollens that cause hay fever can also cross-react with the fruits or vegetables to which they are related. Latex, which is commonly associated with allergy in the health care industry (Editorial, 2000) can also cross-react with pollens and has been associated with allergic reactions to bananas, kiwi fruit and avocados (Mahler *et al.*, 2000). A number of other cross-reactions between pollen and fruit and vegetable allergens are now recognised, for example between ragweed, melon, cucumber and other 'gourds', or between birch pollen and apple, cherry, pear and peach (Lahti *et al.*, 1980). Cross-reactions between fruits and vegetables are not infrequently involved in the *oral allergy syndrome* (Section 6.4.5). For further information on cross-reactions see Section 6.5.

## 6.3  Diagnosis

Food allergy must be distinguished not only from food poisoning but also from non-immunological causes of intolerance (Chapter 1). One of the reasons for the slow acceptance of food allergy as a clinical entity has been the long history of misunderstandings, bogus claims, false diagnoses and quack remedies that have been associated with the

subject, often encouraged by the media. A growing interest in food allergy has nevertheless developed, both because of recent scientific advances and because of public concern about a number of fatal or life-threatening reactions. However, there are still relatively few trained practitioners, and very few clinical posts, to deal with what is now a growing health problem. For many years, allergy has been a 'Cinderella' discipline in the UK, and it has often been left to less conventional practitioners to offer to patients a service that is underprovided within the NHS.

While the patient's history can indicate the food that is involved, the key to the firm diagnosis of food allergy or of other forms of food intolerance usually lies in a clear demonstration of a relationship between the food and symptoms (Chapter 10). This demonstration should involve the exclusion of the suspect food until the symptoms subside, followed by evidence that the symptoms recur after reintroduction. When more than one food is involved the problem may be more complicated and, particularly in childhood, it can be useful to keep a 'diet diary' and to note the appearance of symptoms. When there is still a strong suspicion of an unidentified food allergy, it may be necessary to give a very restricted 'exclusion' diet for a limited period (Chapter 11). If symptoms subside, this is followed by the slow reintroduction of suspect foods. Further investigation may involve the 'double-blind placebo-controlled food challenge' (DBPCFC), in which neither the patient nor the investigator can identify the suspect food (therefore 'double blind') or the innocent placebo with which it is to be compared. In this way, psychological reactions or the side effects of overbreathing (Section 6.3.1) can be excluded.

The diagnosis of food allergy can receive support when skin prick tests or blood tests, such as the radioallergosorbent test (RAST), are used to check for the presence of IgE antibodies to the food concerned (Table 6.2) (Chapter 10, Section 10.2.3). In either case, a positive result can suggest the need for further assessment, but neither type of test can provide definitive evidence that there is a clinical problem. Cross-reactions are common, for example between cereal foods and grass pollen (Bindsley-Jensen & Poulsen, 1997) (see Section 6.5). In patients with a past history of a food allergy, positive tests may persist long after the clinical problem has subsided (Lessof *et al.*, 1980a). Nevertheless, when high values of food-specific IgE levels are shown by a technique that gives a reliable quantitative response, strongly positive results have been reported to give an almost certain diagnosis. This approach can be of value in everyday practice, especially in allergies to egg, milk, peanut or fish, in which there has been a correlation of greater than 95% with challenge test results (Sampson & Albergo, 1984).

For practical reasons, the rule concerning a double-blind challenge is not always followed. For patients who have had a severe reaction with clearly recognisable allergic features, a further challenge may be avoided on safety grounds. In other cases, patients who develop hives or vomiting and diarrhoea after eating a food may simply avoid it on future occasions without ever consulting a doctor. Nevertheless, the importance of establishing a diagnosis in doubtful cases is considerable. When food allergy is incorrectly diagnosed, for example on the basis of a history of tingling or faintness after food (Section 6.3.1) or as a result of commercial laboratory tests of blood or hair, one unfortunate result has been that arduous diets may be prescribed for individuals who do not have an allergy to food at all (see Chapter 10, Section 10.5).

### 6.3.1 Misdiagnoses and misconceptions

Misconceptions about the nature of food allergy have had many repercussions, and a number of patients – including children – have been subjected to isolation in a closed environment because they were told they were suffering from 'total allergy'. Very severe, multiple allergies certainly do occur, but it is frequently the case that the 'diagnosis' of allergic disease has been based on spurious evidence. A few of the children so diagnosed have even been shown to be the victims of a form of child abuse, in which parents fantasise about the need to restrict a child's activities (Taylor, 1992).

Mistaken diagnoses can arise also when people who suspect that they have a food allergy develop anxiety symptoms whenever the particular food is put before them. In such stressful situations, many people overbreathe without realising that they are doing so, and their blood level of carbon dioxide falls as a result. Those who react sensitively to this metabolic change then develop sensations of

**Table 6.2** The diagnosis of food allergy.

| Procedure | Comments |
|---|---|
| *Clinical* | |
| History | May need a diary record of diet and symptoms |
| Skin prick tests | Usefulness limited by the availability of effective test allergens |
| Exclusion diet | Useful when allergy (or other form of food intolerance) is strongly suspected but the food unidentified |
| Open challenge | Especially useful in *excluding* allergy |
| DBPCFC | Cumbersome, requires expertise, and may require a series of tests |
| | |
| *Laboratory* | |
| Specific tests for IgE antibody | Uses RAST or other quantitative methods |

tingling, weakness, giddiness, stiffness and a general malaise, which they may attribute to the food itself (Selner & Staudenmayer, 1997). Even the sight of the food can sometimes cause this reaction, but when given in a disguised form that same food can be eaten without causing any problems. It is the overbreathing that causes the symptoms and not the food.

## 6.4 Clinical features of atopic disease

Reports on the prevalence of eczema and other atopic diseases indicate that they have become substantially more common during the past 50 years (Taylor *et al.*, 1984; Hanifin, 1987). As is discussed in more detail in Chapter 4 (Section 4.7), repeated cross-sectional studies in school children in Aberdeen have shown a progressive increase over the period 1964 to 1994 in the prevalence of hay fever, atopic eczema and asthma. Although no such published data exist for food allergy, there is a generally held view among paediatricians that the prevalence of food intolerance and food allergy have increased in Europe and North America (see Section 4.5).

Whatever the causes of the increase in atopic disease, reports of asthma deaths and of food allergic reactions have led to a heightened public awareness of the problem.

### 6.4.1 Clinical features of food allergy

Although the symptoms of food allergy have sometimes been analysed in more detail in adults (Section 6.4.4), they follow much the same pattern in childhood as in adult life. Compared with adults, children, and infants in particular, are more likely to develop eczema, other skin reactions and gastrointestinal reactions, such as diarrhoea, colic and vomiting, but the range of presentations is the same. These have been summarised in Table 6.3.

### 6.4.2 Childhood eczema

Characteristically, eczema consists of a recurrent or persistent red rash, involving the face and cheeks, the inner surfaces of the elbows, knees, hands, feet and, in the infant, the napkin area. It causes severe itching and often weeps and crusts. It does not appear acutely, like 'immediate' allergy, but 80% of

**Table 6.3** Clinical features of food allergy.

*Oral*
Itching, redness and swelling of the lips and within the mouth

*Gastrointestinal*
Vomiting and diarrhoea
Abdominal pain and colic

*Skin reactions*
Eczema
Hives (urticaria) and skin swellings (angioedema)

*Respiratory*
Nasal symptoms (rhinitis) and conjunctivitis
Throat swelling (laryngeal oedema)
Asthma

*General reactions*
Anaphylaxis – any or all of the above, often with shock and a fall in blood pressure. Anaphylaxis is a potentially life-threatening condition

affected infants have positive skin tests or RASTs as evidence of allergy to environmental agents or to foods (Sampson *et al.*, 1992a). In addition, it is associated with high circulating IgE levels and with an increase in specialised, IgE-bearing Langerhans cells in the skin, suggesting that it may be the late consequence of an IgE mediated allergic reaction in which the lymphocytes, which are also present, have been attracted through Langerhans cell activity (Dolovich *et al.*, 1973; Mudde *et al.*, 1995).

Although about a third of children with eczema are allergic to one or more foods (Burks *et al.*, 1988), this is not usually the only factor, and the rigours of an exclusion diet can give disappointing results. When, for example in children with egg sensitivity, the food causes an obvious and immediate relapse, dietary exclusion is likely to be adhered to. However, when cows' milk exclusion results in only a modest improvement in a baby who has been shown to be mildly sensitive, many parents are reduced to continuing with cows' milk formula, or with a protein hydrolysate formula milk, and relying on other measures such as the avoidance of woollen clothing, the use of aqueous cream or oatmeal preparations instead of soap, and the use of emulsifying ointments after a bath.

### 6.4.3 Childhood asthma

Childhood asthma is characterised by breathing difficulty, usually with wheezing or cough, and is associated with a variably increased resistance in the lung airways due to muscle spasm, thickening of the mucous membranes and/or plugs of mucus secretions. It is another condition in which food allergy can be a factor in precipitating an attack even if it was not the original cause of the asthma; indeed with few exceptions the cause of asthma is unknown. When children attending a hospital asthma clinic were surveyed, three-quarters of them said they could recall attacks provoked by at least one type of food, including milk, egg, fish and nuts. After a double blind challenge test 67 (24%) of 279 children with a history of food-induced asthma were found to wheeze after a specific food challenge (Bock, 1992).

It is recognised that a number of factors can combine to provoke or exacerbate asthmatic attacks, including throat and chest infections, allergies to dust mites, pollens, pets, emotion (perhaps by causing overbreathing, see Section 6.3.1), acid reflux from the stomach, and irritants such as smog, cigarette smoke, or toxic effects of sulphite food preservatives (see Appendix 1), so that food is seldom the only factor. In these circumstances, while food exclusion diets have a role in selected cases, treatment is more likely to require such aids as corticosteroids and bronchodilator inhalers rather than a reliance on diet.

### 6.4.4 Clinical features in adults

Food allergy does not commonly develop for the first time in adult life, although it can on occasion result when adults are exposed to new foods, *e.g.* kiwi fruit. In such circumstances, many features are the same as those observed in children. But the clinical pattern of response may sometimes differ both in the target organs affected and in the way in which attacks may be precipitated. In one detailed study of 45 patients (Atkins *et al.*, 1985a,b), most reactions involved the gastrointestinal tract, either alone or in combination with the skin or respiratory tract. In that series, the allergic reactions began at an average age of about 20 years, and most had persisted for 10 years or more. They occurred in patients with a previous allergic history, although few could remember reactions to food in childhood. Diarrhoea, colic or vomiting accounted for the most common problems, sometimes combined with skin reactions or respiratory symptoms. In many,

the reactions were provoked by more than one food but were mostly mild and self-limited.

A range of predisposing factors may help to determine which parts of the body form the principal target for the allergic response. For example, asthma sufferers who then develop food allergy are more likely to have a bout of asthma during a food reaction, just as eczematous subjects are likely to react with an exacerbation of their eczema or with hives. Hourihane (1997a) has reviewed the factors that may make severe reactions more likely. They include the presence of asthma, cardiovascular disease (especially if treated with beta-blockers or ACE inhibitors), exercise, the consumption of alcohol with food, delay in treatment and anxiety.

Characteristically, allergic symptoms (ranging from skin reactions to swelling of the lips, mouth or throat, breathing difficulties, vomiting or diarrhoea) develop within an hour after the food is taken. A severe and even life-threatening reaction may be provoked some hours later, however, in a condition known as food-dependent exercise-induced anaphylaxis. In the first reported case of this kind, severe anaphylactic symptoms developed in a shellfish-sensitive long distance runner who exercised the day after he had eaten shellfish. He had had several food-related anaphylactic attacks, but it was noted that he never had problems if he took exercise without the food or if he took the food but did not exercise (Maulitz *et al.*, 1979). This story is now regarded as typical of a danger that needs to be publicised among food-allergic subjects. As in childhood, the availability and use of adrenaline may be crucial for those food-allergic subjects who have a history of food-induced anaphylaxis or asthmatic attacks.

### 6.4.5 The oral allergy syndrome

The oral allergy syndrome (OAS) is a reaction which begins when the food makes its first contact with the mucous membrane of the mouth and throat. The most striking features are oral itching, lip swelling, redness, and swellings inside the cheeks, but a tightness of the throat can also result from swelling of the glottis and there may be a more generalised anaphylactic reaction. It was first described as a reaction to apple and hazelnut in patients who had become allergic to birch pollen (Tuft & Blumstein, 1942) and, although any food can cause it, it is most commonly reported to occur in reactions to fresh fruit and vegetables in those who also have pollen allergy. In such cases, it is often preceded by the development of hay fever.

Although cross-reactivity may not be a precondition in all cases, the syndrome provides an example of the way in which cross-reacting allergic reactions are provoked by similar proteins in different foods; in this case by tree or grass pollens on the one hand and fruit or vegetables on the other. Well documented 'clusters' of hypersensitivity have been reported, usually but not always to foods in the same botanical family. There have, for example, been reported associations between allergy to: apple and pear; kiwi fruit and avocado; potato and carrot; parsley, celery, carrot, mugwort and spices; celery, cucumber, carrot and watermelon; and rubber latex, chestnut and banana (see Section 6.5).

Oral allergy can also occur in patients who are sensitive to eggs or shrimp, as the first phase of a more severe, generalised reaction (Amlot *et al.*, 1987). Patients who react to fruit and vegetables rarely have anaphylactic reactions, although these have been recorded in reactions to foods as diverse as peach, apricot, walnut, cherry, tomato, apple, hazelnut, pear, fennel, plum, pea, chestnut, maize, lettuce and lentil (Ortolani *et al.*, 1993).

## 6.5 Foods that cause allergic reactions

Table 6.4 lists the foods that are recognised as being causes of allergic reactions in children and adults. The most common trigger foods for allergy (IgE and non-IgE) are considered to be cows' milk, eggs, peanuts, tree nuts, soya beans and soya products, fish, shellfish and wheat (and other cereals containing gluten) (see Chapter 12). Some of these are more common causes of allergy than others, *e.g.* milk and eggs compared with fruit (*e.g.* citrus fruit, tomatoes) and vegetables, and some are more commonly associated with very severe reactions, *e.g.* peanuts and tree nuts. Some foods are particularly associated with reactions in early childhood, *e.g.* milk, and the sensitivity usually disappears in 12–24 months (see Section 6.5.1). This is not the case with all allergies, *e.g.* peanut allergy is generally life-long.

Table 6.4 also shows foods and other substances, *e.g.* pollen, with which cross-reactions are possible. For example, individuals sensitised to a type of tree nut may also react to other nuts. Allergy to wheat (IgE mediated) has been reported but has to be distinguished from the delayed type of sensitivity to gluten, the latter being the basis of coeliac disease (see Chapter 9). The gluten-free wheat that is given to patients with coeliac disease may not necessarily suit wheat-allergic patients, because it contains various residual wheat proteins to which severely allergic patients could react.

A wide variety of other foods can also cause allergic reactions, including various fruits and vegetables (see Section 6.4.5), seeds, spices and animal products. In some cases the reactions can be severe, for example with celery, mustard and sesame (including sesame oil) (Chiu & Haydik, 1991). (In common with other 'gourmet' oils, sesame oil contains small amounts of sesame seed

**Table 6.4**　Common foods that can cause allergic reactions and their associated cross-reactions.

|  | Foods that can cross-react |
|---|---|
| Cows' milk | Other animal milks |
| Hens' eggs | Eggs of other birds |
| Peanuts | Various tree nuts.* Rarely other legumes |
| Various tree nuts | Cross-react with one another and with peanut* |
| Soya bean | *Seldom* cross-reacts significantly with other legumes |
| Fish | Most (sometimes all) other fish |
| Shellfish | Probably other shellfish |
| Wheat | Wheat products but often *not* oats, rice, rye, barley, maize |
| *Reactions can also occur with:* | |
| Fruits and vegetables | Sometimes birch tree and other pollens |

* Especially on skin testing

protein, which is retained in order to provide the characteristic flavour.)

### 6.5.1 Allergic reactions to food in young chidren

The decline in breast feeding of the past 50 years and changes in infant feeding practices, *e.g.* weaning before the age of 4 months, may well have increased the prevalence of food allergy in infancy (see Chapter 5 for a discussion of these issues). In a prospective follow-up study of 1265 infants over a period of 10 years (non-randomised), Fergusson *et al.* (1990) reported that those who had been given four or more solid foods before the age of 4 months had a three-fold increase in recurrent eczema as compared to those who had received none.

Babies with a family history of allergy are more prone to develop allergy themselves, especially cows' milk allergy, which probably affects as many as 2% of infants and young children in Britain. In some but not all cases this reaction to milk is mediated by IgE antibody production, but it can also be mediated by antigen-specific T cells (*i.e.* type IV hypersensitivity, a more delayed response); see Chapter 2 (Section 2.5.3) for more information about the mechanisms. Cows' milk allergy mediated by IgE and T cell mediated delayed hypersensitivity (sometimes referred to as cows' milk protein intolerance) needs to be distinguished from lactose intolerance (Chapter 8) and collectively remain a cause of considerable ill health in some young children.

In the past, mothers of babies who developed symptoms after the introduction of cows' milk were often advised to change from one milk formula product to another and, even if they avoided the asthmatic and other problems that affect the more severe cases, their babies suffered an avoidable period of ill health. These days, the usual advice is to use an infant formula that contains protein hydrolysates. Hydrolysates may be based on cows' milk, other animal proteins or soya, and have been shown to be less allergenic than foods providing the unhydrolysed (whole) protein (see Chapter 5, Section 5.9, Section 6.6 and Chapter 11).

Fortunately, babies with cows' milk allergy usually lose their sensitivity as they grow older. In a prospective study of 1749 newborn babies in Denmark, Høst and Halken (1990) identified 39 (2.2%) with cows' milk allergy, as demonstrated by skin,

intestinal or respiratory reactions, all of which disappeared with an elimination diet and recurred after a milk challenge. Follow-up challenges established that of the 39, 22 recovered within a year, 30 within 2 years, and 34 (87%) by the age of 3. Recovery rates were least good in those with positive blood or skin test evidence of IgE antibodies to milk.

Høst and Halken (1990) found that 21 of 39 infants who were sensitive to cows' milk developed an allergy to other foods, especially eggs, citrus fruit and tomato, and nine were still intolerant to one or more foods at the age of 3. In 11, a more general allergic tendency was evident and they also developed inhalant allergy. This, and the frequency of an atopic family history, suggests that cows' milk sensitivity is often the first expression of an allergic constitution (Sprikkelman *et al.*, 2000).

Isolated allergies to other foods can occur, often developing at about the time when these foods are introduced into the diet, *e.g.* egg and fish (Fig. 6.1, Esteban, 1992). Another topical example would be peanut allergy (see Section 6.5.2). Esteban also showed that those foods that cause allergy when given in infancy are far less likely to cause problems when they are first introduced in older children. Of all cows' milk allergy in childhood in this study, 97.5% had developed within the first year. For egg allergy, 64.4% of all childhood cases developed within the same time scale, as did 48% of cases of fish allergy. However, this was the case for only 7% of other food allergies. Other foods to which children react include soya (David, 1993b) and are shown in Table 6.4.

### 6.5.2 Peanut allergy

Peanut allergy and tree nut allergy have come into prominence in the last few years, following a number of reports of fatalities and clear evidence that peanut allergy has become more common (Hourihane, 1997a,b). This specific situation has focused media attention on the problems of food allergy in general.

Peanuts are a relatively new food in the UK since World War II. The USA produces 2 million tonnes of peanuts annually, and Britain imports over 100 000 tonnes each year. The scale of these imports has been largely a post-World War II phenomenon, and the opportunities for sensitisation have steadily

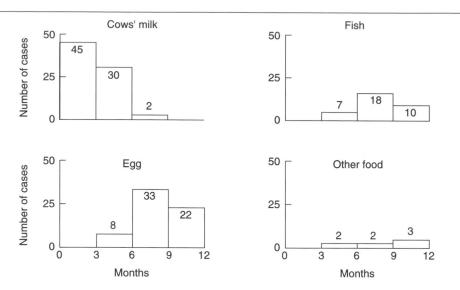

**Fig. 6.1**   The presentation of food allergies in the first year of life. After Esteban (1992).

increased. Interestingly, there is again evidence that while exposure is important it is not the only factor. In parts of Africa, where there are high rates of consumption of peanuts but low rates of allergy, allergic reactions to peanuts are almost unknown. Although tree nuts, notably Brazil nuts, almonds and hazelnuts, can also cause severe reactions, it is peanuts that have caused the most concern because of the severe reactions and deaths that have recently been reported.

Peanuts ('ground nuts') are in fact legumes and therefore related to soya beans, but because of their similarity to tree nuts people often think of them as being related. Indeed, skin test reactivity with one or other type of tree nut has been demonstrated in 12 out of 19 peanut-allergic children (Bock & Atkins, 1989). None of the 12 children reacted to a double-blind challenge with a tree nut, but the potential for cross-reactivity will remain uncertain until more studies are carried out. Meanwhile, it is understandable that children who are allergic to peanuts often avoid tree nuts as well.

The onset of peanut allergy is early and the condition is, in most cases, life-long. The history of reactions is usually so clear-cut that the classical double-blind challenge test may be unnecessary to make the diagnosis and may be avoided on safety grounds. Nevertheless, not all patients considered

by themselves or their parents to be peanut-allergic prove to be so, and challenge tests are more often carried out in order to exclude the diagnosis than to confirm it. Even proven peanut allergy may sometimes remit, and in experienced centres the use of challenge tests under close supervision may, therefore, be an aid to management.

In some highly sensitive individuals, it has been shown that as little as 100 µg of peanut protein provokes symptoms and that 5 mg can be enough to cause a systemic reaction. Even proximity to an open jar of peanut butter can sometimes be enough to provoke wheezing and urticaria (Mudde *et al.*, 1995), and for safety reasons some airlines have stopped giving peanut snacks to their customers (see Chapter 12).

Exposure to peanuts in one form or another can occur at very early ages. Although the evidence that peanut allergy can result from exposure *in utero* is inconclusive, the COT report (Department of Health, 1997) on peanut allergy recommended that

'pregnant women who are atopic, or for whom the father or any sibling of the unborn child has an atopic disease, may wish to avoid eating peanuts and peanut products during pregnancy' (see Chapter 5, Section 5.2.2).

Apart from the possibility of exposure through the mother's diet, either in the womb or via the mother's milk, it has been suggested in France that some infant formulas (that are no longer available) contained unrefined peanut oil and could provoke both eczema and oral reactions to peanuts (Moneret-Vautrin *et al.*, 1991). Eight per cent of over 100 French babies under the age of 4 months showed skin test reactions to peanut, implying sensitisation in the womb or soon after birth. However, the role of oils in provoking reactions is still unclear. Refined peanut oil appears not to contain allergens, but may not be safe if (as in some restaurant cooking procedures) it becomes contaminated with peanut protein. Cold pressed oil, on the other hand, may contain peanut protein (3.3 mg/ml in one study) (Hoffman & Collins-Williams, 1994), and has been shown to provoke reactions in a few highly sensitive peanut-allergic individuals (Hourihane, 1997a) and remains under suspicion as a potentially sensitising agent.

Despite the evidence that the avoidance of peanuts in early childhood can help to reduce early allergic reactions, by the age of one year 18% of a group of American children had been exposed to peanuts although their mothers were specifically advised to avoid them (Zeiger *et al.*, 1989).

The most important information that severely peanut-allergic individuals and their parents require is the knowledge of whether any food they are offered contains peanuts, unrefined peanut oil or tree nuts, either as ingredients or contaminants. Manufacturers have responded to the need for this type of information (see Chapter 12). Restaurant meals may nevertheless involve an unavoidable risk in the most severe cases, and there have even been reactions caused when cooking utensils, which have come into contact with nuts, have then been re-used for preparation or service of a 'nut-free' meal. As discussed in Section 6.6, those who are at risk of anaphylaxis should carry preloaded adrenaline syringes and be trained in their use. It is a matter of concern that many people suffering severe reactions are still inadequately treated (Hourihane, 1997b).

### 6.5.3 Can genetic modification influence allergenicity?

Clearly it is necessary to determine whether food derived from genetically modified plants is allergenic and specifically whether the products of novel genes engineered into crop plants or fruits are potentially allergenic. There are a number of ways in which these safety needs are being addressed and these include: comparing the structure and sequence of new proteins with those of known human allergens, looking for serological identity between novel proteins and known human allergens, examining the stability and other physicochemical features of the new protein and determining whether the new protein is able to induce IgE antibody responses (Dearman & Kimber, 2001; Kimber & Dearman, 2001).

## 6.6 Management of food allergy in childhood

The dietary management of allergy is considered in detail in Chapter 11, and is only summarised here, using cows' milk allergy as an example.

Cows' milk allergy can present in many ways. Some babies are sensitised from birth, but the most common story is for diarrhoea to develop a week or so after cows' milk has been introduced, sometimes with vomiting. Less often, skin itching and eczema appear later on, often accompanied by irritability and sleep disturbance, especially in babies with florid eczema. In a few cases, symptoms develop for the first time after an acute intestinal infection (Gribbin *et al.*, 1976).

When diarrhoea is the principal symptom, it is important to exclude an intolerance to lactose (Chapter 8). Wheezing, coughing and/or eczema make an allergy more likely, especially if symptoms develop rapidly after a feed. A red rash around the mouth may wax and wane or may become a persistent feature.

A diagnosis of allergy to cows' milk or of cows' milk protein intolerance (delayed hypersensitivity) requires the exclusion of cows' milk from the diet. If there is a symptom-free period, then this is followed by challenge tests with milk under close supervision to show that the symptoms recur. If the diagnosis is confirmed, there is the difficulty of replacing cows' milk with other sources of protein, energy (calories), calcium and vitamins. It is therefore a diagnosis that should not be made lightly.

Infant formulas based on heat-denatured and enzymically hydrolysed milk proteins are usually well tolerated, are less sensitising in their own right, and have been recommended not only in proven cases of cows' milk allergy but also for allergy prevention in the infants of atopic parents when a substitute for breast feeding is needed (Businco *et al.*, 1993) (see Chapter 5, Section 5.9). Their poor taste and smell are, however, a disadvantage. Soya milk is also well tolerated as a staple food in most children but can itself cause hypersensitivity (see Section 6.5) (Giampietro *et al.*, 1992). A number of well-formulated infant milk formulas use soya protein and are now available on prescription. However, other soya products are available which are not designed for infant feeding and should not be used because they lack sufficient amounts of essential nutrients, especially calcium.

Assuming the successful dietary control of symptoms, an interval of up to a year may be needed in severe cases before trying to assess whether a child's cows' milk sensitivity has subsided. The reintroduction of milk will again have to be closely supervised in order to avoid provoking a more serious reaction. The same applies to other foods responsible for allergic reactions.

After early infancy the dietary problems diminish. By the age of 2 there are no foods which cannot be replaced, albeit with difficulty. Half a litre of cows' milk can provide all the protein, a quarter of the energy (calories), and all the daily calcium and riboflavin that a young child requires. Should cows' milk have to be discontinued, there are few disadvantages in the use of other sources of nutrients, including meat, vegetables, fish and fruit, provided that all the necessary nutrients are present in the diet in adequate amounts. If there is any doubt, supplements should be considered so that growth will not be compromised. When bread and cereals need to be replaced, the possible substitutes include gluten-free wheat or maize, rice and potato products.

Two of the most difficult problems that parents of affected children face is the need to scan the contents of shop products and to supervise an exclusion diet in older, more mobile children who are of the party-going age. For the shopper, lists are now available of commercial foods which are 'free from' various ingredients (Chapter 12). However, because of the risks inherent in an unbalanced diet which lacks essential components, the advice of a dietitian is needed whenever substantial dietary restrictions are envisaged (Chapter 11). Furthermore, the 'free-from' lists in circulation cannot be relied upon to be up to date. Particularly where the allergy is severe, the best advice is to check labels carefully and, if in any doubt, to speak directly with the manufacturer's Customer Services Department (see Chapter 12).

Not only in children with cows' milk allergy but in other children too, it is the most severe allergic or anaphylactic reactions that are the least likely to remit. The only proven treatment is to avoid the food concerned, and the role of diet is discussed in Chapter 11. A number of claims have been made for unproven therapies such as rotating diets, but the claims for success are often highly suspect when the initial diagnosis of food allergy has been made by methods which have never been validated (see Chapter 10, Section 10.5).

Although there is a tendency for food allergy to diminish or remit with time (Chapter 4, Section 4.3.1), a lower remission rate has been reported for those with allergies to egg, milk and wheat, and lowest of all for peanut (Sampson & Scanlon, 1989). Inevitably, foods are sometimes reintroduced inadvertently and, if they are found to be well tolerated, dietary restriction may no longer be needed. The reintroduction of foods that have caused severe reactions can be hazardous, however, and normally requires close medical supervision.

In the most severe cases of childhood food allergy, in which the child has severe asthma or is thought to be at risk of anaphylaxis, it is important that ready-loaded adrenaline (using an appropriate dose for the child) should be available for intramuscular injection together with a liquid antihistamine preparation (Sampson 1996b). Those caring for the child must be trained in the use of adrenaline. Administration of adrenaline may be so crucial that those who care for a child outside of the home, *e.g.* at school, should also have access to it and know how to use it (American Academy of Paediatrics ad hoc Committee on Anaphylaxis in school, 1993). In the USA, it is claimed that no deaths have occurred in patients who received adrenaline immediately, although even a slight delay resulting in the administration of adrenaline within 15 minutes had allowed near-fatal reactions to occur (Sampson *et al.*, 1992b).

## 6.7 Difficulties in diagnosis and management

For the person who has had a bad experience after eating a specific food, a personal decision to eat no more of that food can do no harm even if the diagnosis is wrong, provided that the nutrients the food would have provided are obtained from other food sources. There are other situations, however, in which an incorrect self-diagnosis has led to a more seriously restricted diet or to unpleasant symptoms that are related to anxiety and not to food intolerance. Fashions in diagnosis have certainly played a part, and the literature provided by commercial laboratories or kinesiology enthusiasts may lead vulnerable people first to consider that they may themselves have a food-allergic disease, and then to receive a prompt confirmation of their self-diagnosis through the medium of the laboratory test (sometimes accompanied by a long list of foods to be avoided). For a more detailed discussion, see Chapter 10.

It deserves emphasising that only properly conducted challenge tests can establish a diagnosis of food allergy beyond doubt and that, taken alone, even the finding of a high specific IgE level is not totally conclusive. Indeed, many commercial laboratories, using a variety of other methods, have produced discrepant results even when reporting on pairs of coded blood samples from the same patient. It has even been claimed that food allergy can be diagnosed by testing hair samples, a claim which has been discredited (Sethi *et al.*, 1987). In addition, some laboratories offer dietary advice after measuring IgG antibodies to food. These antibodies are easily measured but have no relevance to the diagnosis of food allergy (Lessof *et al.*, 1991).

The distinction between allergy and other forms of food intolerance can provide further problems, especially when the symptoms involve the stomach or affect bowel function. The response may then occur only with large quantities of food or when the challenge is repeated on more than one occasion. A convincing blind challenge test may then be difficult or impossible, and this has caused confusion in the past. Furthermore, symptoms may be affected by dietary adjustments which increase or decrease the passage of food residues to the lower bowel, for example by increasing the bran content of the diet or by alcohol, coffee, tea or smoking. As with asthma and skin reactions, more than one contributory factor may combine to provoke adverse reactions to food in the intestinal tract.

Symptoms that are clearly food related but which are mild and are prevented by avoiding a single food (or wine) may not need the attention of a doctor. However, those with symptoms that lead them to attempt a seriously restricted diet need to be sure that their symptoms are appropriately investigated. If, then, a diagnosis of food allergy is established, avoidance of the food is the mainstay of treatment and, as in childhood, the advice of a dietitian can be invaluable. A dietary approach must, of necessity, be combined with other medical treatment for associated asthma, skin reactions or intestinal symptoms. It is also important to make sure that, if stress is a factor, its importance is recognised. Desensitisation may well have a future role but has as yet had little success (see Chapter 13).

Finally, for those who are at risk of developing anaphylactic reactions, information concerning their medical condition should be available to others at all times; for example, through the wearing of a Medic-Alert bracelet. While the immediate injection of adrenaline can be life-saving, symptoms can recur as the effect of the adrenaline wears off, and it is therefore important that this is followed by a period of medical observation.

## 6.8 Key points

- Allergy can be defined as the adverse health effects that may result from the stimulation of a specific immune response. In the context of food allergy, the allergic sensitisation is induced to food proteins, substances that in non-sensitised subjects are tolerated fully.

- Allergy is not the most common result of adverse reactions to food; 2% of infants and young children are affected. In severe cases, allergy can be life threatening. In some cases (for instance peanut allergy), food allergy can persist to later life. Adult onset food allergy is less common.

- Individual susceptibility to a particular food allergy appears to be determined by a number of factors including: genetic make-up and heritable factors; the local environment, and in particular the environment during infancy; the age at which first exposure to the food occurs and the nature, extent and duration of that exposure; and the integrity of the gastro-intestinal tract.

- Although an anaphylactic reaction or a strongly positive IgE antibody test is prognostic of food allergy, appropriately conducted challenge tests (preferably double-blind and placebo-controlled) are an important means to diagnose or refute food intolerances. The use of non-validated tests may lead to the neglect of other treatable conditions, and to unnecessary and often harmful dietary restrictions.

- Common foods that can cause food allergic reactions in the UK are hens' eggs, cows' milk, peanuts, various tree nuts, soya beans, fish, shellfish and wheat. Reactions to some fruits and vegetables can also cause problems.

- Allergic cross-reactions occur in some people. For example, people sensitised to birch pollen sometimes also react to apple and hazelnut; people sensitised to rubber latex may also react to bananas, chestnuts, kiwi fruit and avocados. Cross-reactions can also occur in people sensitised to clusters of substances, for example mugwort, parsley, celery and spices; or celery, cucumber, carrot and watermelon.

- Food allergic symptoms can affect all organ systems but often affect the skin, gastro-intestinal tract and respiratory tract.

- Treatment of food allergy depends upon the use of a nutritionally balanced diet that nevertheless excludes the offending food, and the availability and proper use of emergency measures for severe cases.

# 7
# Other Manifestations of Food Intolerances

## 7.1 Introduction

The terms 'food intolerance' or 'adverse reactions to foods' cover a wide variety of immediate and late onset reactions (Chapter 1), which can be caused by immunological mechanisms or triggered by non-immunologically mediated responses.

Toxins, enzyme deficiencies and a variety of medical conditions, such as inflammatory bowel disease, neurological and psychiatric conditions, peptic ulcers and pancreatic insufficiency, can mimic clinical symptoms of allergy.

These differential diagnostic possibilities must be borne in mind, particularly in adulthood, when the diagnosis of a non-IgE mediated food intolerance is made or entertained.

The major target organs affected by clinical reactions to foods are the gastrointestinal tract, the skin and the respiratory system (see Chapter 2, Figure 2.9, which shows the reactions associated with allergy). Many different clinical features can arise from non-toxic adverse reactions to food. Adverse reactions may be manifested by symptoms and clinical signs that are confined to a single organ system but often more than one system is involved.

## 7.2 Reactions affecting the skin

### 7.2.1 Urticaria and angio-oedema

Urticaria occurs in acute and chronic forms: acute urticaria is defined as lasting for less than 6 weeks, whereas chronic urticaria lasts for longer periods

(Hannuksela & Haahtela, 1987; Zuberbier et al., 1996)

### Acute urticaria

In general, children suffer more often from acute urticaria than do adults. Acute urticaria is also more common than chronic urticaria. Episodes generally occur within an hour of contact and often fade within 3 hours. Initially there are localised symptoms of itching and burning, which develop into erythema and urticaria at the site of contact. Contact urticaria to foods is common and may progress to a more widespread urticaria, angio-oedema and occasionally to severe life-threatening reactions (i.e. anaphylaxis) (Greaves & Lawlor, 1991). A detailed description of food allergy and information on anaphylaxis can be found in Chapter 6.

Urticaria/angio-oedema occurs in 15–20% of the population at some time in their lives with an estimated prevalence at any one time of 0.05 to 0.1% (Juhlin, 1980). In one study, food was implicated as a cause of acute urticaria in 15% of 163 children experiencing symptoms (Kauppinen et al., 1984). Most acute food-related urticarial reactions occur in atopic subjects. Many different foods or food components can cause urticaria (Moneret-Vautrin et al., 1996; Zuberbier et al., 1996; Jarisch et al., 1999) and the role of allergen-specific IgE as a triggering mechanism is unclear.

In food-allergic subjects, urticarial wheals may develop within minutes of a precipitant such as raw egg white or cows' milk touching the skin.

Immediate lip swelling may occur in patients on contact with peanuts or peanut butter, or as a result of being kissed by someone who has recently eaten peanuts, cows' milk or egg. Urticaria may occasionally be associated with oral allergy symptoms and/or anaphylaxis. This most commonly occurs in people who are allergic to peanuts, tree nuts or shellfish (Amlot *et al.*, 1987; Rance *et al.*, 1999).

In a cross-sectional UK questionnaire survey of adverse reactions to foods, 6.2% of individuals claimed problems with urticaria, 6.3% with angio-oedema and 49% claimed a reaction to foods (Young *et al.*, 1994). This could suggest that the prevalence figures for food related urticaria have previously been underestimated. Alternatively, these figures could reflect perception rather than reality.

Given the possible progression of urticaria to an anaphylactic shock, it is of concern that some people are unaware of the potential severity of their reactions. This is of particular relevance to individuals suffering from shellfish, peanut or tree nut allergies. Individuals need to be aware of this possibility and may be putting themselves at risk by not seeking medical and dietetic advice on appropriate avoidance of allergens and by not having available emergency self-medication and training in its use.

Drugs such as aspirin and other non-steroidal anti-inflammatory drugs can at times exacerbate food induced urticarias (Cant *et al.*, 1984; Genton *et al.*, 1985). Vasoactive amines, including histamine, and histamine releasing agents may cause or aggravate urticaria, and the condition has been linked with ingestion of tartrazine and other food additives (see Appendix 1) (Antico & Di Benardino, 1995; Wüthrich, 1998) and alcohol (see below).

### Chronic urticaria

The incidence of atopic disease appears not to be increased in patients with chronic urticaria (Champion *et al.*, 1969). In a study of 94 children with chronic urticaria, 20 reported a history of reactions to food, but when challenged with the food (open challenge), only two children reacted (Harris *et al.*, 1983). Chronic urticaria is only rarely associated with IgE-mediated food allergy. However, azo-dyes and benzoic acid have been

implicated as triggers (see Appendix 1) (Greaves, 1995).

### Other forms of urticaria

Rarely, exercising soon after eating certain foods, such as wheat, shellfish or nuts, can induce urticaria/angio-oedema, whereas neither that particular food nor exercise alone causes any reaction (McNeil & Strauss, 1988) (Chapter 6, Section 6.4.4). Urticarial reactions can be elicited by a variety of non-immunological, non-food-related causes, such as drugs, infections, physical triggers. They can also be a symptom of hereditary diseases, *e.g.* hereditary angio-oedema.

### Atopic dermatitis

Atopic dermatitis is a disease that affects children and adults. The prevalence of atopic dermatitis in the UK is increasing (see Chapter 4). Cohort studies have identified a prevalence of atopic dermatitis of 5.1% in those born in 1946, 7.3% in those born in 1958 and 12.2% in those born in 1970 (Taylor *et al.*, 1984). There is evidence for a higher prevalence (~16–17%) in certain ethnic groups, for example in black Caribbean children born in the UK and in Asian patients (Sladden *et al.*, 1991; Williams *et al.*, 1995). There is a paucity of prevalence data in adults.

The role of food allergy in the aetiology of atopic dermatitis is unclear, although the likelihood of a food-related trigger being involved is highest in early infancy. Atopic dermatitis is a clinical diagnosis and many other factors may contribute to or aggravate the disease.

Positive and immediate skin-test reactions to foods are commonly observed (Atherton, 1984) and CD4$^+$ T cells are the predominant infiltrating cell type in skin lesions (Beyer *et al.*, 1997). Dietary eliminations on the basis of skin tests in patients with atopic dermatitis are often unhelpful. The value of dietary eliminations needs to be confirmed by a food challenge protocol (Chapter 11).

Reactions to food challenges can be demonstrated in some patients with atopic dermatitis (Sampson & Scanlon, 1989) and atopic dermatitis may be exacerbated within a day of ingestion of a food allergen (Sampson, 1988). Since patients may have multiple allergies, the dietary exclusion of single foods does not necessarily benefit the management of atopic dermatitis. The foods commonly implicated in atopic dermatitis are shown in Table 7.1.

**Table 7.1** Some foods and ingredients commonly associated with causation or exacerbation of atopic dermatitis in the UK.

| | |
|---|---|
| Cows' milk | Chocolate |
| Hens' eggs | Fish |
| Peanuts | Citrus fruits |
| Tree nuts | Meat (chicken, pork, beef) |
| Soya | Shellfish |
| Wheat | Food additives (benzoate, glutamate, metabisulfite, tartrazine) |

On isolated occasions, other foods have been reported to cause or exacerbate atopic dermatitis, *e.g.* chickpeas and tomatoes

**Table 7.2** Symptoms of adverse, food-related* reactions affecting the gastrointestinal tract.

Vomiting
Gastro-oesophageal reflux
Abdominal pain
Abdominal distension and flatulence
Diarrhoea
Constipation
Specific syndromes:*
    Oral allergy syndrome
    Cheilitis/oral granulomatosis
    Enteropathies:
        Cows' milk sensitive enteropathy
        Coeliac disease (gluten intolerance)
    Allergic eosinophilic gastroenteropathy
    Dermatitis herpetiformis
    Infantile colic
    Irritable bowel syndrome

*The level of scientific evidence for these food-associated disorders and syndromes is variable.

There is little published evidence that food additives aggravate or cause atopic dermatitis. One small DBPCFC study in 25 children with severe atopic dermatitis (Van Bever *et al.*, 1989) suggests that food additives (tartrazine, sodium benzoate, glutamate and metabisulfite) (see Appendix 1) and/or acetylsalicylic acid may have caused pruritus and erythema of the skin in 6 out of the 25 children challenged.

## 7.3 Reactions affecting the gastrointestinal tract

Adverse reactions to foods can affect any part of the gastrointestinal tract and its normal function. The aetiology and symptomatology of these are variable (see Table 7.2). The mechanisms involved and the site of the reaction influence the time taken for symptoms and clinical signs to develop after eating the offending food.

The role of foods and food ingredients as precipitants in some diseases of the gastrointestinal tract (for example irritable bowel syndrome) remains unresolved (Bischoff *et al.*, 1996). Moreover, a favourable response to food elimination procedures in a patient with a well-characterised inflammatory bowel disease (such as Crohn's disease) does not necessarily imply that particular foods play a role in the aetiology of the disease. A change in microbial bowel flora, for example, could

be the cause of temporary improvement in this context.

### 7.3.1 Vomiting

Vomiting, alone or in combination with acute or chronic diarrhoea, is a common feature of adverse reactions to food (Walker-Smith *et al.*, 1984; Walker-Smith, 1995; Sicherer, 1999; Eigenmann & Calza, 2000). It results from inflammation of the mucosa of the stomach and oesophagus. Bleeding may be caused by the inflammatory response or as a result of small tears in the mucosal lining caused by repeated retching.

### 7.3.2 Gastro-oesophageal reflux

Gastro-oesophageal reflux can occur as an adverse reaction to food, particularly in infants with allergic gastroenteropathy and a constituent eosinophilic oesophagitis (Hill *et al.*, 1984; Ford & Walker-Smith, 1987). Gastro-oesophageal reflux, as measured by oesophageal pH monitoring, can be detected soon after a cows' milk feed, although features of an eosinophilic oesophagitis take longer to develop. Coffee drinking and smoking may contribute to reflux by relaxing the gastro-oesophageal sphincter (Locke, 1999).

### 7.3.3 Abdominal pain, distension and flatulence

Significant gas production within the gastro-intestinal tract is a normal occurrence. Under conditions of impaired digestion and absorption of carbohydrates from the diet and subsequent fermentation, pain, distension and increased flatulence may occur. Lactase deficiency (see Chapter 8) is possibly an underlying aetiology in the susceptible individual.

These relatively non-specific symptoms can also be associated with diarrhoeal diseases, irritable bowel syndrome and inflammatory bowel disease. Misdiagnosis is, therefore, possible unless appropriate tests are performed (see Chapter 10). These symptoms are seen sometimes as isolated instances of adverse reactions to foods and are usually associated with impaired digestion and absorption resulting from damage to the functional integrity of the intestine.

### 7.3.4 Diarrhoea

Frequent loose stools can result from impaired absorption of nutrients and water, or from intestinal secretion of fluid as part of an inflammatory response, or from a combination of both. The inflammatory response may also cause bleeding, so an additional feature would be blood in the stools (see Section 7.4.1).

### 7.3.5 Bacterial overgrowth

Problems such as small bowel bacterial overgrowth syndromes and fermentative diarrhoea may arise from gastrointestinal functional disturbances, following conditions such as gastroenteritis and surgery. Such syndromes are often self-limiting but may occasionally need treatment and abdominal pain may be the only feature.

### 7.3.6 Constipation

Constipation can be the consequence of inflammatory responses of the lower bowel. In children, cows' milk is a cause of a food-induced constipation. In a double-blind cross-over study of 65 children aged between 1 and 6 years with chronic constipation, 68% improved when their customary intake of cows' milk was replaced by soya milk.

Many of those who responded had evidence of other atopic manifestations. It was suggested that the resultant painful defaecation induced stool retention and constipation (Iacono *et al.*, 1998). These important observations need to be confirmed in other studies. It remains to be established clearly whether the improvement was the result of the reduction in cows' milk intake, the change in diet, an increase in the dietary fibre intake, or some other factor not measured directly in the study.

## 7.4 Enteropathies

A major feature of the enteropathies is a loss of the normal structure of the intestinal mucosa, which impairs mucosal digestive and absorptive function (Kuitunen *et al.*, 1975; Walker-Smith *et al.*, 1978). Enteropathies have been reported in response to wheat gluten (coeliac disease), other cereals, cows' milk, soya, eggs, rice, fish and chicken. The immunological mechanisms involved are described later. The most recognised food induced enteropathy is coeliac disease (see Chapter 9).

### 7.4.1 Allergic eosinophilic gastroenteropathy

Allergic eosinophilic gastroenteropathy represents a spectrum of conditions, which predominantly affect infants and young children, and in which there is inflammation of the gastrointestinal mucosa, with eosinophilic infiltration. The symptoms and signs reflect the site and extent of damage. Involvement of the stomach or oesophagus may present with vomiting. Damage to the small intestine and colon can cause significant loss of protein and nutrients, as well as impaired digestion and absorption. Consequently, the range of symptoms includes bloody diarrhoea, impaired weight gain and growth. Protein-losing enteropathy, enterocolitis and/or another form of colitis that mimics inflammatory bowel diseases may occur in severe cases.

Sometimes, children present only with an anaemia, associated with an occult loss of blood in the stools. Some patients have atopic features but otherwise other organs are not directly involved. Most cases present in the first 3 months of life and resolve spontaneously in early childhood (Moon & Kleinman, 1995).

The causes and mechanisms of these conditions

are not well understood. Some cases are associated with atopic clinical features. These patients, for example, show an increase in the number of blood eosinophils and exhibit positive RASTs and skin prick tests, recognised as indicators of possible IgE mediated reactions; however, others may not show these features (Min & Metcalfe, 1991; Moon & Kleinman, 1995). These are rare diseases and it is thought that between a third and a half of cases may be caused by food allergy, most frequently to cows' milk or soya (Pfaffenbach *et al.*, 1996).

Eosinophilic colitis can occur in an exclusively breast fed infant (Wilson *et al.*, 1990) and in such circumstances the mother should go onto an exclusion diet (Isolauri, 1995; James & Burks, 1996) if she wishes to continue to breast feed. (See Chapter 11 for information on alternative milks.)

### 7.4.2 Infantile colic

Sometimes known as 3-month colic, this is a common problem in babies and a condition that is often managed by parents rather than by health professionals. It is an ill-defined syndrome of intermittent episodes of inconsolable crying, drawing up of legs, some abdominal distension and excessive gas. A study in babies and older children, who had each been shown via challenge tests to be allergic to cows' milk, found that 75% reacted with colic during a challenge with capsules containing whey protein (Lothe & Linberg, 1989) and IgE mediated hypersensitivity may play a role in some babies. However, not all children with colic respond to dietary measures such as cows' milk exclusion. It has been suggested that psychosocial factors may also be involved, such as a disturbed maternal–infant interaction and/or periodic overexcitement of the child, *e.g.* lots of lively attention when a parent returns home in the evening.

It is unclear whether the features of a disturbed infant–mother (infant–parents) relationship are primary or caused by the highly disruptive and often distressing features of this syndrome.

Mechanisms have not been investigated in a prospective way and the relationship of infant colic with cows' milk and other foods or food components, which might be present in maternal breast milk or milk formulas, needs further study. Infants with colic could initially be managed by reducing the overall stimulation that parents and carers

might be giving the baby, particularly noisy and exuberant behaviour such as 'throwing' the child up in the air. If this is unsuccessful, then a therapeutic trial of cows' milk exclusion could be considered (Lucassen *et al.*, 1998). When adopting this strategy, breast-feeding mothers also need to exclude milk from their diet (with adequate calcium supplementation, in particular) (see Chapters 5 and 11).

### 7.4.3 Irritable bowel syndrome

The diagnosis of irritable bowel syndrome (IBS) should be considered in patients with ill-defined gastrointestinal symptoms, where there are no endoscopic, histopathological or other abnormal findings (Fotherby & Hunter, 1985). IBS may be experienced by 10–20% of adults in the western hemisphere and is twice as common in women as in men. There is some evidence that abnormal colonic fermentation and gas production may be involved in the pathogenesis (King *et al.*, 1998). There is also some evidence that mucosal inflammatory mechanisms, similar to those involved in immunological reactions (Collins, 1999; Collins *et al.*, 1999), may be contributing to the syndrome. There is a lack of well-designed, appropriately powered, randomised clinical trials to study possible precipitants and the cause of exacerbations in IBS.

There can be no single explanation for IBS, in which the patient, without evidence of organic disease, complains of abdominal pain, bloating and constipation, or diarrhoea, or an alternation between the two. When questioned, 30% of apparently healthy British adults admit to bowel disturbances, which are similar to those that in others are so disturbing to the individual that they have led to more consultations than any other gastroenterological condition (Thompson & Heaton, 1980). The evidence suggests that, in many cases, the symptoms of disordered intestinal motility are strongly conditioned by a person's perceptions and sensitivity.

Symptoms of IBS are seen in any condition in which unabsorbed food residues reach the lower bowel, where they are fermented. A classical example is seen in lactase deficiency (Ramirez *et al.*, 1994), in which a lack of the enzyme allows unabsorbed milk lactose to pass through the bowel and be fermented in this way (see Chapter 8). It has also been reported that antibiotics can precipitate irritable bowel symptoms, for example after the prophylactic use of metronidazole before gynae-cological operations (Alun Jones, 1985). Since the bacteria eliminated by antibiotics can in some cases consume hydrogen rather than produce it (Levitt *et al.*, 1974), an increase in unabsorbed gas products may explain these findings.

Following the pioneering studies of Burkitt *et al.* (1972), the harmful effects of low fibre diets became a cause for concern. The preferred treatment for diverticulitis changed completely and high fibre diets were prescribed freely, not only for diverticular disease but also, notably, in IBS. Despite the recognised general benefits of a high fibre diet, 55 out of 100 patients with IBS in one clinic said that a high fibre diet made them worse and only 10 benefited (Francis & Whorwell, 1994). While this study may be of relevance only to selected patients (Editorial, 1994) or to patients with particular symptoms, there have been other, more detailed claims that various specific foods can provoke symptoms in patients with IBS, and that dietary measures can provide effective treatment in at least some of these cases (Hunter *et al.*, 1982; Bentley *et al.*, 1983; Farah *et al.*, 1985).

It has also been suggested that IBS is frequently the result of a specific intolerance to one or more foods (Alun Jones, 1985). A review of published double-blind, placebo-controlled challenges suggests, especially in patients with diarrhoea, that problem foods were identified in between 6% and 58% of cases (Niec *et al.*, 1998). These included milk, wheat, eggs and foods with a high salicylate or amine content. In constipation-prevalent IBS, a high fibre diet with increased physical activity may be helpful (Evans *et al.*, 1998).

Despite these findings, many investigators have failed to find a positive response to dietary manipulation, only a poor and non-specific response, or there were features of anxiety or depression in patients with IBS (Bentley *et al.*, 1983; McKee *et al.*, 1988). Patients with IBS may have a reduced pain barrier to normal intestinal distension (Farthing, 1998). These findings suggest that there may be more than one subgroup in what is, in fact, a syndrome of symptoms rather than a specific disease. A variety of spasmolytic and other gut selective agents have been used in the treatment of IBS (Battaglia *et al.*, 1998).

## 7.5 Respiratory system effects

Foods or ingredients reported to act as secondary triggers for respiratory effects, *e.g.* asthma and rhinitis, include seafood, meat, eggs, cereals, additives and other food items. Respiratory features normally accompany eczema, urticaria, oral allergy syndrome or other gastrointestinal symptoms (Novembre *et al.*, 1987; Bousquet *et al.*, 1992; Moneret-Vautrin *et al.*, 1996).

### 7.5.1 Asthma

In a study of 107 adults with perennial bronchial asthma, 15 out of 21 patients with a history of food allergy developed bronchial responses to food challenge (Pelikan & Pelikan-Filipek, 1987). Nevertheless, it is difficult to be sure how many patients with asthma have genuine food-related bronchial hypersensitivity reactions (Moneret-Vautrin *et al.*, 1996); the incidence has been estimated to be 8.5%. Other studies in children (Oehling & Baena Cagnani, 1980; Novembre *et al.*, 1988) and in patients of all ages (Onorata *et al.*, 1986) have suggested that 2.0–8.5% of asthmatics show bronchospasm in response to food challenge. Food-induced respiratory symptoms were produced by DBPCFC in 205 children with atopic dermatitis (James *et al.*, 1994).

Mannino (2000), using different methodologies, suggested that 10–25% of asthma cases in adults may be related to occupation. Occupational asthma attacks can be due to food particle inhalation or result from sensitisation to cross-reacting pneumo-allergens, such as pollen, feathers and latex. An occupational history of exposure, usually by the respiratory route, to allergens present in food is sometimes found in those who work in the food industry and who acquire adverse reactions to the food when it is consumed (Mannino, 2000). On the other hand, a number of individuals with occupational asthma react to inhalation of the allergen but have no clinical symptoms after oral intake (Lopez-Rubio *et al.*, 1998; Daroco *et al.*, 2000; Rodriguez *et al.*, 2000). The surveillance of work-related and occupational respiratory disease in the UK (SWORD 97) (Ross *et al.*, 1998) found the highest incidence among workers in the manufacture of wood products, textiles and food, particularly grain products and foods derived from crustaceans. It highlights a marked increase in occupational asthma attributed to latex among health care workers, laboratory technicians and shoe workers.

A survey of 177 asthmatic children suggested that the prevalence of adverse reactions to food varied according to the season and severity of asthma at the time of ingestion (Wilson & Silverman, 1985; Wilson, 1988). A possible basis for such observations is that food allergens may create, in some patients, a background bronchial hyperreactivity that primes or exacerbates the response to other precipitants of asthma. Thus, although these allergens (egg, milk, soya, wheat and fish, identified on the basis of history and positive skin prick test) do not themselves cause symptoms, their elimination might in some patients improve their symptoms and their response to standard pharmaceutical agents (James *et al.*, 1996). The effects of an elimination diet must be confirmed by objective measurements of respiratory function. There is no good evidence that elimination of milk reduces mucous or phlegm production in the normal individual or in individuals who believe that they may suffer from a milk-induced increase in mucus production (Pinnock & Arney, 1993).

### 7.5.2 Rhinitis and conjunctivitis (hay fever)

Rhinitis (runny nose, nasal itching, sneezing and nasal congestion), with or without conjunctivitis, is associated with the intake of specific food items, although usually less frequently than asthma-type symptoms (Oehling *et al.*, 1992). Open food challenges of 107 adult patients with asthma caused immediate nasal obstruction in 6% and conjunctivitis in 2% (Pelikan & Pelikan-Filipek, 1987). These reactions are most probably caused by an IgE mediated mechanism comparable to grass or tree pollen induced hayfever.

### 7.5.3 Serous otitis media

Serous otitis media has been reported as an adverse reaction to certain foods, *e.g.* cows' milk, wheat and egg white, but the relationship is unclear (Bernstein, 1992). It has been claimed that serous otitis media improves after elimination diets and that recurrence occurs after open food challenge with the trigger food (Nsouli *et al.*, 1994). DBPCFC studies, including the demonstration of transient

hearing loss, are necessary to assess whether a dietary approach to treat serous otitis media in childhood is warranted.

### 7.5.4 Milk-induced pulmonary haemosiderosis (Heiner's syndrome)

Heiner's syndrome is a rare multi-system disorder in children, characterised by recurring episodes of lung inflammation with pulmonary infiltrates of haemosiderin-laden macrophages, blood eosinophilia, haemosiderosis, gastrointestinal blood loss, iron deficiency anaemia and failure to thrive. The patients may have IgG antibodies to cows' milk (Barnes *et al.*, 1988; Fossati *et al.*, 1992) and other reactivities have also been reported. However, the immunological basis of this rare syndrome is not understood fully (Lee *et al.*, 1978). Laboratory tests such as identifying precipitating antibodies to cows' milk (or other allergens involved) may be useful in diagnosis. Resolution of symptoms follows the elimination of relevant allergens.

## 7.6 The central nervous system and behaviour

### 7.6.1 Migraine and food intolerance

Although headache is perceived to be very common it is difficult to obtain accurate overall prevalence rates because most sufferers do not seek medical treatment. Moreover, headaches are of different clinical pictures ranging from the usually one-sided throbbing incapacitating migraine headaches to episodic tension-type headaches. Based upon a number of investigations, population prevalence rates for headaches, defined as very severe, incapacitating or migraine, appear to be in the ranges of 2–9% for males and 4–20% for females.

### 7.6.2 Migraine and diet

It is clear that a variety of factors is associated with the risk of migraine headaches and the precipitation of an attack. Among these are changes in the menstrual cycle and hypoglycaemia. Diet is believed by many clinicians and patients to represent an additional trigger for migraine headache. As a consequence, dietary interventions are widely used, with much of the attention focusing on foods with components that have vasoactive properties.

In an examination of 429 consecutive patients with migraine headache, many reported that symptoms could be precipitated by one or more foods. In 16.6% of cases, at least two of the following foods were implicated: cheese, chocolate and citrus fruit. Additionally, 18.4% reported sensitivity to all alcoholic drinks, while another 11.8% were sensitive to red (but not white) wine and 28% found that beers could precipitate headaches. Individuals who were sensitive to cheese and chocolate often also reported reactions to red wine and beer. In contrast, none of 40 patients with tension-type headaches were sensitive to any of these foods and only one subject reported a reaction to alcoholic drinks (Peatfield, 1995). The implication is that cheese, chocolate and red wine may be causally related to migraine headaches, but not to tension-type headaches, and that separate mechanisms contribute to headache associated with alcoholic drinks.

### 7.6.3 Food allergy and migraine

Although food preparations used for skin tests are not always reliable, there is evidence that food allergy (as defined by positive skin prick test reactions) may be associated with migraine headaches. Mansfield *et al.* (1985) described investigations of 43 adult patients with migraine, referred from a neurology clinic. In all subjects, skin prick testing was performed with a total of 83 foods. Those patients who displayed positive reactions were placed for one month on an elimination diet that excluded the foods that had provoked skin test responses. The remaining subjects, with negative skin prick tests, were placed on a diet that eliminated wheat, corn, egg and milk for the same period. Of the 43 subjects, 13 (approximately 30%) experienced a two-thirds or greater reduction in the frequency of headaches while on the elimination diet. These subjects underwent a series of single-blind challenges with capsules containing specific foods or a placebo. Those with positive challenges then received full double-blind placebo-controlled challenges. Of these 7 subjects, 5 experienced migraine with the active food challenge and none responded to placebo. In these investigations it was found that 11 out of 16 subjects with positive skin

prick tests responded to dietary manipulation, whereas only 2 of the 27 subjects who were skin test negative responded. The conclusion drawn is that food-related migraine headaches may in some instances be associated with food allergy (as defined by skin prick test reactivity). The mechanistic basis for this association is unclear, although inflammatory mediators (and in particular prostaglandins and vasoactive amines) released from mast cells by IgE mediated degranulation (see Chapter 2, Section 2.5) are likely candidates. What is not clear, however, is why the release of such mediators should cause migraine in some subjects but not in others. In relation to induction of migraine by diet, the variable results obtained with skin prick testing indicate, firstly, that skin testing with food will yield both false positive and false negative results and, therefore, should not be used as the sole diagnostic criterion and, secondly, that other probably non-immunologic mechanisms are also important.

Significantly, food-triggered migraine cannot always or necessarily be excluded when a food challenge, under controlled conditions, fails to provoke an attack. This is because there may be a requirement for other factors in addition to food to provoke a response, as occurs in food allergic exercise-induced anaphylaxis (see Chapter 6).

### 7.6.4 Migraine and non-immunologic effects

It was reported by Hanington (1971) that foods containing tyramine are frequently implicated by migraine patients as causing headaches. However, subsequent studies have yielded equivocal results, with evidence both for and against an important role for this vasoactive amine (Moffett *et al.*, 1972; Ziegler & Stewart, 1977), and tyramine-free diets have been found not to affect the frequency of headaches (Medina & Diamond, 1978).

Foods traditionally associated with migraine (such as chocolate, cheeses and red wine) may lack tyramine, but contain appreciable amounts of phenylethylamine, a vasoactive amine that is able to cross the blood–brain barrier and which is known to disrupt cerebral blood flow. In a single-blinded study reported by Sandler *et al.* (1974), 36 subjects who believed that chocolate precipitated symptoms received either phenylethylamine or placebo. A significantly higher number of individuals reported headache following exposure to the amine compared with the placebo. However, subsequent studies suggested that many brands of chocolate may contain very much lower levels of phenylethylamine than those assumed by Sandler *et al.*, and concluded that either chocolate-induced migraine is not attributable to phenylethylamine, or that some migraine patients are sensitive to very low levels of the amine (Schweitzer *et al.*, 1975). The picture is clouded further by doubts that chocolate *per se* is necessarily able to provoke migraine. A double-blind placebo-controlled study of patients with a history of cocoa- or chocolate-induced migraine was reported by Moffett *et al.* (1974). Of 25 test subjects, one reported headache with both chocolate and cocoa, 8 only with chocolate, 5 with placebo and 11 with neither. The conclusion drawn by the authors was that chocolate alone is rarely able to precipitate migraine.

Assessment of the possible role of adverse reactions to food and food additives in migraine has been difficult for some of the same reasons noted below in relation to behavioural reactions (Section 7.7). In a controlled provocation trial involving 88 children with severe frequent migraine referred to a specialist centre, 93% recovered on oligoantigenic diets; sequential reintroduction of foods and subsequent DBPCFC in 40 of the children identified causative foods (Egger *et al.*, 1983). Most patients responded to elimination of several foods: cows' milk caused symptoms in most of the children and many deteriorated when egg, chocolate, orange or wheat were reintroduced.

Associated symptoms experienced by the children, including abdominal pain, behaviour disorders, fits, asthma and eczema, had also improved with the elimination diet. However, the degree to which these data can be generalised to the migrainous population as a whole is limited because only a highly selected group of subjects was investigated.

Histamine has also been considered. Although it has been reported that improvement of symptoms is associated with a histamine-reduced diet (Wantke *et al.*, 1993), other studies have failed to confirm an important role for vasoactive amines among children with migraine (Salfield *et al.*, 1987).

Taken together, it would appear that although some patients with migraine are sensitive to various vasoactive amines, this is not a general rule as witnessed by the difficulty in demonstrating

appreciable numbers of reactors under controlled conditions.

Alcohol has frequently been cited as a precipitating factor in migraine. Alcohol has little impact on cerebral blood flow so intracerebral vasodilation is not thought to be implicated. An important question is whether it is the alcohol itself within alcoholic drinks that is the cause of headaches. Littlewood *et al.* (1988) investigated 19 subjects with migraine who believed symptoms were provoked by red wine, but not by any other alcoholic drink. Preparations of red wine or vodka, of equivalent alcohol content, were consumed in blinded fashion. It was found that a headache was provoked in 9 of 11 subjects given red wine, whereas in contrast no subjects receiving vodka had an attack. Neither red wine nor vodka caused symptoms in controls. The authors concluded that neither alcohol nor tyramine was responsible for the headaches precipitated by red wine and suggested that other substances such as phenolic flavonoids might be possible triggers.

### 7.6.5 Foods commonly associated with migraine

Food components are frequently associated with attacks of migraine. The available evidence suggests that both immunological and non-immunological mechanisms may be involved, but in neither case are the pathogenetic mechanisms clearly defined. The foods most commonly cited are:

*Chocolate:* There is good evidence that patients frequently cite chocolate as inducing migraine attacks. As discussed above, however, there is some doubt that chocolate alone is able to trigger a reaction.

*Coffee:* Both the excessive consumption of coffee and coffee withdrawal have been reported to cause unpleasant effects akin to anxiety, which frequently include headaches (Greden, 1974).

*Alcohol:* Many migraine sufferers believe that alcoholic beverages precipitate attacks. As cited above, there is good evidence that red wine may be a trigger.

*Monosodium glutamate:* Clinical reactions associated with presumed intake of monosodium glutamate (Chinese restaurant syndrome) were first described by Kwok in 1968 (Schaumburg *et al.*, 1969). Among the reported symptoms were a sensation of burning, warmth, pressure and tingling confined to the face, neck, upper chest and shoulders after eating certain foods. Although still widely reported, the notion of a specific pattern of symptoms after ingestion of monosodium glutamate has not been confirmed in a variety of trials, including a DBPCFC study of six patients believed to be sensitive (Kenney, 1986).

## 7.7 Evidence of reactions to food in teenagers and adults with mental disorders

Food intolerances *per se* resulting in mental disorders are not common, but dietary deficiencies are frequently found alongside mental illness in adults. The role of poor nutrition, institutional diets, alcohol abuse and poverty all make it likely that deficiencies often result from mental illness rather than that a mental illness is caused by a deficiency. A deficiency, however, can still have its harmful effects, including those affecting mental function. Deficiencies are still reported in spite of advances in the care of the mentally ill. For example, the average plasma vitamin C concentration was lower in 885 psychiatric in-patients (0.51 mg/100 ml) than in 110 reference individuals (0.87 mg/100 ml) (Schorah *et al.*, 1983). Few patients had values as low as those found in clinical scurvy (less than 0.1 mg/100 ml), but 32% had concentrations below the threshold (0.35 mg/100 ml) at which some detrimental effects on health have been reported. Clinically-evident deficiencies of other vitamins have also been described. Three patients with Wernicke's encephalopathy and three with wet beri-beri, all accompanied by gross thiamin deficiency, were found during normal psychiatric practice in England (Carney & Barry, 1985). Deficiency states can cause psychiatric conditions such as Wernicke's encephalopathy and can also be a secondary feature. Thus, although dietary deficiencies are known to be associated with mental illness, it is probable that the deficiencies that have been observed in psychiatric inpatients result from mental illness and the impact of hospitalisation, rather than *vice versa*.

### 7.7.1 Children and adolescents

Specific nutritional deficiencies can be induced by nutritionally imbalanced food intake. It has been hypothesised that delinquent behaviour and offending could be associated with a poor diet. The literature on nutritional changes in delinquent youngsters and criminal adults gives much less guidance for practice and is more controversial. Evidence, largely confined to the work of Schoenthaler and others (*e.g.* Schoenthaler, 1994; Schoenthaler & Bier, 2000; Schoenthaler *et al.*, 2000) is difficult to appraise. In these studies, the impact of interventions such as reducing intake of foods and beverages high in sucrose or low in food additives, or both, or use of vitamin and mineral supplementation, was studied mostly in juvenile delinquents in young offenders' institutions. Although improvements in behaviour as measured by decreases in disciplinary offences were noted, in many cases, double-blind placebo-controlled designs were not adopted. There is also some scepticism raised about the lack of experimental rigour and the omission of challenge procedures. It is nevertheless feasible that food ingredients and food additives might have pharmacological effects and that vitamin and other nutrient deficiencies might influence behaviour, although this explanation seems less plausible.

## 7.8 Hyperactivity and attention deficit hyperactivity disorder (ADHD)

Attention deficit hyperactivity disorder (ADHD) is a psychiatric disorder, affecting more than 1% of children and perhaps as many as 5%; estimates of prevalence vary according to the exact definition that is used (Taylor, 1999). The diagnostic features (Conners *et al.*, 1997, 1998) are:

- *Inattentiveness:* very short attention span, over-frequent changes of activity, distractible.
- *Overactivity:* excessive movements, especially in situations expecting calm such as classroom or mealtimes.
- *Impulsiveness:* won't wait his/her turn, acts without thinking, thoughtless rule-breaking (detailed diagnostic criteria have been defined by the American Psychiatric Association, 1996 and by the international classification of disease, ICD-10).

In order to make the diagnosis, the severity of the problem has to be outside what would be expected for the developmental level of the child, and the problem behaviour has to be present in more than one situation, *e.g.* both at home and at school. All three problems (inattentiveness, overactivity, impulsiveness) have to be present together for a diagnosis of the category known as hyperkinetic disorder to be made, while ADHD can be diagnosed on the basis of one of them (Conners *et al.*, 1980, 1998).

The problems almost always start at an early age and individuals are at a serious risk for later mental health. There is a strong heritability, estimated at about 80–90% from twin studies (Faraone *et al.*, 1999). However, the exact pattern of inheritance is not known and these studies make it plain that there are also important environmental factors (Tucker *et al.*, 1999). There is plausible evidence for structural and functional abnormalities underlying ADHD (Castellanos, 1997). Several genes coding for neurotransmitter receptors or transporters are known to have variant allelic forms that are more common in ADHD than in the general population and evidence is accumulating for abnormalities in genes related to dopaminergic systems in the CNS, preferential transmission of alleles at polymorphisms of the dopamine transporter, dopamine-$\beta$-hydroxylase and dopamine D4 and D5 receptors (Daly *et al.*, 1999; Swanson *et al.*, 2000). However, this characterises only a minority of children and is also seen in about 10% of the normal population.

### 7.8.1 Studies on attention deficit hyperactivity disorder

There are reports of more than 100 randomised controlled trials of specific treatments, including stimulant medication and behaviour therapy, and a number of meta-analyses that have themselves been quantitatively assessed (Connor *et al.*, 1999). Pharmaceutical treatments, although effective in some cases, are not widely accepted in the UK because of the potential risks, and this is one reason why dietary therapies are preferred by many parents, teachers and health visitors. However, recently there has been concern about the increasing use of stimulant therapies in very young children, which is inconsistent with current guidelines (Angold *et al.*, 2000).

Whether diet affects ADHD or is involved in its aetiology is, therefore, clearly a matter of great importance.

Studies investigating potential links between diet and the aetiology of ADHD face a number of methodological problems, some of which may be unavoidable. Case identification has frequently been poor, and as a result studies are based on subjects defined by different criteria and thus it is hard to generalise from the findings. Studies have also often been strongly dependent on subjective measurements and, consequently, interpretations have been susceptible to the effects of observer expectation and possible suggestion (observer bias).

Apart from maintaining the blindness of controlled studies, there is also an unavoidable presence of many other potentially confounding and uncontrolled factors within the social environment.

No one study has been able to overcome all the problems. It is, therefore, necessary to consider the wide range of studies of dietary manipulation, population surveys and trials using diets that eliminate some foodstuffs and also those that utilise confirmatory food challenges.

### 7.8.2 Studies on the Feingold diet

The Feingold diet excludes artificial food colours and flavourings (see Appendix 1), as well as foods containing salicylates, which Feingold thought were contributing to hyperactivity in children by a pharmacological rather than an immune mechanism (Feingold, 1975).

Some studies on groups of children suffering from hyperactivity used such an elimination diet or a variation thereof, mostly incorporating a challenge with food additives such as tartrazine, other colours and natural and synthetic salicylates (Conners *et al.*, 1980; Mattes & Gittelman, 1981; Rowe, 1988; Pollock & Warner, 1990). Challenge studies have generally involved controlled exposure to food colourants, often in biscuits in comparison with a placebo. Despite common public support for the diet's effectiveness, it is difficult to draw overall conclusions. The studies comparing dietary treatments suggest that a large number of children with ADHD do not benefit from dietary intervention. Conners *et al.* (1980) have suggested that the positive outcomes, reported in a small proportion of the subjects investigated in challenge studies, could be explained by a combination of placebo effects and a positive effect of diet. Studies on single cases, which allow individual hypotheses to be tested, add some support to this view and it may be concluded that a small number of cases of ADHD may indeed be sensitive to food colourants.

### 7.8.3 Clinical studies of wider food exclusions

A series of studies has suggested that among hyperactive children there is more evidence of an atopic propensity, such as positive RASTs, than in a reference group (Tryphonas & Trites, 1979). Removing the allergens from the diets of these children, particularly allergens from meat and cereals, produced a small improvement in behaviour. Egger *et al.* (1985) describe a controlled trial, in which a range of possible dietary precipitants were removed by a radical exclusion diet (known as a few-foods diet) (see Chapter 11, Section 11.4.3), and were then reintroduced one at a time, and the effects finally compared with a placebo. The results were clearly positive, and clinical improvement was largely confined to parental ratings. This type of rating is the most likely to be sensitive to any failure of the maintenance of 'blind' status, on the one hand, but is also the most relevant indicator of the diet's effectiveness. In a similar study using a less highly selected series, 78 children started on the diet; of these, 59 improved in open trial and 19 were selected for a double-blind crossover challenge because the foods to which they appeared to be intolerant could successfully be disguised. Cows' milk, wheat flour, citrus fruits and food colourants were among the most commonly incriminated foods. There was a significant effect of the provoking foods, by comparison with the placebo, on behaviour ratings; and also on behaviour as observed by an independent psychologist and on some psychological tests of abilities related to attention (Carter *et al.*, 1993). In a similar study, 19 out of 26 children responded in open trial conditions; 16 of the 19 went on to undergo a double-blind challenge, and rated behaviour was worse on challenge days than on placebo days (Boris & Mandel, 1994).

Kaplan *et al.* (1989) applied a random-allocation design and found that the behaviour ratings of children with ADHD were better during a period of treatment with the exclusion diet than during a period on a comparison diet. The test diet excluded food additives, including colours, preservatives and monosodium glutamate (see Appendix 1), as well as chocolate- and caffeine-containing foods, and any food that families thought might affect their own child.

A community survey has suggested that the great majority of children whose parents believe them to be intolerant of foods do not show any adverse reactions when the food is given under controlled, blind challenge conditions (Amlot *et al.*, 1987). The numbers of individuals undergoing a challenge procedure were small (Fossati *et al.*, 1992) and other potentially provoking foods were not excluded while the incriminated food was being given, so that the multiple-intolerance theory was not truly tested.

An immunisation/desensitisation approach was used in one study. The authors claimed a reduced sensitivity, after using this method, when the offending food item was introduced in a subsequent challenge (Egger *et al.*, 1985). However, the methodological problems in this study are marked; in particular, the outcome measures were too weak and open to bias to sustain reliable conclusions.

There is, therefore, sufficient consistency in the findings to suggest that some commonly eaten foods, though not the same foods for all children, can induce problem behaviour in a subgroup of children with ADHD. The size of this subgroup is unknown.

However, there is a need for further prospective trials comparing the effects of dietary therapy with other treatment modalities, such as stimulant and behavioural therapy. Moreover, it is important to know how far these results can be generalised to less specialised treatment settings, because this therapy is difficult to manage and could potentially cause nutritional deficiencies and failure to thrive.

### 7.8.4 Mental illness and gluten sensitivity: schizophrenia

There has been persistent speculation in the literature that mental illnesses, especially schizophrenia, might be exacerbated or even caused by an abnormal sensitivity to gluten. One such hypothesis (Dohan, 1988) proposes genetic abnormalities (see Section 7.8.5) that would permit exorphins (the opioid peptides derived from food proteins such as gluten) to reach the cerebrospinal fluid in harmful amounts and/or to interact abnormally with brain opioid receptors, influencing dopaminergic and other neurons. Although high opioid-like activity in isolated peptides from wheat gluten hydrolysates has been reported in rat brain tissue, using techniques to determine competitive binding to opioid receptor sites, this by itself does not prove the hypothesis (Huebner *et al.*, 1984).

A number of challenge studies using gluten has been carried out in schizophrenic patients. Only one provides any support for gluten as an aetiological factor in schizophrenia (Singh & Kay, 1976, 1983); however, several randomised controlled trials have not confirmed this. The value of these randomised controlled trials is limited by the small numbers of subjects (Potkin *et al.*, 1981; Storms *et al.*, 1982), and it remains an open question as to whether there are really subgroups of patients who respond in different ways. The data suggest that sensitivity to dietary gluten is generally not characteristic of young chronic schizophrenic patients. In family members of patients with coeliac disease there seems to be a greater prevalence of mental illness, and single case reports have demonstrated a possible reduction of SPECT (single photon emission computer tomography) abnormalities in these coeliac patients on a gluten-free diet.

A double-blind controlled trial of a gluten-free versus a gluten-containing diet was carried out in 24 inpatients in a maximum security hospital. Most suffered from psychotic disorders, particularly schizophrenia. There were beneficial changes in the whole group of patients, between the pre-trial and gluten-free periods, in a number of psychotic parameters. The changes, however, were maintained during the gluten challenge period and it seemed that they could be attributed to the increased level of attention the patients received (Vlissides *et al.*, 1986).

### 7.8.5 Autism

The concept of the autistic syndrome is currently broadening and genetic influences (Auranen *et al.*, 2000; Hoh & Ott, 2000) (see Section 7.8.4), as well as effects of viral infections and bowel abnormalities, are currently under discussion as potential triggers for this syndrome (Berney, 2000). As discussed in Section 7.8.4, it has been suggested that food-derived proteins, in association with genetic abnormalities, may be implicated. A simple trial was undertaken on seven patients with infantile autism who were given a gluten-free diet; three were subsequently provoked with gluten/placebo in a double-blind study. No beneficial effects of the gluten-free diet were seen; rather, it was one more negative factor leading to further social isolation in this group of highly socially handicapped patients and families (Sponheim, 1991). In contrast, another study found evidence of an improvement of autistic symptoms in 36 children on diets in which cows' milk or other skin-test-positive foods were eliminated for 8 weeks (Lucarelli *et al.*, 1995).

### 7.8.6 Cot death (sudden infant death syndrome, SIDS)

Cot death or sudden infant death syndrome (SIDS) refers to a sudden unexpected death in infancy and remains a diagnosis by exclusion, which leaves few clues to its aetiology. The widespread search for a cause has included assessment of potential links with diet, but an association between SIDS and allergic sensitisation has not been found. For example, cot death has been linked to an allergic sensitivity to cows' milk and anaphylaxis following cows' milk consumption by some authors (Turner *et al.*, 1975; Coombs & Holgate, 1990), although the association has subsequently been rejected on the basis of the findings of a study with a larger sample size (Ford *et al.*, 1996). Postmortem examinations and estimations of tryptase, a secretory component of mast cells with a long half life (Hagan *et al.*, 1998), or the measurement of allergen-specific IgE antibody (Mirchandani *et al.*, 1984) also failed to support the allergy/anaphylaxis hypothesis. Holgate *et al.* (1994) suggested that mast cell degranulation may be occurring around the time of cot death in some cases, possibly as a result of anaphylaxis, but an alternative explanation could be the release of tryptase by an hypoxaemic stimulus (Edston *et al.*, 1999).

In general, allergy is not associated with an increased risk of cot death and a major reduction of SIDS in the UK has been achieved by educating parents to lie infants on their backs, when placing them in their cots to sleep, and to avoid overheating through the use of warm duvets, especially during periods of intercurrent illnesses (Jeffery *et al.*, 1999; Mehanni *et al.*, 1999; Sheridan, 1999; Cullen *et al.*, 2000).

## 7.9  Other clinical symptoms that may be related to adverse effects of foods

### 7.9.1  Enuresis and cystitis

Claims that enuresis in children may respond to dietary elimination of cows' milk, chocolate, citrus fruits and cola, amongst other things, have not been systematically evaluated. However, there have been case reports of eosinophilic cystitis accompanied by these features. In this disorder, the bladder mucosa has an eosinophilic infiltrate that responds to antihistamines, steroids and dietary manipulation (Littleton *et al.*, 1982).

Interstitial cystitis is a non-bacterial cystitis, which is commoner in women; it is possibly an autoimmune disorder occasionally aggravated by foods. The Interstitial Cystitis Support Group has issued nutritional advice in its publications (Interstitial Cystitis Support Group, 1998) and advises sufferers to avoid certain drinks, including alcohol, carbonated beverages and drinks containing caffeine, and foods such as all fruits (except melon and pears), all spicy foods, vinegar, tomatoes, cheese, chocolate, mayonnaise, all tree nuts (except almonds), onions and yoghurts. The relationship of this condition to eosinophilic cystitis is not clear and neither is the scientific basis for the effectiveness of the dietary advice given (Lundeberg et al. 1993; O'Leary *et al.*, 1997; Propert *et al.*, 2000). Systematic DBPCFCs are needed to demonstrate a rationale for this treatment in this condition.

### 7.9.2  Vaginitis/vaginal discharge

Egger *et al.* (1983), in their paper on headache and elimination diets, report that a proportion of the girls studied had a vaginal discharge, which resolved while they were on an elimination diet.

IgE mediated vaginal immune responses have been reported in relation to ingested substances, and it has been suggested that such substances, primarily medications but also possibly foods, could induce an allergic vaginitis in susceptible women (Witkin, 1993). Systematic studies would be needed to elucidate whether or not adverse reactions to foods or food ingredients could contribute to the pathogenesis of this not uncommon problem.

### 7.9.3  Arthropathy, arthritis

There has long been speculation that an association exists between diet and arthropathies and that relief from arthritis (probably rheumatoid) can be obtained by the use of exclusion diets (Gudzent, 1935; Lewin & Taub, 1936; Turnbull, 1944). Some of these case reports and series suggest a link between arthropathy and foods, particularly milk, other dairy products or eggs (Panush *et al.*, 1986; Golding, 1990). However, there is little unequivocal evidence of a link between diet and arthritis, perhaps because of a relative paucity of controlled studies.

There have been relatively few randomised controlled trials in this area. An exception is the study by Van de Laar and Van der Korst (1992), in which 116 patients who fulfilled at least six of the American Rheumatology Association criteria, including a positive rheumatoid factor test for the diagnosis of rheumatoid arthritis, were randomly assigned to one of the two groups. During the first 4 weeks of the study the subjects followed their normal diet, then one group received a diet which was 'allergen'-free while the other group received a diet which was allergen-restricted. No difference was seen between the clinical effects of the two diets. Nine patients, three in the allergen-restricted group, six in the allergen-free group, showed favourable responses, followed by marked exacerbation of disease during rechallenge. Dietary manipulation also induced some changes in objective measures of disease activity in these patients. Of the nine who showed signs of improvement, six rheumatoid factor positive patients participated in a further study. Placebo controlled rechallenges showed adverse reactions to specific foods in four of them. In three of these patients, biopsies of both the synovial membrane and of the proximal small intestine were carried out before and during allergen-free feeding. In two patients, both with raised total serum IgE concentrations and specific IgE antibodies to certain foods, a marked reduction in mast cell number in the synovial membrane and proximal small intestine was demonstrated (Van de Laar & Van der Korst, 1992).

From the above data it may be concluded that

food intolerance exists in a minority of patients with rheumatoid arthritis. Long term therapeutic effects are rare and dietary manipulation in the treatment of rheumatoid arthritis must still be considered experimental and should be performed as part of a DBPCFC protocol until it becomes possible to identify patients who are likely to benefit from dietary therapies.

---

### 7.10 Key points

- In an individual with an apparently strong clinical history of food intolerance, it is important to consider and prove or refute whether specific foods are really triggering factors causing ill health.
- There is good evidence that particular foods and their constituents can affect the well-being of some individuals. While there is reliable evidence in conditions such as food-induced anaphylaxis and food-induced gastrointestinal diseases such as colitis, the evidence in other conditions, such as autism, cot death and rheumatoid arthritis, is far less convincing.
- There are also a number of conditions, including asthma, migraine and irritable bowel syndrome, in which food is merely one of the factors which may be capable of triggering symptoms without necessarily playing a fundamental part in the cause of the disease.
- Well-controlled prospective studies, addressing the question of food-related triggers systematically, are rare but are clearly needed.
- The role of diet and associated factors in the pathogenesis of migraine warrants further study.
- There is no good evidence that foods play a causative role in mental disorders.
- A subgroup of children with ADHD may show signs of food-induced behavioural changes. The size of this group of affected children is unknown.

# 8
# Enzyme Defects and Food Intolerance

## 8.1 Introduction

Defects in the production of enzymes may affect the digestion and absorption of carbohydrates, fats or proteins. Sometimes these occur as inborn errors of metabolism and sometimes they can be acquired. In some situations the effects of the enzyme defect are primarily gastrointestinal, as occurs in non-congenital lactase deficiency (Section 8.3). In other cases, the enzyme defect is associated with systemic effects. Examples of inborn errors of metabolism with systemic effects are aldehyde dehydrogenase deficiency (with its associated alcohol intolerance) and the rare disorder of hereditary fructose intolerance (Section 8.9). Other inborn errors of carbohydrate metabolism that respond to life-long dietary modification include the glycogen storage diseases. Inborn errors of metabolism that involve disordered amino acid metabolism include phenylketonuria, hypertyrosinaemia and maple syrup urine disease (Scriver *et al.*, 2001). These also respond to life-long dietary modification. In addition, a variety of disorders exist that respond to vitamin therapy.

Acquired enzyme defects of the gastrointestinal tract are usually transient and often remain undiagnosed. Apart from those induced by therapeutic drugs, of which there are many, the most frequently recognised are those caused by damage to the intestinal mucosa and microvilli, usually as the result of infection. Rotavirus infections are a frequent cause of infantile diarrhoea (see Chapter 1), and although the damage that they cause is patchy, it is associated not only with poor absorption of sodium, glucose and water but also with depressed levels of lactase, maltase and sucrase

(Haffejee, 1991). The effects are usually very transient, but it has been noted that children with late (1–24 hours) vomiting or diarrhoea after cows' milk challenge have high levels of rotavirus antibodies and that, unlike those who react to cows' milk within 40 minutes, they show no evidence (in the form of a positive IgE antibody test to cows' milk) that allergy is the cause of their symptoms.

Two examples of carbohydrate-related enzyme defects are provided below. Firstly, lactose intolerance (Section 8.2), which is localised to the gastrointestinal tract, and secondly, hereditary fructose intolerance (Section 8.9) which has more generalised symptoms as the defect occurs in the liver.

## 8.2 The nature of lactose intolerance

Lactose intolerance is the most common form of carbohydrate intolerance and the main topic of this chapter. Lactose or milk sugar is a disaccharide consisting of glucose and galactose. It is found only in the milk of mammals and is the main carbohydrate found in milk and other dairy products. It cannot be absorbed without prior digestion to its component sugars, glucose and galactose. Lactase, produced in the brush border of the mucosa of the small intestine, is required for this process. Lactase is one of several disaccharidases contained in the brush border of the small intestine's epithelial cells (enterocytes). In humans, lactase activity is detectable in the fetal gut as early as 8 weeks of gestation (see Ferguson & Watret, 1988). In most mammals, lactase activity decreases after weaning but, in some human ethnic groups such as western European Caucasians, lactase activity can persist into adult life, enabling total digestion of large quantities of dietary lactose. Family studies suggest that the ability to express lactase in adult life is inherited at a single gene locus (Ferguson & Watret, 1988). Consequently, within a family, the dual inheritance of the gene for lactase absence leads to very low or absent lactase activity in homozygotes, intermediate levels result when one gene for lactase persistence is inherited and high intestinal lactase activities are present when the individual inherits two genes (*i.e.* is homozygous) for lactase persistence.

Recent studies have suggested that sequences in the lactase gene and the transcription factors that bind these sequences play a role in regulating the expression of the lactase gene (Troelsen *et al.*, 1997) but it remains uncertain whether these sequences play a role in human late onset lactase decline (Lee & Krasinski, 1998).

On rare occasions, lactase deficiency or absence can be congenital, but typically it occurs either transiently, for example after a bout of viral gastroenteritis, or in early or mid childhood in populations that experience a genetically-determined reduction in lactase secretion and activity after weaning. Maldigestion of lactose, and the associated symptoms known as lactose intolerance, results; this condition is population-specific, being particularly common in non-Caucasian populations (Section 8.4). Symptoms develop in mid-to-late childhood as a result of a progressive reduction in the amount of enzyme produced. The terms used to describe this condition can be found in Table 8.1.

## 8.3 Types of lactose intolerance

### 8.3.1 Congenital lactase deficiency

Congenital lactase deficiency is a very rare, autosomal recessive condition present from birth, in which active lactase is absent or at very low levels (Rings *et al.*, 1994). In this condition, lactase levels at birth are 0–2% of reference levels (Savilahti *et al.*, 1983). Severe symptoms may lead to advanced dehydration and neurological damage. Unless treated with a lactose-free formula with progression onto a totally lactose-free weaning diet, this condition may be fatal.

**Table 8.1** The terminology used in describing adverse reactions to lactose.

**Lactose** is the main carbohydrate in milk products, and comprises a disaccharide consisting of glucose and galactose.

**Lactase** is an enzyme located in the small intestine that hydrolyses lactose to its components: glucose and galactose. This process is necessary in order to digest lactose and subsequently absorb its component sugars.

**Lactase deficiency or lactase non-persistence** is a decreased secretion and/or activity of lactase in the small intestine.

**Lactose maldigestion** occurs as a result of lactase deficiency or non-persistence. Lactose cannot be fully hydrolysed (digested) and its component sugars absorbed, via the portal circulation, from the small intestine. Undigested lactose passes into the colon.

**Lactose intolerance** comprises adverse gastrointestinal symptoms caused by undigested lactose passing into the colon. The nature of symptoms varies widely among individuals and the likelihood of developing symptoms depends on the amount of residual lactase activity and the quantity of lactose ingested.

### 8.3.2 Late onset lactase deficiency/lactase non-persistence

Low lactase activity is a condition found normally in most adult humans and adult mammals, and is the most common carbohydrate intolerance. It is genetically inherited and presents as an age-related decrease in lactase activity, which normally becomes apparent between the ages of 5 and 20 years. It is not a condition of early childhood. The loss of lactase activity is rarely total, but decreases to 10–30% of the initial level of the enzyme activity can occur. The prevalence of lactose non-persistence increases with age within a population and nearly all affected individuals could digest lactose when they were young children (Kleinman, 1998). It is particularly common in Africans, Asians, black Americans, Greek Cypriots, Indians, Chinese and Australian aborigines (Scrimshaw & Murray, 1988; Sahi, 1994). In fact, it is estimated that as many as 70% of adults worldwide experience a decrease in their ability to produce lactase after early childhood (Section 8.4). In contrast, however, it is not common in populations of northern European descent, *e.g.* in Ireland, the UK, Scandinavia and in white North Americans, and is relatively uncommon in white Australians and New Zealanders.

### 8.3.3 Secondary lactose intolerance

Secondary lactose intolerance is caused by injury to the intestinal mucosa and is secondary to various gastrointestinal diseases and conditions, such as rotavirus infection, parasitic gastroenteritis (giardiasis), coeliac disease, cows' milk protein intolerance, immunodeficiency syndromes (*e.g.* HIV), protein-energy malnutrition, small intestinal resection and other neonatal gastrointestinal surgery (Walker-Smith, 1988). It is the villi lining the intestinal mucosa that are affected first by the type of damage caused by gastroenteritis. Lactase is particularly vulnerable, therefore, as unlike other disaccharidases most of the enzyme activity is present in the mid part of the villus and at the villus tip (Ferguson & Watret, 1988). Secondary lactose intolerance is usually transient, lasting from a few weeks to a few months, and is treated with a lactose-free diet. It is not a foregone conclusion that it will develop in children who experience gastroenteritis. In a study in London, Trounce and Walker-Smith (1985) found that only 7.5% of children admitted to hospital with gastroenteritis had lactose intolerance, and a further 8% had a monosaccharide intolerance.

## 8.4 Prevalence of lactose intolerance

Scrimshaw and Murray (1988) and Sahi (1994) have reviewed the prevalence of lactose maldigestion around the world. It is estimated that about two-thirds of the world's population shows lactase non-persistence. In South America, Africa and Asia the prevalence is above 50%, reaching almost 100% in some Asian countries, where milk is not traditionally consumed as part of the typical adult diet. In contrast, studies indicate that there is only a small decrease in lactase activity in people living in or originating from north west Europe, *e.g.* British, Irish, white Americans and Scandinavian people. For example, in the UK, Sweden, Holland, Belgium and Ireland, only 5% of the population are thought to suffer any degree of lactose maldigestion. In other European countries, the prevalence of low levels of the lactase enzyme is higher, ranging from 15 to 75%, although the exact figures are difficult to determine. In Jordan and Saudi Arabia, the prevalence of low levels of lactase activity is thought to be less than 25%. Within countries there is

considerable variation depending on genetic inheritance. For example, in the United States, the prevalence of low levels of lactase activity is 15% among whites, 53% among Mexicans and 80% among the black population. The white population of Australia and New Zealand have prevalences of 6% and 9%, respectively, but the prevalence is far higher in the Australian aboriginal population.

It has been speculated that the ability of northern Europeans to digest lactose is associated with the fact that the climate in such countries is conducive to dairy farming and consequently milk and dairy products have been part of the adult daily diet for centuries. In times of food shortage, this situation encouraged the spread in the population of a mutant gene that allowed lactase persistence after early childhood. The post-weaning drop in intestinal lactase may occur as early as 2 years of age in some races, or at 5 years in Caucasians (Ferguson & Watret, 1988; Sahi, 1994).

Ferguson *et al.* (1984) estimated the prevalence of lactose maldigestion in UK adults to be 5%. In a study conducted in Birmingham (Iqbal *et al.*, 1996), primary lactase deficiency was present in 10% of white subjects, 51% of Asians and 81% of African-Caribbeans, as determined by biopsy of the distal duodenum (the subjects were under investigation in relation to dyspepsia). However, a questionnaire revealed that lactose intake did not differ between lactase-persistent and lactase-deficient subjects, both within each racial group and between groups. Furthermore, diarrhoea, bloating and cramps were not more significantly common in lactase-deficient than lactase-persistent individuals.

It should be noted that lactase non-persistence is not synonymous with lactose intolerance because of the variation in ability to digest lactose amongst maldigesters. A number of studies have now indicated that many of those individuals with reduced levels of lactase can consume the amounts of lactose commonly present in habitual diets without experiencing symptoms (Rosado, 1997). When consuming the quantities of lactose typically encountered in habitual diets, symptoms of lactose intolerance are present in only 30–50% of lactose maldigesters (Suarez *et al.*, 1995; Vesa *et al.*, 1996a, 1997), and even this group can usually ingest smaller amounts (1–5 g) without symptoms. As a result, it has been estimated that the proportion of lactose intolerant individuals in the UK, as opposed to lactose maldigesters, is closer to 2%. Suarez *et al.* (1997), in a study in the United States, demonstrated that symptoms were trivial following ingestion of two 'cups' of milk per day (one with breakfast and one with dinner). This level of milk consumption (equivalent to 25 g of lactose, with a 'cup' providing about 250 ml of milk) is typical of the average milk intake in the USA, and about double the current average in Britain (of just over 250 ml a day).

Several recent well-controlled studies (Suarez *et al.*, 1995, 1997; Hertzler *et al.*, 1996) have shown that both lactose digesters and lactose maldigesters report experiencing symptoms after ingestion of very low lactose and lactose-free milks, which suggests that some of the symptoms experienced by lactose maldigesters are not related to lactose digestion. It has been suggested that some self-diagnosed sufferers of lactose intolerance may in fact have irritable bowel syndrome (IBS).

Because the symptoms of lactose intolerance and IBS are very similar, misdiagnosis between the conditions is common (Shaw *et al.*, 1998). In double-blind controlled studies, self-diagnosed lactose intolerant individuals were found not to suffer significantly more from intolerance symptoms when they were consuming ordinary milk containing 15 g lactose per day compared to lactose-hydrolysed milk (*i.e.* low lactose milk). Vesa *et al.* (1998) reported that although the incidence of lactose maldigestion in IBS is no more common than in the whole population, those with IBS were more likely to report subjective intolerance. Other studies have demonstrated that not all patients with suspected lactose intolerance improve with a lactose-free diet, and therefore are more likely to suffer from IBS than lactose intolerance (Shaw *et al.*, 1998). However, an individual can have lactase deficiency and also suffer from IBS, in which case the symptoms associated with lactose consumption can be aggravated.

## 8.5 Clinical features of lactose intolerance

The main symptoms of lactose intolerance include colic, abdominal distension, nausea, flatulence and abdominal pain; watery, foamy, acid stools; and failure to thrive. The symptoms vary widely amongst individuals and depend to some extent on the amount of residual lactose activity and the quantity of lactose ingested. However, it is thought that the inter-individual variability in colonic flora may to some extent account for inter-individual differences in symptoms. In lactose maldigestion, lactose passes into the colon where it is fermented by the resident bacteria, producing short chain fatty acids and gases ($CO_2$, $H_2$, $CH_4$). Gas production may result in flatulence, bloating and distension pain. Unabsorbed lactose also has an osmotic effect in the gastrointestinal tract, drawing fluid into the lumen and causing diarrhoea.

Excessive gas production and accumulation are strongly related to subjective symptoms (Hermans *et al.*, 1997), although in a study of lactose maldigesters, the reports of symptoms did not correlate with the amount of maldigested lactose or the volume or rate of gas production *per se*, but rather with altered intestinal transit rate and increased perception of luminal distension (Hammer *et al.*, 1996). Women seem more likely than men to report symptoms in response to similar amounts of maldigested lactose (Krause *et al.*, 1997).

## 8.6 Diagnosis of lactose intolerance

Useful investigations include: testing liquid stool for reducing substances, the hydrogen breath test (there is an increase in expired breath hydrogen after lactose) and the measurement of lactase activity in a jejunal biopsy specimen.

### 8.6.1 Lactose maldigestion – reducing substances in stools

In infants with diarrhoea, unabsorbed lactose can easily be detected using paper chromatography. A simple test for faecal reducing substances, using Clinitest tablets, is a useful way of testing for unabsorbed lactose in a child with diarrhoea (Ferguson & Watret, 1988). The test is regarded as positive if reducing substances are present at a concentration of 0.5% or more (1% or more in neonates), whilst the child is on a lactose-containing feed (Trounce & Walker-Smith, 1985).

### 8.6.2 Lactose maldigestion – breath test

Breath tests, being non-invasive tests, are very useful in population screening and other clinical investigations of carbohydrate digestion. The principle of the test is that normal mammalian cells do not produce hydrogen; however many bacteria, including the normal gut flora, generate hydrogen if a suitable substrate is available. Such a substrate is lactose, which would usually not reach the colon where the bacteria reside, as it would be fully digested and absorbed in the small intestine. The presence of such a substrate in the colon results in a sudden burst of metabolic activity and the production of hydrogen. The gas is absorbed into the blood and can be detected and measured as it is excreted in the breath.

### 8.6.3 Tissue lactase activity

The jejunal biopsy is the critical diagnostic investigation, but obtaining a biopsy from the correct site is important. The normal values for tissue lactase in the first and second parts of the duodenum are substantially lower than the normal reference values for the jejunum.

### 8.6.4 Other tests

Other tests include the classic lactose tolerance test, in which the profile of blood glucose, after an oral loading dose of glucose, is compared with that which follows a similar loading dose of lactose. Striking differences between the curves may be attributable to lactose maldigestion. The problem with this type of test is that it requires quantities of lactose that far exceed those typically consumed as part of a meal. Similar problems exist with the test of clinical lactose intolerance, which is based on assessment of clinical symptoms following the ingestion of a 50 g oral load of lactose (equivalent to about 1 litre of milk), compared with a similar dose of another carbohydrate. The problem lies in the fact that 10% of healthy individuals will develop gastrointestinal symptoms, dizziness, nausea and palpitation after eating 50 g of any carbohydrate as a single oral load (Ferguson & Watret, 1988). For comparison, a 200 ml glass of milk provides about 8 g of lactose.

The conventional lactose load, 50 g, used in tolerance tests, produces symptoms in 70–80% of lactose maldigesters, whereas 10–15 g of lactose, equivalent to half a pint of milk, will produce symptoms in only 30–60%.

## 8.7 Treatment of lactose intolerance

This depends on the severity of the lactose intolerance, but requires either complete or partial removal of lactose from the diet.

### 8.7.1 Secondary lactose intolerance

Treatment of secondary lactose intolerance is by temporary exclusion of lactose from the diet until the bowel has recovered lactase activity. Post-gastroenteritis lactose intolerance in infants is now thought to be less common (Trounce & Walker-Smith, 1985). This is probably due to better treatment protocols for diarrhoea management, thus reducing the severity of bouts of diarrhoea (Brown *et al.*, 1994). If, following an episode of gastroenteritis, the introduction of normal feeds causes watery diarrhoea and lactose intolerance, a return to an oral rehydration solution for 24 hours followed by a further introduction of normal feeds is usually successful (Booth, 1997). Parents should be reassured that it takes a while for diarrhoea or looseness of stools to disappear after the lactose intolerance has resolved.

Where lactose intolerance persists, a low lactose, nutritionally complete infant formula (*e.g.* SMA LF, Enfamil lactose-free, Galactomin 17 or AL10) or a lactose-free soya infant formula (Isomil, Infasoy, Wysoy, Prosobee or Farley's soya) may be given. Use of low lactose formulae will fail if lactose intolerance is secondary to cows' milk protein intolerance as such products contain whole cows' milk protein. All weaning foods should be both milk-free and lactose-free.

### 8.7.2 Late onset lactase deficiency

The tolerance of lactose is very variable, but many adults can tolerate about 12 g/day (equivalent to 250 ml of cows' milk) or more of lactose. Few people need to avoid all lactose and quickly learn how much lactose they can tolerate. For older children and adults, nutritional therapy can involve the following measures either singly or in combination:

- reducing or avoiding lactose intake,
- use of lactase derived from bacteria,
- use of lactase pre-treated dairy products.

## (i) Reducing or avoiding lactose intake

Foods that contain lactose include all mammalian milks and products made from them. In addition, use of lactose as an ingredient in the food industry is widespread because of its physiological properties, making its avoidance particularly difficult. It provides good texture, binds water and is a carrier for colour. It is also less sweet than most sugars, *e.g.* it is less than half as sweet as glucose and considerably less sweet than sucrose. It can be present in chocolate, ice cream, margarine and many manufactured foods such as sausages, breaded meats or fish, soups, crisps, puddings and sweets. Even tablets such as aspirin may contain lactose as a filler. Hard cheeses, such as Cheddar, Leicester, double Gloucester, Stilton and parmesan, and cheeses such as Edam, Brie and Camembert have a negligible lactose content and are generally well tolerated.

Several studies have demonstrated that yogurt, despite its lactose content (about 6 g/100 g in plain yogurt), is better tolerated than ordinary (unfermented) cows' milk (4.8 g/100 g) by individuals with lactose intolerance (Rosado *et al.*, 1992; Shermak *et al.*, 1995). This effect was initially assumed to be the result of the inherent β-galactosidase activity present in yogurts containing live bacteria, but the reality may not be so clear-cut. In the studies of Marteau *et al.* (1990) and Savaiano *et al.* (1984), the tolerance of heat treated yogurt, with no viable bacteria, was not significantly inferior to that of yogurt containing viable bacteria. Similarly, digestion and tolerance of lactose were equivalent after ingestion of four different fermented dairy products that collectively had a four-fold difference in their β-galactosidase activity (Vesa *et al.*, 1996b). These effects do not seem to be the result of differences in fat or lactose content (Rosado *et al.*, 1992). It has been suggested that the effects of yogurt consumption on lactose tolerance may be linked to delays in gastric emptying and a lengthening of transit time (Arrigoni *et al.*, 1994), or to changes in colonic fermentation (see below).

In principle, the symptoms of lactose intolerance are dose-dependent: the larger the amount of lactose administered, the more pronounced the symptoms are likely to be. However, the gastrointestinal symptoms caused by lactose maldigestion can vary between individuals and other factors can also affect the degree of intolerance. Slow gastric emptying and long intestinal transit time have been shown to improve lactose absorption. Therefore, for sufferers, it helps to have lactose as a part of a meal rather than between meals. The metabolic activity of colonic flora varies greatly between individuals and is thought to play an important role in the appearance or absence of intolerance symptoms, which are independent of lactase activity in the intestine. Unabsorbed lactose increases the acidity of the colon contents, potentially causing changes in the composition of the colonic bacteria and their metabolic activities. Over time, some adaptation of bacterial flora might lead to improved tolerance of lactose, despite maldigestion (see below).

Probiotics have been used in the treatment of lactose intolerance with varying degrees of success (Goldin, 1998; de Roos & Katan, 2000). A probiotic is defined as 'a live microbial feed supplement which benefits the host animal by improving its microbial balance' (Fuller, 1992). Lactobacilli produce β-galactosidase, effectively lactase, which hydrolyses the lactose in dairy products. Fermented milk, containing lactobacilli, given to lactose intolerant patients has been found to reduce breath hydrogen significantly (Kim & Gilliland, 1983). More recently, however, *Lactobacillus acidophilus* BG2FO4, a strain of lactobacilli, failed to change breath hydrogen excretion after lactose ingestion (Saltzman *et al.*, 1999). Non-fermented milk containing bacteria (*Bifidobacterium longum* B6) grown on lactose (as opposed to other substrates) also significantly reduced breath hydrogen in a study by Jiang *et al.* (1996). More work is needed before it can be judged whether there is a role for the use of probiotics *per se*, as opposed to yogurt in general, in lactose intolerance.

## (ii) Use of lactase derived from bacteria

It is possible to improve tolerance of lactose-containing foods with the use of commercial enzyme preparations, based on microbial β-galactosidase. These preparations are taken before meals or snacks, sprinkled on food or added to milk 24 hours before consumption. As glucose is sweeter than lactose, enzyme treatment imparts a slightly sweet taste to milk. This treatment is popular in the USA (DiPalma & DiPalma, 1997) and there is some evidence to support effectiveness and safety in adults (DiPalma & Collins, 1989; Lin *et al.*, 1993). These products are less popular in the UK, but can be purchased over the counter. There is as yet no evidence to support their use in infants and young children.

### (iii) Ingesting lactose-treated dairy products

Alternatively, it is possible to purchase commercially pretreated lactose-reduced milk from supermarkets and health food stores. The hydrolysis of milk is approximately 90%. It is a treatment not advocated in infants and young children. For this age group, there are few data to support the use of such products and there are plenty of alternative nutritionally complete ACBS (Advisory Committee for Borderline Substances) prescribable, low lactose formulas available.

### 8.7.3 Potential for adaptation

There is no evidence that lactase can be induced in those with lactase non-persistence. However, there have been some reports suggesting that tolerance to lactose can be developed (Johnson *et al.*, 1993; Hertzler & Savaiano, 1996; Briet *et al.*, 1997) or induced to totally unabsorbable carbohydrates such as lactulose (Florent *et al.*, 1985; Flourie *et al.*, 1993), perhaps via gradual modification of the bacterial profile present in the colon. Hertzler and Savaiano (1996) found an increase in faecal β-galactosidase activity, and improved breath hydrogen concentration and symptoms, after daily ingestion of lactose over a period of two weeks (increasing from 0.6 to 1.0 g lactose/kg per day, subdivided into three equal doses). Another suggestion is that tolerance can be induced through changed acidity in the colon brought about by unhydrolysed lactose, which reduces the rate of gas production (Perman *et al.*, 1981; Holtug *et al.*, 1992).

Adaptation has recently been reported in a carefully controlled 3-week study of African-American adolescent girls, who consumed 33 g lactose per day, as milk, with meals (Pribila *et al.*, 2000). This represented a doubling of their previous habitual intake of milk.

## 8.8 Nutritional adequacy of low lactose diets

As milk and milk products are important sources of many nutrients, such as protein, calcium and riboflavin, avoidance of dairy products is not advised without good reason, and then appropriate dietary modifications need to be made to ensure that nutrient deficiencies do not arise. For example, if alternative sources of calcium are not consumed, intake may be sufficiently low to compromise bone health.

Milk is a major source of nutrition in the diets of infants and young children, and a nutritionally adequate replacement for milk is essential. If dietary restriction is required, *e.g.* in secondary lactose intolerance, the diets of young children should routinely be supervised and assessed by a dietitian. Even in older children, if they are unable to drink adequate quantities of calcium-enriched low-lactose formula, they should take a suitable lactose-free calcium supplement.

It has been suggested that lactose maldigestion is a risk factor for developing osteoporosis, a condition characterised by low bone mass, microarchitectural deterioration of bone tissue leading to enhanced bone fragility and a consequent increase in fracture risk. A study in Italian women (Corazza *et al.*, 1995) demonstrated that both bone mineral density and calcium intake were significantly lower in women with both lactose maldigestion and intolerance (*i.e.* suffered symptoms) than in those with maldigestion alone. This finding supports other studies that have shown that women with osteoporosis have a significantly higher prevalence of lactose maldigestion and milk intolerance, and lower daily calcium intakes than age-matched controls of similar ethnic origin (see Lee & Krasinski, 1998). The prevalence of osteoporosis has been steadily increasing in recent years, even when account is taken of the fact that the average age of the population is increasing. The aetiology is multifactorial; nevertheless, the importance of achieving an adequate calcium intake in the presence of lactose maldigestion should be emphasised. Among lactose digesters, the complete avoidance of dairy products is rarely necessary, and hard cheese and yogurt are usually better tolerated than milk. Also, there is some evidence that gradual re-introduction of lactose can promote a change in the gut microflora, such that entry of lactose into the colon is better tolerated.

## 8.9 Hereditary fructose intolerance

In this rare inherited autosomal recessive condition, a deficiency exists of the liver enzyme 1,6-biphosphate aldolase, which results in accumulation of fructose-1-phosphate in liver cells. Fructose-1-phosphate acts as a competitive inhibitor of the enzyme phosphorylase, responsible for the conversion of glycogen to glucose. The result of this inhibition is hypoglycaemia. Affected babies are symptom-free while they are solely breast fed. However, once they receive infant formula or weaning foods containing fructose, they develop hypoglycaemia. They may also be jaundiced or have an enlarged liver, and progressive liver disease sometimes results. Treatment requires total elimination of fructose from the diet for life.

## 8.10 Key points

- Lactose maldigestion is the most common form of carbohydrate intolerance caused by an enzyme defect, although others do exist. Low levels of the intestinal enzyme lactase prevent the digestion of the disaccharide lactase to its component sugars (glucose and galactose) and hence lactose cannot be absorbed and passes undigested into the colon, causing a range of characteristic symptoms.
- Lactose maldigestion is uncommon in northern Europe, although it is widespread in most other parts of the world. When milk is consumed, symptoms are typically experienced to varying degrees in people of Asian, African, Jewish and Hispanic descent. Lactose maldigestion can occur after gastroenteritis, but this is also uncommon in the general population. The degree of lactose intolerance, the duration and the symptoms experienced vary widely and treatment should be individualised.
- It is essential that any treatments used for lactose intolerance are safe, nutritionally adequate, closely monitored and have been adequately tested in relevant age groups.
- Lactase levels do not seem to be inducible in those with lactase non-persistence, but there is limited evidence that gradual reintroduction can lead to greater tolerance.
- Complete avoidance of dairy products is not usually necessary. Moderating milk intake, taking milk with meals and, where possible, replacing fresh dairy products with fermented dairy products, which are usually better tolerated, might be enough to keep the intolerance symptoms under control. Hard cheeses, *e.g.* Cheddar, contain only trace amounts of lactose and so are well tolerated even by those who experience symptoms with very small amounts of lactose (2–3 g lactose/100 g food). Such strategies enable calcium intake to be maintained.
- The tolerance of yogurt is, at least in part, thought to occur because the bacteria used in its production contain an enzyme that can aid lactose digestion in the human gut.
- Lactose-reduced milks are now widely available. Commercial lactase preparations also exist, both in a liquid form to be added to milk products before consumption and as tablets to be taken before eating lactose-containing meals.
- People who are very sensitive to lactose should be aware that lactose is widely used as an ingredient in ready-made meals and other food products. Such individuals are advised to check the ingredients labels of foods for lactose and to look for other ingredients that might contain lactose as a component, such as whey powder and dried skimmed milk.

# 9
# Coeliac Disease and other Gluten Sensitive Disorders

## 9.1 Gluten

The strict chemical definition of gluten is the visco-elastic mass which remains when a wheat flour dough is washed exhaustively in tap water. The term has now been extended to include all those proteins that are deleterious to individuals with the conditions described below, *i.e.* the storage proteins of wheat, rye, barley and possibly oats. Within wheat gluten the gliadin fraction is known to be disease activating, and has been extensively studied.

## 9.2 Manifestations of gluten sensitivity

It is becoming clear that gluten sensitivity may manifest itself in a number of ways. Most experts now agree that, in genetically susceptible individuals, the immune system reacts inappropriately to dietary gluten, triggering a variety of problems. In coeliac disease the target organ is the gut, particularly the small intestine, whereas in dermatitis herpetiformis the skin is the organ primarily affected. Recently, evidence has emerged that in a few individuals the nervous system may bear the brunt of gluten sensitivity.

## 9.3 Gluten sensitive enteropathy

Coeliac disease is a permanent intolerance to dietary gluten, which manifests as gastrointestinal disease (enteropathy), affecting mainly the small intestine. The condition is triggered by the ingestion of wheat, rye, barley and traditionally oats,

although the disease activating properties of oats are now very much in doubt (see Section 9.20). The condition is characterised by malabsorption of nutrients, which is secondary to structural damage to the small intestinal mucosa. Biopsies of the small intestines of patients with untreated coeliac disease show disorganisation and stunting of the normal villous architecture, with elongation of the crypts. There is a lymphocytic infiltration of the surface epithelium and an inflammatory cell infiltrate of the lamina propria, that is the layer underneath the epithelial surface. These abnormalities revert towards normal on removal of dietary gluten.

It is now recognised that gluten sensitivity causes a spectrum of small intestinal mucosal lesions (Marsh, 1992). The type 1, infiltrative lesion, comprises a normal villous architecture. However, the epithelium contains an increased number of lymphocytes. This lesion is found in patients with dermatitis herpetiformis and reverts towards normal on removal of dietary gluten. It is often accompanied by no gastrointestinal symptoms. A proportion of relatives of patients with coeliac disease has this lesion in the absence of clinical signs of the condition.

The hyperplastic type 2 lesion has lymphocytic infiltration extending into deepened crypts. Crypt hyperplasia occurs prior to villous flattening, and not as a secondary compensatory effect, as was previously thought.

The destructive type 3 lesion is the classical flat mucosa, seen in symptomatic untreated coeliac patients. It has the typical features of a fully developed cell mediated immune response: hypertrophic crypts, lamina propria swelling and a flattening of the small intestinal villous architecture. The features of a cell mediated immune response in the small intestine are listed below (Table 9.1). These features are not specific to coeliac disease and can be seen in other conditions.

**Table 9.1** Features of an advanced cell mediated immunological inflammation in the small intestinal mucosa.

Increased microvascular permeability
Increased populations of:
  Plasma cells
  Neutrophils
  Eosinophils
  Basophils
  Mast cells
Increased secretion of inflammatory mediators/cytokines
Lymphocyte infiltration:
  Surface epithelium
  Crypt epithelium
Upregulation of MHC (major histocompatibility complex) class II expression.

Source: Marsh, 1992.

There are two further lesions at either end of the gluten sensitive enteropathy spectrum. These include a pre-infiltrative or type 0 lesion that has been identified in some patients with dermatitis herpetiformis whose small intestinal biopsies are structurally normal, but whose small intestinal mucosal secretions contain high levels of coeliac-specific antibody (Section 9.12.1). Individuals with this lesion are now known as latent coeliacs (Section 9.3.2) (Holm, 1998).

The type 0 to type 3 lesions are reversible by dietary management. However, a type 4 hypoplastic lesion is seen in some unresponsive coeliac patients and is considered to represent a failure of mucosal regeneration. This lesion occurs in those with enteropathy-associated T cell lymphoma, which complicates some cases of coeliac disease. The lesion does not respond to gluten withdrawal and the prognosis is poor.

### 9.3.1 Subclinical or silent coeliac disease

It is now recognised that the clinically apparent forms of coeliac disease may form what has become known as the tip of an iceberg, underlying which there is a much greater base of silent gluten sensi-

tivity (Catassi *et al.*, 1994; Ferguson, 1999). Silent coeliac disease occurs where there is histological evidence of enteropathy but with no clear signs or symptoms.

### 9.3.2 Latent coeliac disease

There is a subgroup of patients who have positive serological tests for gluten sensitivity (Section 9.7.2), but in whom a small bowel biopsy appears normal. The term latent coeliac disease means that a person carries the so-called markers of coeliac disease, has a normal jejunal mucosa while taking a normal gluten-containing diet, but will develop a gluten sensitive enteropathy later in life. Symptoms are rarely present while the disease is latent, and the individual is not treated with a gluten-free diet, although this policy may change in the future (Holm, 1998).

### 9.3.3 Transient gluten intolerance

The idea that coeliac disease might not be permanent in all individuals emerged in the 1960s, when it was noted that not all coeliac patients relapsed clinically when gluten was added to their diets. This led to the unfortunate misconception that 'children can grow out of coeliac disease'. However, when diagnostic criteria were tightened, it became apparent that almost all the so-called transient cases in fact showed histological relapse, when gluten was re-introduced to the diet. Today these cases would be known as silent coeliac disease (Maki, 1998). It is unfortunate that the myth of transient coeliac disease still persists. Certain alternative practitioners have been known to advise young adult coeliacs to rely on positive thought rather than a gluten-free diet. The long term consequences of this practice could be very serious (Sections 9.8.3, 9.13).

## 9.4 Dermatitis herpetiformis

This skin condition manifests as an itchy blistering rash on the knees, thighs and elbows and is diagnosed by the finding of granular IgA deposits at the dermo-epidermal junction of unaffected skin. The condition is almost always associated with a degree of gluten sensitive enteropathy, although it may be less severe than coeliac disease. The rash usually responds to the drug dapsone but can also be treated with a gluten-free diet, although dietary treatment may take up to a year to achieve results. Even though the enteropathy may be clinically silent, a gluten-free diet is advisable (reviewed by Fry, 1992).

Neurological manifestations of gluten sensitivity will be dealt with in section 9.8.4.

## 9.5 Prevalence of coeliac disease

Older literature suggests that coeliac disease has a prevalence of around 1 case in 1500 people in the UK. However, the advent of sensitive serological screening tests (Section 9.7.2) has allowed studies which suggest that the true prevalence may be higher, both in the UK (although a population-based study has yet to be conducted) and abroad (see Chapter 4, Section 4.2.1). Studies in Italy (Catassi *et al.*, 1994), the USA (Not *et al.*, 1998) and the Netherlands (Rostami *et al.*, 1999), have suggested that 1 in 300 of the general population in these countries may be gluten sensitive. For example, the Italian study included 3351 school children and found the prevalence to be 3.28 cases per 1000 children. A study from Belfast has suggested a prevalence of 1 in 120 (Johnston *et al.*, 1998). In the UK, 1000 patients who presented to their general practitioner with tiredness, bowel problems or a variety of other symptoms, were serologically screened for gluten sensitivity (Hin *et al.*, 1999). As a result, 30 patients screened positive, and coeliac disease was confirmed in all of these by small bowel biopsy (see Section 9.7.1).

The prevalence of adult coeliac disease appears to be higher in women than men (reviewed by Logan, 1992a and b). However, this may partially reflect a higher rate of diagnosis in women. For example, a woman with undiagnosed coeliac disease that has led to a subclinical deficiency of, for example, iron, might develop clinical symptoms of iron deficiency as a result of blood loss at menstruation or the nutritional stress of pregnancy; subsequent investigation might then lead to diagnosis of coeliac disease.

## 9.6 Presentation of coeliac disease

### 9.6.1 Infants and children

The presentation of coeliac disease in infants and children has been reviewed by Schmitz (1992) and Anderson (1992). The earlier the introduction of gluten to the infant diet, the shorter the delay between gluten ingestion and the onset of symptoms. The relationship appears to be related to the duration of breast feeding. The classical features of coeliac disease are usually seen in infants aged between 9 and 18 months. There is diarrhoea, failure to thrive and abdominal distension. Anorexia is common, and the infant is frequently irritable, or miserable and depressed. Weight gain is more affected than height, with muscle wasting. However, the pattern of age and mode of presentation varies from country to country, and changed in the latter part of the last century. In a multi-centre study in Europe, it was shown that there has been an overall rise in the age of diagnosis from 2 years in 1975 to 4 years in 1990 (Greco *et al.*, 1992). It is now becoming more usual for diagnosis to occur later in childhood (Maki, 1998), associated with less florid symptoms. Decreased appetite and abnormal stools may have been present for years but assumed by the child (and parents) to be normal. Constipation may be present. The child may present, via the endocrinologist, with short stature. There may be a significant number of children who are asymptomatic or display atypical symptoms such as arthritis. The nutritional consequences of coeliac disease in infancy and childhood include iron deficiency anaemia and moderate hypoproteinaemia. Some degree of osteoporosis is common but rickets is rare except in subtropical countries.

The introduction of a gluten-free diet in young children usually gives rapid and gratifying results. Behavioural disorders subside in days and appetite is restored. Weight gain is rapid and, later, height starts to catch up. Where diagnosis has been delayed until the teens, gluten exclusion may trigger a late puberty. There is seldom permanent short stature.

### 9.6.2 Adults

Diagnosis of coeliac disease may be delayed until adulthood (Cooke & Holmes, 1984; Howdle &

Lowsowsky, 1992). This may be because of a clinically silent lesion, or because symptoms such as bowel frequency may come to be accepted as normal. In some, an acute gastrointestinal infection may trigger the onset of bowel symptoms. There have been reports of individuals who have had a previously normal small bowel biopsy, later developing a lesion, leading to the suggestion that in some individuals, the condition may be latent. Adults typically complain of weight loss, diarrhoea and lassitude. However, some patients may present with a variety of symptoms resulting from the deficiency of single specific nutrients, such as folic acid or calcium, in the absence of weight loss or loose stools. Indeed some patients may be constipated and a few are obese. Findings at presentation may include osteomalacia, anaemia, neurological signs or various skin disorders. Depression and infertility may be features. Some patients may have suffered ill health for decades (Hankey & Holmes, 1994). Anti-depressants and nutrient supplements may have given transient relief, merely delaying or confusing the diagnosis. Individuals complaining of diarrhoea may be referred to a surgeon who will investigate the colon for inflammatory bowel disease and, finding no pathology, may diagnose irritable bowel syndrome. The patient may finally reach the gastroenterologist through a variety of different hospital departments. There is a great need to increase awareness amongst health professionals of the range of symptoms and the frequency of gluten sensitivity within the population.

## 9.7 Diagnosis of coeliac disease

### 9.7.1 Small intestinal biopsy

Biopsy of the small intestine is the gold standard for diagnosis of gluten sensitive enteropathy. There must be defined histological abnormalities of the small intestinal mucosa in a patient consuming a gluten-containing diet, which revert towards normal on the removal of dietary gluten. Clinical symptoms and abnormal biochemical and serological tests should normalise. If there is any doubt about the diagnosis, the patient should later be challenged with gluten. In adults it is usual to ask the patient to consume 10 g of gluten per day for 4 weeks. This is most conveniently taken as 4 slices of bread per day, or less for children. Gluten powder is available but is most unappetising in texture and appearance, and is therefore not recommended. A return of the mucosal abnormalities, following gluten challenge, confirms the diagnosis (Walker-Smith *et al.*, 1990; British Society of Gastroenterology, 1996).

Microscopy reveals that the normal finger-like characteristics of the villi, which provide the vast surface area normally available for absorption, may be lost completely (total villous atrophy) or the lesion may be partial, known as subtotal villous atrophy. The lamina propria and the epithelial layer are heavily infiltrated with inflammatory cells.

Structural measurements may be made. The normal villus height/crypt depth ratio is between 5:1 and 3:1. Coeliac disease is diagnosed when there is a villus height/crypt depth ratio of below 3:1 (Fig. 9.1).

As mentioned in Section 9.3, many individuals with gluten sensitivity may have milder lesions, so that the diagnosis may rely on the demonstration of a raised intra-epithelial lymphocyte count, in the absence of any other morphological change. However, these changes are non-specific and must be shown to be gluten dependent.

Conditions other than coeliac disease may cause destruction of the villous architecture. Table 9.2 shows some of the possible causes of abnormal villous architecture.

### 9.7.2 Serum antibody tests

Patients with coeliac disease and dermatitis herpetiformis have raised serum anti-gliadin antibodies, as do individuals with other conditions including Crohn's disease. Measurement of anti-gliadin antibody, while still considered to give some information (British Society of Gastroenterology, 1996), is being superseded by more specific tests. Individuals with untreated coeliac disease display serum antibodies to components of connective tissue, such as reticulin and endomysium. The smooth muscle bundles of monkey oesophagus or human umbilical cord contain typical endomysial connective tissue surrounding the muscle cells. By incubating the serum from a patient, with untreated coeliac disease, on sections of oesophagus or umbilical cord, the anti-endomysial antibody present in the serum

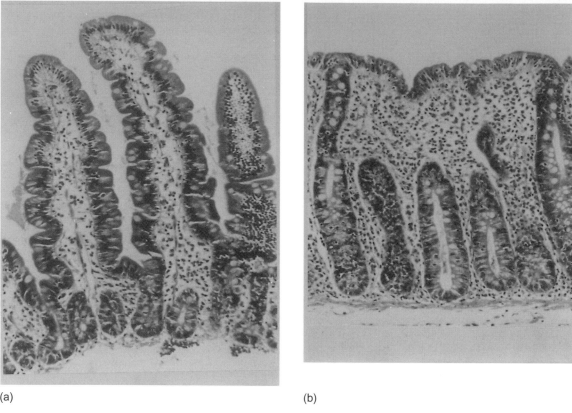

(a)                                                        (b)

**Fig. 9.1**   Photomicrograph showing (a) normal small bowel mucosa and (b) the classic flat lesion of untreated coeliac disease, × 400 magnification.

is allowed to react with the exposed antigen. By using a fluoresceinated secondary antibody, the pattern of staining of the serum antibodies around the smooth muscle cells can be seen. It is now recognised that, within the endomysial tissue, the target antigen is the enzyme tissue transglutaminase (tTG) (Dieterich *et al.*, 1997). This has allowed the development of a simple and cheap enzyme-linked immunosorbant assay (ELISA) for IgA-tTG (Sulkanen *et al.*, 1998).

It is important to note that the reliability of screening tests is highly dependent upon the competency of laboratories performing them (see Ellis *et al.*, 2001 for a review). There is, at present, no standardised procedure for any of the coeliac serological tests. The EMRC/ESPGHAN Working Group 'Serological Screening For Coeliac Disease'

has defined robust non-commercial test protocols for IgG and IgA anti-gliadin (AGA), IgA anti-endomysial (AEA) and IgA-tTG antibodies. These protocols have been used by several laboratories and the overall sensitivities and specificities have been reported (Stern, 2000), as shown in Table 9.3.

The IgA-tTG ELISA should prove invaluable in population and family screening. Testing of all children through GP surgeries could lead to early diagnosis and treatment. At least 1 in 50 patients with coeliac disease have selective IgA deficiency (Cataldo *et al.*, 1998), so these serological tests will never have 100% sensitivity. Individuals with a family history or symptoms suggestive of gluten sensitivity should be screened additionally for IgA deficiency. Those who are found to be IgA deficient

**Table 9.2** Causes of an abnormal small intestinal mucosa.

Coeliac disease, including:
  Non-responsive coeliac disease (refractory or collagenous sprue)
  Complications of coeliac disease (ulceration, malignancy)
Cows' milk protein intolerance
Soya protein intolerance
Immunodeficiency syndromes
Eosinophilic gastroenteropathy
Mediterranean lymphoma
Protein-energy malnutrition
Intractable diarrhoea of infancy
Gastroenteritis in children
Infections:
  Parasites, for example giardia
  Human immunodeficiency virus
Small bowel bacterial overgrowth syndrome
Whipples disease
Tropical sprue
Arterial disease of the small intestine
Drug and radiation damage
Zollinger-Ellison syndrome

Source: Howdle & Lowsowsky, 1992.

in the presence of normal IgG levels should be considered for jejunal biopsy. Measurement of IgG$_1$ AEA may prove useful in these cases (Cataldo *et al.*, 2000).

The results of serological tests for gliadin, endomysium and tTG rapidly revert towards normal on removal of gluten from the diet, suggesting that these antibodies are not primary to the pathogenesis of coeliac disease, but rather are by-stander phenomena (Sollid *et al.*, 1997). Patients who embark upon a gluten-free diet prior to thorough investigation by a gastroenterologist risk misdiagnosis or a lengthy diagnostic process.

## 9.8 Disease associations

### 9.8.1 Dermatitis herpetiformis

This condition is strongly associated with coeliac disease and has already been considered in Section 9.4.

### 9.8.2 Type I (insulin dependent) diabetes and other autoimmune disorders

Type I diabetes affects 10% of patients with coeliac disease. There are weaker associations with other conditions, such as autoimmune thyroid disease and primary biliary cirrhosis. Co-existing coeliac disease should be suspected in patients with these conditions who display symptoms suggestive of malabsorption. A recent report suggests that the prevalence of associated autoimmune disorders in coeliac disease increases significantly with age at diagnosis (Ventura *et al.*, 1999). In those individuals diagnosed before the age of 2 years, the prevalence of autoimmune disease was significantly lower, particularly if the subjects were not given a gluten challenge as part of their diagnostic process.

### 9.8.3 Malignancy

Perhaps the most worrying disease association with coeliac disease is malignancy, particularly the so-called enteropathy associated lymphoma (EAL) (reviewed by Holmes & Thompson, 1992; Holmes, 1998) but also other cancers. Patients with coeliac disease appear to be at greatly increased risk of developing small bowel lymphoma, compared to the normal population. The precise frequency of malignancy associated with gluten intolerance is unknown, and appears to vary amongst different

**Table 9.3** Sensitivities and specificities for IgG and IgA anti-gliadin (AGA), IgA anti-endomysial antibody (AEA) and IgA-tTG antibody.

|                 | IgA-AGA | IgG-AGA | IgA-AEA | IgA-tTG |
|-----------------|---------|---------|---------|---------|
| Sensitivity (%) | 83      | 86      | 90      | 93      |
| Specificity (%) | 82      | 76      | 99      | 95      |

Source: Stern, 2000.
*Note:* The sensitivity means the number of cases that would be detected out of 100 individuals with the disease. The specificity means, out of 100 people testing positive, the number that would actually have the disease.

populations. In one study, 210 coeliac patients, who had attended Birmingham General Hospital over a number of years, were studied at the end of 1974. There had been 21 deaths from malignancy, where the expected number would have been 5, and 13 of these were due to lymphoma when the expected frequency for the general population would be 0.1. When the surviving members of the series of patients were reviewed at the end of 1985, it was demonstrated that those who had taken a strict gluten-free diet for a least 5 years had no greater risk of developing cancer than the general population.

Enteropathy associated lymphoma appears to be T cell in origin (Isaacson *et al.*, 1985), suggesting that chronic stimulation of gluten sensitive T cells has progressed to malignant change. Some individuals may first present with EAL, having no previous diagnosis of coeliac disease. Whether these individuals have harboured a clinically silent lesion or have ignored mild symptoms is unknown. It does again underline the importance of detection of all cases of gluten sensitivity at an early stage. Once gluten sensitivity is diagnosed, a strict gluten-free diet is the best insurance against malignancy. Greater awareness of the situation should help to reduce the incidence of malignancy in the future.

### 9.8.4 Neurological disorders

Patients with coeliac disease may suffer from any of a large number of neurological or psychiatric disorders (Cooke & Holmes, 1984). Some of these are associated with nutrient deficiencies, others do not appear to be.

Recent reports (Hadjivassilou *et al.*, 1999) have shown that there is a very large excess of positive anti-gliadin antibodies in patients with neurological disorders of unknown origin, which may or may not be associated with a finding of enteropathy on biopsy. The authors suggest that there may be a distinct subgroup of patients with gluten sensitivity, where the brunt of the disease is borne by the cerebellum or peripheral nerves. They suggest routine screening for anti-gliadin antibodies in neurology clinics.

Anecdotal accounts of treatment of multiple sclerosis with a gluten-free diet have existed for many years. In fact there is little evidence to support such treatment. Small bowel biopsies from

11 patients with multiple sclerosis, consuming a normal gluten-containing diet, were identical to those of control subjects without the disease (Bateson *et al.*, 1979). Another series of 14 patients showed no morphological or biochemical changes to the small bowel consistent with gluten sensitivity (Jones *et al.*, 1979). Only 1 of 36 patients with multiple sclerosis had detectable serum anti-gluten antibody, and this was of low titre (Hunter *et al.*, 1984). These and other authors (Hewson, 1984) find no evidence to support the role of a gluten-free diet in treatment of multiple sclerosis.

One might speculate that some patients, misdiagnosed as suffering from multiple sclerosis, may in fact have been suffering from a neurological deficit secondary to nutritional deficiency caused by coeliac disease. Alternatively, some individuals may have belonged to the subgroup described by Hadjivassilou *et al.* (1999), in whom gluten had induced peripheral neuropathy or cerebellar ataxia. In either situation, instigation of a gluten-free diet may resolve the neurological deficit. Cases of this sort may have given rise to anecdotal accounts of the value of a gluten-free diet in the treatment of multiple sclerosis.

The possibility that there might be a connection between gluten sensitivity and autism has attracted some interest. Eight autistic patients with fat malabsorption and alleged behavioural improvement on gluten restriction were given ordinary diets and 20 g per day of gluten for 4 weeks. There was no change in bowel habit, and no histological abnormalities were detected in small bowel biopsies (McCarthy & Coleman, 1979). Pavone *et al.* (1997) assessed 120 coeliac patients for signs of autism, using standard procedures; no child tested positive. These authors also studied 11 patients with infantile autism who were shown not to have antibody profiles consistent with coeliac disease. Thus the small amount of scientific literature available does not support a connection between autism and coeliac disease *per se*.

However, anecdotally parents report that children diagnosed with autism show dramatic improvement in behaviour within days when placed on a wheat- and dairy-free diet. The explanation offered in a popular magazine covering this story was that food peptides, which have opiate properties, are addictive, interfere with brain neurotransmitters and leak into the circulation. There are, indeed, studies in high quality journals to suggest that both gluten and casein peptides, released during normal digestion, may have opiate qualities (Zioudrou *et al.*, 1979; Fukudome *et al.*, 1997). A study of 21 autistic children, who had no clinical findings consistent with known intestinal disorders, demonstrated that 43% had altered intestinal permeability. The authors postulated that this might be a possible mechanism for increased passage through the gut mucosa of peptides derived from foods (D'Eufemia *et al.*, 1996). Unfortunately there is little in the literature to either confirm or refute the role of diet-derived opiate peptides in autism, making informed comment difficult. Gillberg (1995), reviewing the literature, found there was insufficient evidence to suggest the use of opiate antagonists in the treatment of autism.

Dietary intervention studies have given equivocal results. A single autistic child (O'Banion *et al.*, 1978) was shown to have deterioration in behaviour in response to a number of food substances, including wheat, dairy products and sugar. It is unlikely that sugar could have opiate properties. In a study in Italy (Lucarelli *et al.*, 1995), 36 patients with autism were given diets which eliminated milk products and the patients showed a marked improvement in behaviour. On the other hand, in another study of 7 autistic patients given a gluten-free diet with double blind gluten/placebo challenge (Sponheim, 1991), there was no connection between gluten ingestion and behaviour. If anything, the rigours of the diet led merely to further social isolation of the patients and their families. Autism is a spectrum of disorders, there may only be subsets of sufferers who respond to specific dietary interventions. It is clear that carefully controlled behavioural studies using larger numbers of cases are needed in order to clarify this issue. Only after such studies will health professionals be able to give informed advice to anxious parents.

For information on research into autism and diet contact the Autism Research Unit, University of Sunderland at www.autism99.org.com.

### 9.8.5 Down's syndrome

Down's syndrome patients have a far greater prevalence of coeliac disease than the general population. The reason for this is unknown. Down's syndrome is characterised by the presence of three copies of chromosome 21; however, no association has been found between chromosome 21 and coeliac disease (Morris *et al.*, 2000).

### 9.8.6 Epilepsy

Epilepsy appears to be associated with coeliac disease. In one recent study, 1 in 44 patients attending a seizure clinic was found to have previously undiagnosed coeliac disease (Cronin *et al.*, 1998).

## 9.9 Genetics

The precise mode of inheritance of coeliac disease is unknown (Tighe & Ciclitira, 1995). At least 10% of first degree relatives of affected individuals also suffer from the condition; use of reliable screening tests may reveal higher figures. There are conflicting reports of concordance among monozygotic twins with proportions ranging from 70 to 100% (it should be noted that some early reports failed to show that the twins were definitely identical).

In the UK, 95% of coeliac and dermatitis herpetiformis patients possess the human leucocyte antigen (HLA) class II DR3, DQ2 haplotype. It is now known that it is the DQ2 molecule that is associated with gluten sensitivity and that a common allele, rather than a rare mutant, confers susceptibility (Brett *et al.*, 1999).

Since HLA (also known as MHC) molecules are responsible for presenting antigens to the immune system (Chapter 2, Section 2.4.4), the hypothesis evolved that DQ2 allows gliadin peptides to be presented to the immune system, leading to damage to the host tissue. Moreover DQ2, but not DR3, binds a peptide that has been shown to be disease-activating in coeliac small intestine (Johansen *et al.*, 1996; Shidrawi *et al.*, 1998).

Of the UK population, 25–30% have the DQ2 molecule, but only a tiny proportion of these individuals are gluten sensitive. In fact HLA class II appears to contribute only 30% to the total genetic susceptibility. In an attempt to identify other susceptibility loci, genome wide searches are currently being undertaken by a number of groups. No definite answer is likely to be available for some time (King *et al.*, 2000).

and carboxypeptidases, which cleave at various sites. It is, therefore, unlikely that deficiency of a single peptidase could result in the accumulation of a toxic product (Peters & Bjarnason, 1984). This theory has received little attention recently.

## 9.13 Treatment

Coeliac disease is treated with a gluten-free diet, with total exclusion of wheat, rye, barley (and possibly oats) (Section 9.20). The clinical symptoms of the condition should quickly revert toward normal. A study of patients who received a gluten-free diet for 2 years showed a significant increase in body weight, fat mass and bone mass (Smecuol *et al.*, 1997). Similarly, children treated with a gluten-free diet for one year showed an almost total return to normal body composition (Rea *et al.*, 1996). However, for patients not diagnosed until after the third decade (the normal period for achieving maximum bone density), peak bone mass is never achieved, and subsequent physiological decline may cause a rapid progression of osteoporosis. Therefore, some authors suggest that the existence of osteoporosis be actively sought in all coeliac disease patients, using bone mineral densitometery (Weaver & Robertson, 1999).

The British Society of Gastroenterology (1996) has produced guidelines for the treatment of coeliac disease. The commonest nutritional deficiencies found at the time of diagnosis are of iron, folic acid, calcium and vitamin $B_{12}$. These should resolve spontaneously on instigation of a gluten-free diet, but dietary supplementation is considered reasonable, especially in severe cases. There is some evidence that there may be a permanent derangement of vitamin $B_6$ metabolism in some coeliac disease patients, even on a gluten-free diet (Cooke & Holmes, 1984).

Strict life long adherence to a gluten-free diet, which may include wheat starch, abrogates the risk of malignancy (Section 9.8.3) which exists in patients who take a partial or 'gluten-reduced' diet (Holmes & Thompson, 1992).

Cereal proteins are frequently used as binders and extenders in a wide variety of manufactured foods. Lists of ingredients may not always make this clear. For example 'hydrolysed vegetable protein' or 'modified starch' might well mean gluten or wheat flour. Patients with coeliac disease must be wary of all processed foods, unless specifically told that they are gluten-free.

A large number of processed gluten-free products, such as bread, biscuits, cakes and pasta, are now available commercially for coeliac patients; some are available on prescription for those with a definite diagnosis of coeliac disease. Some of these products are based on 'naturally gluten-free' cereals, such as rice and maize, or on non-grass plants such as potato, soya or buckwheat. However, the baking qualities of these substances are poor and the resultant product may be unpalatable. Therefore, many manufacturers rely on 'rendered gluten-free' wheat starches. These are prepared by washing flour so that the water-insoluble gluten is removed and only the starch remains. In practice, some gluten proteins are partially water-soluble, and some will inevitably remain to contaminate wheat starch (Skerritt & Hill, 1992).

The clinical significance of the trace quantities of gluten remaining in 'gluten-free' products based on wheat starch is unclear, since individual responsiveness and relapse rates with small amounts of gluten vary considerably. A recent Scandinavian study suggested that regular use of wheat starch containing products over a number of years was not deleterious to health (Kaukinen *et al.*, 1999).

The UK Coeliac Society liases with food manufacturers to produce a regularly updated list of foods, which do not contain gluten as an ingredient; however, unless the product is labelled as gluten-free, it need not conform to the regulations cited in Section 9.15.

## 9.14 Compliance with a gluten-free diet

As more information emerges, and a greater choice of gluten-free manufactured food is available, it becomes easier to select a nutritious and palatable gluten-free diet. Manufacturers need to be aware that gluten sensitivity occurs amongst many racial groups, all of whom require gluten-free fare to suit their different cultural requirements.

Mothers of young children may find it difficult to control what goes on at school or at children's parties. There is a need to keep all those who come into contact with the child informed, without causing social isolation to the young patient. The UK Coeliac Society and dietitians can help with these issues.

When adolescence is reached it becomes almost impossible to monitor food and drink intake. It is not uncommon for teenagers to drop the gluten-free diet. A study of Italian coeliac adolescents showed that almost half consumed gluten-containing foods. Those who consumed a strict gluten-free diet were making poor food choices, and consuming large amounts of fat rather than carbohydrate, and were thus more likely to be overweight and have low intakes of fibre, iron and calcium (Mariani *et al.*, 1998).

A proportion of patients fail to respond to a gluten-free diet (O'Mahony *et al.*, 1996), the commonest cause being voluntary or inadvertent gluten ingestion. If thorough investigation of the diet eliminates this as a cause, there is a need to consider other food intolerances, for example milk or soya, pancreatic insufficiency or lymphoma.

## 9.15 Legislation relating to gluten-free food

Legislation relating to gluten-free foods has been reviewed by Janssen (1998). The WHO/FAO Codex Alimentarius Commission sets standards for European food legislation. Any food claiming to be gluten-free must contain no more than 0.3% protein derived from wheat, rye, barley or oats, as measured by Kjeldahl nitrogen (Codex Alimentarius Commission, 1981). This may represent from 10 to 30 mg gliadin/100 g (Hill & Skerritt, 1990; Skerritt & Hill, 1992). Measurement of Kjeldahl nitrogen does not discriminate between the coeliac-activating gluten protein and other wheat proteins, which include albumins, globulins and non-gluten starch granule proteins.

Many manufacturers of gluten-free foods also make foods for other special dietary requirements, so their factories are not necessarily gluten-free. In addition to the technical difficulties in producing high quality wheat starch that is free of gluten, there is the potential for contamination during preparation and processing of gluten-free foods (Ellis *et al.*, 1998a).

There have been moves recently to restrict further the amount of residual gluten allowed in nominally gluten-free foods, and to alter the method by which it is measured. The proposed new Codex Standard suggests a tiered definition of gluten-free: an upper limit of 10 mg gliadin/100 g

product (200 ppm gluten) for 'rendered gluten-free' products and 1 mg gliadin/100 g (20 ppm gluten) for naturally gluten-free substances (Codex Alimentarius Commission, 1998).

## 9.16 The cereals: taxonomy and chemistry

The taxonomy and chemistry of cereals has been reviewed by Shewry *et al.* (1992). The cereals are members of the grass family or *Gramineae* (see Fig. 9.2). Wheat, rye and barley are closely related, whilst oats are more distant. The major tropical cereals, maize, millet and sorghum, belong to a different subfamily.

Bread wheat, *Triticum aestivum*, has three genomes, each with seven pairs of chromosomes. Durum wheats (pasta) have two genomes. These genomes encode separate but related proteins. As a result there are large numbers of very similar but not identical storage proteins, which constitute gluten.

### 9.16.1 Definition of prolamins

The prolamin storage proteins of the main food cereals account for approximately 40% of the protein content of the seeds except for oats and rice, which have a prolamin content of approximately 5–10%. Figure 9.3 shows how the prolamins were defined originally, on the basis of their solubility, by Osbourne (1907).

Wheat gluten is the cohesive visco-elastic mass that remains after dough is washed exhaustively in tap water, the low salt concentration of which facilitates removal of not only the starch granules, but also the albumins and globulins. Gluten can be further subdivided into those proteins that are soluble in dilute ethanol solution, termed prolamins, and those that are not, the glutelins. For wheat, these groups of proteins have been given the trivial names gliadins and glutenins. The alcohol soluble prolamins in other cereals have been named as follows: barley – hordeins; rye – secalins; maize – zeins; sorghum – kafirins; millet – kafirins; oats – avenins; rice – oryzins.

The amino acid compositions of the alcohol soluble prolamins are unusual, being high in glutamine and proline, which together account for between 30 and 70% of the total. It is now understood that a considerable proportion of cereal seed proteins, which have related or similar amino acid

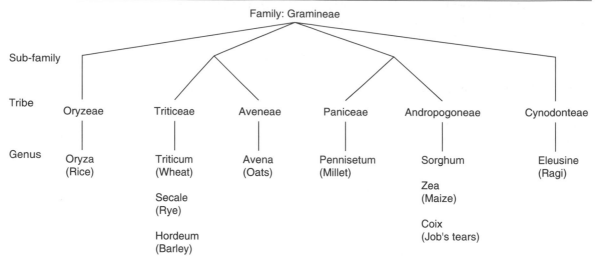

**Fig. 9.2** The taxonomy of the *Gramineae* (source: Shewry *et al.*, 1992).

compositions to the alcohol soluble proteins, are themselves insoluble in aqueous alcohol as a result of the formation of interchain disulphide bonds. The resultant high molecular weight proteins present in wheat are known as glutenins. Once these disulphide links are reduced the monomers are soluble in alcohol/water mixtures.

In wheat, about 80% of the protein is gluten, of which 40% is gliadin and 40% glutenins. The

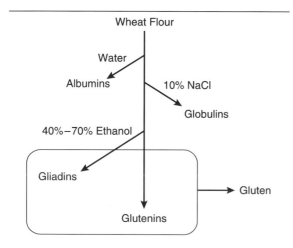

**Fig. 9.3** The Osborne classification of wheat proteins (source: Osbourne, 1907).

remainder of the protein comprises albumins, globulins and starch granule proteins.

Wheat glutenins are very important because their polymeric structure and elastic nature act together to trap carbon dioxide released by yeast during leavening of dough, giving bread wheat its characteristic baking qualities.

## 9.17 Methods for assessing suitability of cereal proteins for gluten sensitive individuals

### 9.17.1 *In vivo* gluten challenge

The *in vivo* gluten challenge remains the gold standard for assessment. Before any protein or peptide can be claimed to be either disease activating or safe for coeliac patients, feeding experiments must be performed in several volunteer patients, with small intestinal biopsies prior to and at least one time point after the challenge. Morphometric analyses of the biopsies will finally prove the safety or otherwise of a given cereal protein or peptide (Ciclitira *et al.*, 1984; Sturgess *et al.*, 1994).

### 9.17.2 *In vitro* tissue culture

This technique involves the culturing of coeliac jejunal biopsy specimens in the presence or absence of gluten protein and peptide, followed by histological assessment. Results analogous to the *in vivo* gluten challenge have been obtained (Shidrawi *et al.*, 1995).

### 9.17.3 Tests based on non-human tissue

There is no animal model for coeliac disease; however, some groups have utilised the more undifferentiated tissues of the non-human fetal gut to provide material that appears to be in some ways susceptible to damage by gluten. There is no evidence that the effect of gluten on these tissues has anything to do with coeliac disease pathogenesis. Results should be viewed with great caution.

## 9.18  Which cereals contain gluten?

The cereals that contain gluten are wheat, which includes bread wheat, pasta or durum wheat, and spelt (*Triticum Spelta* — ancient or wild wheat); rye; barley; and triticale (a hardy hybrid of wheat and rye).

Although gluten is an endosperm (flour) protein, other fractions of these cereals become heavily contaminated with flour during milling so that, for example, wheat germ and bran or husk are not acceptable in a gluten-free diet. Wheat starch, if specially prepared to legal standards, is acceptable in a gluten-free diet. Spelt, durum, emmer and einkorn wheats have as much gliadin as bread wheat and must be avoided by coeliac patients (Wieser, 1998). Spelt has been marketed in the USA as 'safe for coeliacs and those with gluten allergy'. Scurrilous companies have attempted to bring this cereal into the UK accompanied by such claims. Other bizarre claims have included the assertion that Russian rye bread is 'safe for coeliacs because it is organic'! This quote appeared courtesy of a food writer in the *Financial Times*, and serves to illustrate the level of confusion that exists (Davenport, 1996).

## 9.19  Which cereals are gluten-free?

Gluten-free cereals include rice, millet, maize and sorghum. Other flour products that are gluten-free are buckwheat; flours made from legumes, *e.g.* garam from chick peas and soya flour; and potato flour.

## 9.20  What about oats?

While substantial evidence implicates wheat, rye and barley in coeliac disease, controversy exists over the toxicity of oat prolamins (Shewry *et al.*, 1992). Several recent studies suggest that quantities of oats of up to 50 g/day are harmless to the majority of gluten-sensitive individuals (Janthuinen *et al.*, 1995). However, these studies excluded 'severe coeliacs' and children. The UK Coeliac Society has produced a discussion document which is available to all interested professionals. In essence, they recommend that most adult coeliacs may consume reasonable quantities of oats. Preliminary studies in children now suggest that they may also safely consume oats, although further confirmation is required (Hoffenberg *et al.*, 2000). Care should be taken to purchase oats destined for coeliac patients from a dedicated oats miller, as contamination with wheat during harvesting, storage and milling is a strong possibility.

## 9.21  Other problematic substances

### 9.21.1 Malt, malt extract, beer and lager

Other substances that contain gluten, and so may be potentially problematic, include malt, malt extract, malt flavouring, beer and lager.

The toxicity to coeliac patients of partial hydrolysates of wheat gluten is well established (Shewry *et al.*, 1992). Confusion exists as to whether foods based on malted barley are suitable for patients with coeliac disease. Malting enzymes do not completely break down barley gluten (Ellis *et al.*, 1990) and the residual partial hydrolysates contain gliadin-like epitopes (Ellis *et al.*, 1994). Both malt and beer contain measurable quantities of hordein, which is difficult to measure and therefore likely to be underdetected. Malt extract, the water soluble fraction of malt, is frequently used as a flavouring agent, *e.g.* in some breakfast cereals. Enzymic partial hydrolysis renders prolamins highly water soluble and so they are likely to be present in malt extract. A major manufacturer provided the malt extract used to flavour cornflakes, for analysis. This contained 1.9 g barley hordein/100 g (Ellis *et al.*, 1998b) and the cornflakes themselves contained 16 mg hordein/100 g, which is above the acceptable level for individuals intolerant to gluten. It must be stressed that cornflakes are not marketed as gluten-free and malt extract is clearly stated as an ingredient. However, until recently this product was included in the UK Coeliac Society's gluten-free list and is consumed in large quantities by many coeliac patients as a palatable and convenient carbohydrate snack. Anyone treating a patient who is not responding well to an apparently strict gluten-free diet should enquire carefully about the use of breakfast cereals, many of which contain malt extract.

### 9.21.2 Communion wafers

Communion wafers are made of wheat and there have been isolated reports of problems associated with their consumption by coeliac patients. Gluten-free wafers based on wheat starch are available, but are not considered appropriate by some sections of the Church. Patients need to be aware of the potential risk so that they can make their own decisions on this issue.

### 9.21.3 Glutenins

These proteins, which provide the baking qualities of wheat, have traditionally been regarded as non-disease-activating in coeliac patients, although evidence is sparse. The high molecular weight subunits have sequences unrelated to gliadin and may well prove not to be disease activating. The low molecular weight subunits of wheat glutenins have similarities to some gliadins and, therefore, coeliac toxicity of the former must be considered a possibility, until further experiments are performed.

## 9.22 Methods of measurement of gluten in foods

A recent meeting of the relevant Codex Committee concluded that there remains no acceptable way of measuring gluten, so it is not possible to formulate new legislation (Codex Alimentarius Commission, 1998). Additionally, the controversy over oats made it difficult to agree exactly what the specificity of the proposed assay should be.

Therefore, there is a need for a sensitive assay, which can measure levels as low as 1–2 mg gliadin/100 g without spurious cross-reactivities with non-gluten-containing cereals, such as maize. Such an assay should be capable of detecting the prolamins of rye, barley (and possibly oats). A major difficulty in achieving this aim has been the lack of a gold standard, since the precise nature of the epitope(s) that exacerbates coeliac disease is unknown. There are varying degrees of cross-reactivity between the prolamins of wheat, rye, barley (and oats), all of which may exacerbate coeliac disease. This makes measurement and detection of prolamins from the other coeliac-activating cereals, using antibodies raised against wheat, difficult. Conversely, non-disease activating cereals, such as maize, contain prolamins that can, in some cases, cross-react with antibodies raised against wheat gliadin.

There are numerous methods available in the literature for measurement of gluten. However, they are either too specific to gliadin, and therefore do not detect all relevant prolamins, or they are not sufficiently specific and therefore give spurious cross-reactivities with, for example, maize or are unsuitable for use with cooked foods.

The use of monoclonal antibodies to target known toxic epitopes may lead to assays that are very sensitive to that particular amino acid sequence (Ellis *et al.*, 1998a), but the assay may be too specific and miss other important, but as yet unidentified, toxic sequences. Further, whole unfractionated wheat gliadin used as the standard (in any assay system) may not reflect the balance of residual proteins left after washing of wheat starch.

Papers have reported the use of two commercial kits based on a monoclonal antibody raised against ω-gliadin (see Chapter 9, Appendix A), for the measurement of gluten in foods, for use either in the home or in the laboratory (Skerritt & Hill, 1991a, b). This subfraction is heat stable, rendering the assays suitable for use with cooked or processed foods. Omega-gliadins, having no sulphur-containing amino acid, do not form insoluble complexes during cooking and are therefore the only fraction that can be extracted and measured. Any method based on the measurement of, say, α-gliadins will give very low and unrealistic results in cooked foods (Ellis *et al.*, 1998a). However, the ω-gliadins are the minor component of the gliadins and represent between 6 and 20% of the total gliadin, depending on the species; thus the predicted error associated with measuring this fraction is −44% to +80% (Wieser *et al.*, 1994).

A recent publication has shown that sophisticated mass spectrometry can be used to detect and quantify cereal proteins. The technique can distinguish between the proteins of many different cereals. Using this method it has been shown that the kits based on ω-gliadins, mentioned above, have a number of problems. Thus, a product with a mass spectrometry pattern showing only rice, appeared to be grossly contaminated by wheat gluten when measured by a kit based on ω-gliadins. Furthermore, at least two versions of the kit, based on the same antibody, are available from different companies. These have given measurements for wheat gluten that differed by a factor of 50 for the same product, which mass spectrometry had shown to contain only rice (Sorell *et al.*, 1998). Mass spectrometry seems to offer a very promising way of checking the results produced by other methods; however, it is expensive and specialised and therefore not appropriate for routine on-line quality control. The hunt for a simple and reliable method continues.

## 9.23  The gluten-free diet and new technologies

Patients must avoid all products containing wheat, rye, barley (and oats) and their products. Great care must be taken with all manufactured foods. With advancements in food technology have come new perils for coeliac patients. Manufacturers have attempted to use gluten as a cheap coating for apples to make them shine. A biodegradable cling film has been developed that is based on gluten! There have even been moves to replace the traditional wax coatings on Edam cheese with a coating based on gluten. The Association of European Coeliac Societies is closely monitoring such developments and lobbying governments and manufacturers. The recent outcry over genetically modified foods has had the unfortunate consequence of panicking some manufacturers into not using maize or soya as fillers and extenders, because they cannot guarantee that they contain non-genetically modified material. Many are turning to wheat for this purpose, so that the list of gluten-free foods may become shorter, further limiting patient choice.

In contrast, technology used to genetically modify organisms may be helpful to coeliac disease patients. A 10-year multi-centre project is now underway with the objective of producing a cereal with the baking and nutritional value of wheat, which is not harmful to coeliacs. A leading coeliac specialist based in London will be involved at all stages of the project in ascertaining the safety of any product produced.

## 9.24  Does the possibility of immune therapy for coeliac disease exist?

It has been shown, for other T cell driven conditions, that the disease process might be modulated by altering the target antigen. For example, in the mouse model of multiple sclerosis, single point amino acid substitutions in myelin basic protein peptide antigens can downregulate the production of inflammatory cytokines by T cells, leading not only to a halt in the disease process but, in some instances, to the reversal of sclerotic change. Coeliac disease is another example where the target antigen is known so that such therapy might be possible in due course (see Chapter 13).

## 9.25  Conclusion

Gluten sensitivity is relatively common, with a number of manifestations. It has become apparent that there is a large amount of undetected gluten intolerance, which if left untreated can lead to unnecessary morbidity and mortality. There is now a simple, inexpensive and reliable serological screening method, and evidence exists to suggest that early post weaning screening and diagnosis may be advantageous. The gluten-free diet has received much attention and is now well defined, with legislation in place to protect consumers. Routine screening for gluten sensitivity, through general practitioner surgeries, of all infants at 18 months could prove both highly cost effective and of great benefit to many individuals.

It must be remembered that wheat forms a very important part of the diet, providing a cheap and important source of a number of nutrients. The vast majority of the population can only gain from the inclusion of bread in the diet and must not be discouraged from continuing to benefit.

## 9.26 Key points

- It is now recognised that gluten sensitivity may cause a variety of conditions affecting the skin, the gut and possibly in some cases, the nervous system.
- Where the gut is the main organ affected, the condition is known as coeliac disease. This is a permanent condition, requiring a life-long strict gluten-free diet.
- Ingestion of gluten activates T cells in the small bowel, which initiate an immune reaction resulting in release of inflammatory mediators, particularly interferon-$\gamma$. This causes damage to the absorptive surface of the small bowel, which results in malabsorption of nutrients.
- Classically, coeliac disease is characterised by diarrhoea, weight loss and anaemia. However, these may be absent and many individuals may suffer from mild or non-specific symptoms, which may be ignored for many years. Delayed diagnosis can result in osteoporosis, infertility or even cancer.
- Coeliac disease is an heritable condition, with first degree relatives of sufferers having a 10% chance of having the condition.
- The condition is triggered by the ingestion of wheat, rye and barley. Oats are probably safe for consumption by gluten sensitive individuals.

- A strict gluten-free diet, which may include high quality wheat starch, is good protection against the long term complications of gluten sensitivity, particularly cancer.
- Small intestinal biopsy remains the gold standard for diagnosis of coeliac disease. However, use of improved serological tests has aided screening programmes, which indicate that in various countries throughout Europe the prevalence of gluten sensitivity is 1 in 250 to 1 in 300 of the population. There are areas, such as parts of Ireland, where this figure may be as high as 1 in 100.
- The skin can be affected by gluten sensitivity in a condition known as dermatitis herpetiformis. Individuals with this condition almost always have some degree of enteropathy, so a gluten-free diet is recommended.
- Gluten sensitivity may be associated with a number of neurological conditions, such as epilepsy. The nature of the association between gluten and the nervous system remains obscure.
- Measurement of gluten contamination in foodstuffs is difficult. Legislation to protect the consumer is in place, and will be tightened up when improved methods of measurement of gluten are available.

# Appendix A: Cereal chemistry

## Wheat prolamins (gliadins) and glutenins

The chemistry of cereals has been extensively reviewed by Shewry *et al.* (1992). Gliadins have been subdivided, on the basis of their electrophoretic mobility, into the α-, β-, γ- and ω-subfractions which can be further separated into over 30 components on two-dimensional electrophoresis. Omega-gliadins contain no cysteine or methionine and are termed sulphur-free. More recent nomenclature, based on amino acid sequences, recognises only the α-type, γ-type, and ω-type gliadins.

Glutenins are composed of subunits stabilised by interchain disulphide bonds to form polymers. The reduced subunits are classified as high molecular weight (HMW) or low molecular weight (LMW); the LMW subunits resemble α- and γ-type gliadins in amino acid composition, the HMW subunits do not resemble other wheat proteins.

## Rye and barley prolamins

Rye and barley storage proteins have similarities with the γ-type gliadins and ω-type gliadins. They do not form a gluten mass and do not have the baking properties of wheat.

## The prolamins of oats and rice and maize

Prolamins account for only approximately 5–15% of the total seed proteins of these cereals, compared to wheat gliadins that comprise 40% of storage protein.

Oat avenins have some similarities to the prolamins of wheat, whereas the prolamins of rice do not. The maize zeins are rich in proline and glutamine. They bear little resemblance to the structure of gliadins but do contain some short gliadin-like sequences.

*Adverse Reactions to Food*

## Appendix B: Cell mediated immunity and coeliac disease

T cells may be classified phenotypically according to the presence of certain cell surface markers, which are detected by immuno-histochemical methods.

CD3 is the pan-T cell marker. $CD3^+$ cells have a further accessory molecule that may be either $CD4^+$ or $CD8^+$. These molecules are responsible for increased activation of the T cell. $CD4^+$ cells interact with HLA class II molecules in association with exogenous antigen, while $CD8^+$ cells largely respond to class I molecules in association with endogenous antigen (see Chapter 2).

Both normal immune and inappropriate hypersensitivity reactions are mediated by T cells in two ways. Antigen-stimulated T cells secrete cytokines, resulting in the recruitment of effector cells, for example macrophages and granulocytes. This is usually a property of $CD4^+ \alpha/\beta$ cells. Mediators such as the cytokines ILl and TNF-$\alpha$ are released from macrophages, causing local cell damage.

Alternatively, activated T cells, usually $CD8^+ \alpha/\beta$ can recognise peptides presented on cell surfaces in association with MHC molecules and cause cell lysis. Tissue damage is due to direct cell death, although cytotoxic cells can release lymphokines and thus recruit non-specific effector cells. Within the intestine, most epithelial $CD8^+$ cells are cytotoxic and lamina propria $CD4^+$ cells can secrete cytokines (MacDonald, 1992). Mast cells can release cytokines, such as IL2, IL4 and TNF-$\alpha$, and therefore may also participate in cell mediated immune responses. In both coeliac disease patients and dermatitits herpetiformis patients on a gluten-containing diet, the intra-epithelial lymphocytes are of the $CD8^+$ subset, and are significantly increased in number but are not activated. However, in the lamina propria, there is a 50-fold increase in the number of T cells present compared to controls, and of these it is the $CD4^+$ subset that is preferentially activated. A strong case could be made for gluten-induced activation of these lamina propria $CD4^+$ (T helper) cells being the mediators of the enteropathy of coeliac disease. The evidence has been fully reviewed by MacDonald (1992). The 'missing link' was lack of any direct evidence of gluten-reactive T cells present in the small intestinal mucosa of patients with coeliac disease. However, shortly afterwards, the first in a series of papers described the presence of gluten-specific, DQ2 restricted T cells in the gut mucosae of patients with coeliac disease (Lundin *et al.*, 1993), but not in normal controls (Mølberg *et al.*, 1997). Recent evidence suggests that there may be an immunodominant epitope (Arentz-Hansen *et al.*, 2000). When these cells are grown in tissue culture and the cell-free growth medium collected, the medium causes damage to normal human gut biopsies, which is identical to the coeliac disease lesion and can be blocked by antibodies to interferon-$\gamma$, but not IL2, ILl or TNF-$\alpha$ (Przemioslo *et al.*, 1995). This suggests that the T cells from the coeliac disease biopsies secrete INF-$\gamma$, which directly causes the damage seen in coeliac disease. *In vivo*, INF-$\gamma$ may also stimulate the production of TNF-$\alpha$ from macrophages, enhancing the effect.

# 10
# Clinically Validated Diagnostic Tests and Non-validated Procedures of Unproven Value

## 10.1 Introduction

Adverse reactions to foods can be caused by a wide range of precipitating factors; foods, food additives and contaminants need to be carefully considered during the diagnostic process.

Some clinical conditions that may masquerade as food allergy are listed in Table 10.1.

The diagnosis of a food allergy depends mainly on taking a careful history, clinical suspicion and a positive response to therapeutic measures. If an IgE

**Table 10.1** Differential diagnosis of suspected food allergic disease.

Each of the following can result from an adverse reaction to food that is not allergy mediated:

- Enzyme deficiencies causing gastrointestinal and liver disease, *e.g.* lactose intolerance, fructose intolerance, galactosaemia
- Irritable bowel syndrome
- Abdominal migraine
- Inflammatory bowel diseases
- Intermittent intestinal obstruction
- Dumping syndrome
- Pyloric stenosis
- Cyclical vomiting
- Pancreatic insufficiency
- Peptic ulcer disease
- Gall bladder disease
- C1 esterase inhibitor deficiency (hereditary angioedema)
- Toxins (food poisoning)
- Bacterial, viral or parasitic infection
- Reactions caused by food additives (nitrates, nitrites)

antibody-mediated disorder is suspected (see Chapter 6), skin tests and *in vitro* tests of food-specific IgE antibodies are often helpful. As a general rule, diagnostic tests should be based on the reported clinical symptoms (*e.g.* gastrointestinal, respiratory and skin symptoms), must be standardised and the results must be reproducible. Additional information may be gathered from a family history.

Adverse reactions to foods (here excluding toxic reactions due to food additives or contaminants and inherited or acquired enzyme deficiencies) are often not due to allergic mechanisms (Table 10.1). Allergic food reactions are usually IgE mediated, but in some circumstances cell mediated immune processes are also important (*e.g.* in coeliac disease, Chapter 9). Currently, the recommended diagnostic procedure for a food intolerance reaction is the double-blind placebo-controlled food challenge (DBPCFC) (see Chapter 11).

In some circumstances, for example in young infants or in some gastrointestinal disorders, where mucosal biopsies are taken before and after a food challenge (see, for example, Chapter 9), a blinded challenge may not be necessary.

## 10.2 Procedures of proven value

### 10.2.1 Double-blind placebo-controlled food challenge

The double-blind placebo-controlled food challenge (DBPCFC) has been considered the gold standard for the diagnosis of food intolerance reactions (Sicherer *et al.*, 2000). This approach sounds simple; however, the application of this method in daily practice is not as straightforward as it sounds and must be conducted with specialist help (Huijbers *et al.*, 1994) (for a detailed discussion see Chapter 11).

The selection of foods to be tested in the DBPCFC is based on the clinical history, knowledge of the eight most commonly encountered triggering foods (in the UK, Europe and North America), namely milk, egg, peanut, tree nuts, wheat, fish, shellfish and soya, and/or the skin test results obtained during the initial assessment. Foods unlikely to produce allergic reactions may be screened for by giving open or single-blind challenges.

Before the challenge, the suspected food should be eliminated from the diet, antihistamines should be discontinued and other medications should be minimised to levels sufficient to prevent acute symptoms. As a general principle, to control for a variety of confounding factors, an equal number of foods and placebo challenges is advisable and the order of administration should be randomised.

### 10.2.2 Skin prick tests

The principle of the skin test is that the wheal and flare reaction to an allergen introduced into the skin demonstrates the presence of an IgE antibody specific for that allergen. Allergen associates with specific IgE bound to mast cells. This results in cross-linking of surface-bound antibody, the release by mast cells of inflammatory mediators (*e.g.* histamine) and the influx of other cell types, notably eosinophils (see Chapter 2, Section 2.5 for details). The diameter of the resulting wheal is compared with that of a positive histamine control and a negative solvent control. Wheal reactions with a diameter of 3 mm or greater are usually considered positive. A positive test can confirm that the patient is atopic (Isolauri & Turjanmaa, 1996; Burks *et al.*, 1998; Eigenmann & Sampson, 1998), which is usually defined by multiple sensitivity or at least reactivity to two common allergens (see Chapters 6 or 12 for a list). It can also heighten the physician's suspicion as to the probable precipitants (allergenic substances).

Positive skin tests do not always correlate with the clinical picture (Dreborg, 1989). The predictive power of the skin test is affected by factors such as the different quality and potency of allergen extracts, variability in the investigator's technique, patient's use of antihistamines or steroids and the inappropriate choice of test allergen in the particular patient. In addition, patients who have had clinical reactions in the past can have persistently positive skin tests long after they have lost their clinical reactivity. Allergenic cross-reactivities are discussed in Section 10.2.4. Reactions to some fruits and vegetables (apples, oranges, bananas, peas, melons, potatoes, carrots and celery) may not be detectable with commercially prepared reagents, especially in patients with the 'oral allergy syndrome'. Under these circumstances, the 'prick-prick' technique with fresh foods may be used to test for allergies to these items. The above technique is performed by pricking the fresh fruit or vegetable in question and then using the needle to perform a normal skin test in the patient. A lack of standardisation is a serious disadvantage when using this test.

When appropriately standardised test allergens are used, **negative** reactions typically have 95% accuracy in predicting the absence of clinically relevant allergen-specific IgE antibodies, although the negative predictive accuracy of the skin test varies for different allergens (Eigenmann & Sampson, 1998) and is enhanced by measuring serum levels of specific IgE antibodies at the same time.

In some individuals there may be a discrepancy between the skin test result and the allergen-specific IgE level, or *vice versa*, even in patients with a clear history of an allergic reaction. Under these circumstances, credence should be given to the history and, if in doubt, a challenge must be performed under medical supervision.

The **positive** predictive accuracy is about 50–60% and can be increased by measuring the level of allergen-specific IgE at the same time; again it varies with the allergen in question (Eigenmann & Sampson, 1998). Skin tests can be helpful in clinical conditions when the onset has been severe (anaphylaxis) and would not allow an oral challenge for confirmation of diagnosis. Some patients only react to fresh fruit (for example in oral allergy syndrome). In these circumstances, a direct prick test with the food in question needs to be performed (see above).

Although reports of generalised anaphylactic reactions to a skin prick test are rare (a rate of 3 in 10 000 tests) (Valyasevi *et al.*, 1999), care must be taken when testing extremely allergic patients and the number of skin tests causing potential positive reactions should be limited. Tests should be conducted in a clinical setting as a precaution.

### 10.2.3 Radioallergosorbent test (RAST)

The RAST measures the amount of allergen-specific IgE antibodies in the patient's serum. Historically, the levels of allergen-specific IgE in RAST have been classed as 0 (negative) to 6 (strongly positive). Today, allergen-specific IgE levels are generally measured with an appropriately validated test system. High levels of allergen specific antibodies (>100 kUA/l) can be clinically predictive of an immediate reaction against the allergen in question (Moneret-Vautrin *et al.*, 1993; Roger *et al.*, 1994). Medium to low level positive tests correlate less well with the diagnosis since the RAST only measures immunological sensitisation instead of clinical reactivity (Eigenmann & Sampson, 1998).

### 10.2.4 Cross-reactivities

The serum of hayfever sufferers with allergen-specific IgE against birch pollen may also react to apple, peach, cherry and pear allergens, with or without the patient experiencing adverse symptoms when eating these foods (Mandallaz *et al.*, 1988; Crespo *et al.*, 1995; Beezhold *et al*, 1996). Conversely, the serum of food-allergic patients may show reactivities against pollen allergens without clinical symptoms of hayfever in the patient. This type of cross-reactivity seems to be related to IgE antibodies raised against common plant storage proteins (profilins) and sugar (carbohydrate) determinants of allergens (Aalberse, 2000).

### 10.2.5 Summary

High allergen-specific IgE (RAST) scores and positive skin prick tests (well above a histamine control) are diagnostic in patients with anaphylactic reactions and a clear history identifying the possible triggering food. The positive predictive accuracy of skin prick tests and RAST varies in relation to the allergen in question and the patient's symptoms. The tests are often insufficient to identify correctly a delayed reaction in an individual patient. The predictive accuracy also decreases with increasing age (Dreborg, 1989). Under clinical conditions it is often necessary to rule out possible triggers for anaphylactic reactions and negative tests (see Section 10.2.2) are an important diagnostic tool. The combined negative predictive accuracy of both tests (skin prick and RAST) is around 95%, indicating that the patient is highly unlikely to react to that specific food. Individuals who have multiple food sensitisations and have positive RAST and skin tests do not always benefit from food exclusions based on these results, and may need to undergo food elimination and re-introduction procedures (Chapter 11).

## 10.3 Other procedures of proven value for the diagnosis of adverse reactions to foods

### 10.3.1 Endoscopic studies with and without intestinal biopsy

This type of test involves examining a small piece of the intestinal lining, either through swallowing a small tube to which a capsule is attached or via a thin endoscope which allows positioning of the cutting device under direct view. The biopsy is then examined for histopathological changes under the microscope.

Intestinal biopsies are simple to perform and are often used in patients with slow onset gastrointestinal symptoms and other features such as short stature, unexplained iron deficiency, osteoporosis, weight loss or other characteristic features of potential malnutrition. These tests are also used to investigate patients with coeliac disease and their family members, once the serological screening tests have been conducted and shown to be positive (see Chapter 9).

The intestinal biopsy is usually not indicated for the diagnosis of acute IgE mediated gastrointestinal symptoms. If a biopsy is performed under these conditions, the tissue may show a mild eosinophilic infiltration, possible evidence of degranulated mucosal mast cells and infiltration of other inflammatory cells. Other *in vitro* tests are currently under evaluation but have not yet been sufficiently validated under clinical, as distinct from research, conditions.

For the differential diagnosis of inflammatory bowel disease and food intolerance, serological and endoscopic investigations with histological examination of the mucosal lining are essential.

### 10.3.2 Intestinal permeability test

Under normal conditions, the intestinal epithelium forms a tight mucosal barrier preventing gross uptake of undigested antigenic food substances or microbial organisms. Uptake of very small amounts of undigested proteins is, however, commonly observed.

Alterations to the normal mucosal barrier function can lead to increased uptake of allergens, which may then trigger immune reactions. Changes in mucosal permeability can be a primary sign of an underlying inflammatory disease. They can be caused through an immunologically mediated reaction, which has been triggered by the challenge food. Diagnostic tests relying on measuring changes in intestinal permeability to different substances have been used clinically. During elimination and challenge studies in children and adults, non-degradable marker substances, such as the sugars lactulose and rhamnose, polyethyleneglycol (PEG), chromium 51-EDTA and various proteins, have been used as indicators of intestinal permeability (Strobel *et al.*, 1984; Falth-Magnusson *et al.*, 1986; Scadding *et al.*, 1989; de Boissieu *et al.*, 1994).

Usually in the morning after a fasting period, the patient is asked to drink the test substances, after which the urine is collected for a specified period (*e.g.* 5 hours) and then analysed.

Changes in intestinal integrity affect the permeation of these non-degradable marker substances, which are of known molecular weight. By using substances of differing molecular weight, it is possible to establish the size of the pores in the epithelial membrane. Expressing the results with two substances of different molecular weight as a ratio makes the test less sensitive to collection errors or factors related to gastric retention, intestinal dilution or renal excretion of the test substances. In individuals with food-induced gastrointestinal abnormalities, these tests have been

shown to correlate positively with the intake or avoidance of the triggering food (Strobel *et al.*, 1984; de Boissieu *et al.*, 1994). These tests are analytically demanding and require the back-up of an experienced laboratory.

## 10.4 Other tests applied in the diagnosis of food intolerances

Flow cytometric studies with the measurement of antigen-specific cytokine secretion, studies of peripheral blood mononuclear cells and measurement of IgE in faecal extracts may all identify groups of allergic patients, but the usefulness of the tests in diagnosis of food intolerance in individual patients is not proven.

The measurement of inflammatory mediators in stool samples and endoscopic provocation tests, in which allergens are applied directly and a potential mucosal wheal and flare reaction is observed directly, are currently being evaluated.

### 10.4.1 Respiratory function tests

Food-induced wheezing, as a single manifestation of food allergy, is rare. Only about 5% of food-allergic children with asthma suffer from food-induced deterioration of their lung function (Bousquet *et al.*, 1992; Moneret-Vautrin *et al.*, 1996). These tests could be useful where respiratory symptoms and signs are present in immunologically mediated adverse reactions to foods. In about 5% of atopic individuals with asthma and food allergies, the possibility of deterioration in lung function after the intake of a particular food must be considered. Respiratory tests include serial measurements of $FEV_1$ (forced expiratory volume at 1 second) and other indicators of bronchial constriction or obstruction.

## 10.5 Non-validated procedures of unproven value

There are a number of other procedures that have been claimed to be of value in the diagnosis of adverse reactions to food; most of them have not been validated and many are likely to be of no value (for a discussion, see the report from the Committee on Toxicity of Chemicals in Food, Consumer Products and the Environment (COT), published by the Food Standards Agency 2000). COT comments that

> 'there are a number of procedures used to "diagnose" and treat adverse reactions to food ingredients that do not have a sound evidential base. Misdiagnosis of adverse reactions to food and the imposition of inappropriate exclusion diets can seriously compromise a patient's nutrition and health.'

Unfortunately, these non-validated tests are advertised in the national media and on the Internet without any corroborative evidence of their usefulness in predicting allergic or other food intolerance reactions in the individual patient. Diets based on these tests are hazardous, inappropriately chosen and the patient lacks the necessary dietary supervision of a qualified dietitian. Provision of dietary advice by unqualified practitioners, based on the results of non-validated or unproven tests, is particularly hazardous in childhood, and can potentially result in growth failure and nutrient inadequacies that might affect development. Examples of non-validated tests are given below.

### 10.5.1 Food specific IgG and IgG subclass antibodies

Early hopes that measuring circulating concentrations of food-specific antibodies of the IgG class would assist in the diagnosis of food intolerance were unfounded. It was soon demonstrated that these antibodies are found in the normal population and that IgG antibodies simply reflect immunological encounter and are in fact part of the normal immune response, which varies with age and exposure (see Chapter 2, Section 2.6.4). The determination of IgG antibodies to foods has no predictive value for dietary management of patients with food allergic diseases. (In coeliac disease, measurements of IgG antibodies against gliadin may be useful in monitoring the adherence to a gluten-free diet (see Chapter 9), but apart from this have no other value in the management of the disease.)

### 10.5.2 Cytotoxicity tests

In these tests, the food allergen is added to full blood or white cell suspensions *in vitro*. Evidence of cell death and other changes is ascertained. The test relies on the hypothesis that the observed changes indicate sensitivities to the allergens in question. There is little evidence to support the efficacy of these tests. As with other non-validated tests, the incidence of false positives is high indicating that these tests are non-specific (Kay & Lessof, 1992).

### 10.5.3 Sublingual, subcutaneous and intradermal provocation and neutralisation tests

As a principle, in these tests the food extract is given sublingually or injected subcutaneously or intradermally about 30 minutes before the food antigen in question is eaten. This is done in an attempt to neutralise the subsequent exposure to the food that the patient believes is harmful. Careful evaluation of these tests suggests that they are without discriminatory value and potentially dangerous.

### (i) Sublingual or subcutaneous provocation challenge

During this procedure, dilute food allergens are administered under the tongue of the person. The operator then asks the patient if the food allergen has aggravated the usual symptoms experienced by the subject in response to foods containing the allergen. If the response is positive, this food item is then omitted from the diet. While some allergic people may react (*e.g.* to administration of peanut allergen), this procedure cannot effectively diagnose food allergies, is prone to give false positive results and may be dangerous.

### 10.5.4 Immune complex measurements

Immune complex assays are sometimes performed on patients suspected of having food allergies. This test is done to ascertain whether there are circulating complexes in the blood, consisting of antibodies bound to the food allergen. However, it has been shown that formation of circulating (food) immune complexes is a normal consequence of food digestion.

### 10.5.5 Electro acupuncture

In this test, the electrical activity of the skin is

determined at points considered appropriate for the detection of food allergies. There is no clinical or scientific proof of the diagnostic efficacy of this test.

### (i) Modified electro acupuncture (VEGA testing)

This technique is based on the bioenergetic regulatory principles that have their origins in acupuncture and homoeopathy. It is postulated that the first sign of an abnormality in the body is an electrical change. The VEGA machine purports to measure one aspect of these bioenergetic phenomena by recording the change in skin conductivity after the application of a small voltage to the patient. It is assumed that this stresses the patient and will unmask any weakness in the body. The patient, at the same time, grasps the hand electrode. Applying the probe to the patient's finger or toe then constitutes a control measurement. After calibration, the food extract is placed in a circuit and the measurement repeated. Any change above a prescribed level is considered diagnostic. This technique of diagnosis is without any scientific or clinical basis and could result in inappropriate and/or delayed treatment of disease (Food Standards Agency, 2000).

### 10.5.6  Applied kinesiology and the DRIA test

This is a variant of the provocation neutralisation test. It relies on the measurement of the strength of a big muscle, for example the thigh muscle (quadriceps). The proposition is that when a food-sensitive individual comes into contact with the food allergen, a decrease in the strength of the quadriceps muscle results. This test has also not been validated in a prospective manner.

A variation of this test is based on the subjective measurement of muscle strength in one hand of the subject, while the other hand contains the suspected food in a glass bottle. Again, there is no independent validation of this test (Klinkoski & Leboeuf, 1990).

### 10.5.7  Hair analysis

Hair analysis is a test offered for assessment of the mineral content and nutritional metabolism of the individual. This assumes that the content of the hair reflects the current mineral status and health of the body's tissues. It has been claimed that this test can also be used to diagnose allergy and food intolerance; this test has no role in the diagnosis of adverse reactions to foods (Sethi *et al.*, 1987).

### 10.5.8  Urine injections

This test claims that urine collected from sensitive individuals will cause positive skin test reactions when injected into the subject. There is no information on the value of this highly speculative and potentially very dangerous test.

## 10.6  Non-immunologically mediated reactions to foods

Not all reactions to food involve the immune system (Chapters 1 and 7). Because of the variety of different manifestations and mechanisms involved in possible reactions to foods, it is not surprising that there is often no specific *in vivo* or *in vitro* test to confirm a clinical diagnosis.

However, a number of specific tests are available which can help to establish the presence of metabolic abnormalities when this diagnosis is suspected. Food challenges and biochemical tests, for example measurements of the activity of enzymes such as glucose-6-phospate dehydrogenase (*e.g.* in Favism), and methaemoglobin reductase in red blood cells, or measurements of disaccharidases in intestinal biopsy specimens, can be used to substantiate clinical suspicion and guide management.

## 10.7  Costs of inappropriate treatment to the patient and community

Currently, the cost of inappropriate treatment of allergy and food intolerances is difficult to ascertain (Knutsen, 1994; Negro Alvarez *et al.*, 1994; Grant *et al.*, 1999; Phillips *et al.*, 1999). However, considering that 20–30% of the population considers themselves to be suffering from food allergic diseases, despite the reported prevalence of IgE mediated allergy of about 1–2% in children and less than 1% in adults (Chapter 4), costs are likely to be significant. The spread of inappropriate diagnostic and therapeutic allergy services clearly leads to inappropriate treatment and expense to individual patients and the NHS overall.

It is conceivable that the public's reliance on non-validated tests and treatments in the management of adverse reaction to foods is an indicator of the lack of experienced diagnosis and treatment centres within the NHS.

The public's reliance on non-validated and valueless tests and the subsequent application of potentially harmful treatments can only be countered through public education and heightened awareness of the possible dangers associated with such practices and procedures. For example, the public can usefully be alerted to the fact that the type of claim that can be found on the Internet and in the popular press, which is supported by testimonials, should be treated with great caution. Websites now exist which monitor health claims and highlight ones that they feel are spurious. One such site is www.quackwatch.com. National and international allergy and immunology organisations are also a good source of relevant and critically appraised information.

An increase in the number of competent individuals, experienced in the diagnosis (and management) of food allergic diseases, practising in centres within the NHS is clearly a priority and will facilitate greater access to appropriate and evidence-based care.

## 10.8  Key points

- The diagnosis of a food intolerance (including food allergy) depends mainly on taking a careful history, clinical suspicion and a positive response to therapeutic measures. If an IgE antibody mediated disorder is suspected, skin tests and *in vitro* tests of food-specific IgE antibodies are helpful and often diagnostic in patients with immediate reactions.

- The double-blind placebo-controlled food challenge is considered the gold standard for the diagnosis of a (often delayed) food intolerance reaction. This test requires specialist knowledge and clinical supervision.

- Great care needs to be taken when challenging patients suspected to be at risk of anaphylaxis, and tests should be conducted only under supervision in a clinical setting.

- Other specialist tests of proven value and available via hospitals include endoscopic investigations and intestinal permeability tests.

- The value of many other tests offered direct to the public, *e.g.* via the Internet and magazine advertisements, is unproven. The tests quoted have not been validated and advice based on them can be dangerous. Diets based on diagnoses arising from these tests are highly inappropriate and unreliable, and provision of dietary advice by unqualified practitioners is particularly hazardous for children.

# 11
# Diagnosis and Management of Food Intolerance by Diet

## 11.1 Introduction

Diet is the cornerstone of diagnosis and treatment of food intolerance. Used in combination with food challenges, diet is the only dependable method able to identify offending foods. Food(s) or food constituents that are suspected of causing symptoms are removed from the diet for a specified period to see if symptoms improve. This is followed by a series of open and double-blind placebo-controlled food challenges (DBPCFC) in an attempt to reproduce the original reactions and prove the diagnosis (see Chapter 10). Laboratory tests such as skin prick tests or radioallergosorbent tests (RAST) are used in addition to diet to identify suspect foods (see Chapter 10). However, these have their limitations, as they can show that an IgE reaction has occurred but not that the reaction has been enough to cause symptoms or need treatment.

In some cases the relationship between symptoms and a specific food is sufficiently clear-cut to determine the specific investigations that are required. The diagnosis of food intolerance often involves five stages:

(1) history and clinical assessment,
(2) clinical and laboratory tests,
(3) diagnostic exclusion diet,
(4) open food challenges,
(5) double-blind, placebo-controlled food challenges.

## 11.2 History and clinical assessment

The first step in the process of diagnosis includes a full assessment of the symptoms and their frequency, dietary history, past and present treatments and family history of atopic disease. A detailed diary of food intake, symptoms and their severity, and any medication should be recorded for at least 7 days. This may give vital clues as to which foods are precipitating symptoms. A numerical score can be allocated for the severity of each symptom, *e.g.* 1 to 3 for symptoms which are mild, moderate or severe, respectively (Carter, 1994). Sometimes this can be helpful; for example, abdominal pain may only occur on days when potato or potato products are consumed; but often the relationship between diet and symptoms is less clear. It is important that data are collected on baseline anthropometric measurements, nutritional intake and biochemical and nutritional parameters.

## 11.3 Clinical and laboratory tests

Clinical and laboratory tests are discussed in Chapter 10.

## 11.4 Diagnostic diets

There are 5 types of diagnostic diet:

- exclusion
- empirical
- few-foods
- elemental
- rotation.

The type chosen will depend upon the history and severity of symptoms. Most diagnostic diets are difficult; and it is better if other conventional treatments are tried first. All potential dietary hazards should be discussed with patients or their carers at the outset. Unless a relationship with food appears likely from the history, other diseases should be excluded before trying exclusion diets, particularly in infants and young children with severe symptoms. However, severe symptoms should not exclude a diagnosis of food allergy and intolerance.

### 11.4.1 Exclusion diet

This is the commonest and simplest diagnostic diet. It usually involves excluding one or two foods that appear likely from the history to be responsible for symptoms, *e.g.* milk ingestion causing immediate vomiting, strawberries provoking an urticarial reaction. Dietary intervention necessitates complete exclusion of the identified food(s) or else intolerance may be missed. If symptoms disappear, it is likely that food is responsible. However, it should also be recognised that symptom improvement might be coincidental or even due to a placebo effect (David, 1993a).

Some exclusion diets are difficult to adhere to, particularly if the excluded food is a major component of the diet, *e.g.* milk or wheat. The excluded food may also be hidden in the form of food sub-ingredients present in many manufactured foods. Again, milk and wheat are good examples. Dietetic advice and support is essential, ideally from a state registered dietitian, to ensure:

- Excluded foods are replaced by alternative palatable, readily accessible and affordable substitutes, which provide a beneficial nutrient profile where possible (Section 11.6.1).
- Over all, the diet is nutritionally adequate.
- Practical information is given on shopping, food preparation, cooking, school dinners and 'eating away from home'.
- Accurate, comprehensive but understandable information is given on interpreting food labels.

Dietitians have access to the national Food Intolerance Databank (Chapter 12, Section 12.8.1), which issues annual detailed lists of manufactured foods that are free from common food allergens such as in milk, wheat (gluten) and eggs. The Databank lists can direct shoppers to suitable products, but label checks are still necessary in case there have been recent changes in the product formulation.

A diagnostic diet should always be accompanied by plans to reintroduce the omitted foods after a defined period. The duration required before a food challenge is attempted varies. It partly depends upon the type of food excluded, the diagnosis, the severity of symptoms and the age of the patient. For example, milk intolerance in young children is often temporary and 85% have acquired tolerance by the age of 3 years (Høst & Halken, 1990). However, owing to the severity of symptoms in young infants, the first attempt to reintroduce milk may be delayed until after the age of one year, although many young children may accidentally expose themselves to milk first.

If the presenting symptoms are life-threatening, food challenge is inappropriate. Allergy to peanuts is usually severe and often lifelong (Bock & Atkins, 1989), so many units are reluctant to undertake peanut challenges because of the risk of anaphylaxis. Hourihane *et al.* (1998) reported that a small group of children with suspected peanut allergy had no adverse reaction following open challenges; all of these children were challenged because they either had negative results on skin prick tests with peanut, despite a convincing history, or because an exposure to peanut had been uneventful. Children with a history of life-threatening reactions were not challenged in this study.

### 11.4.2 Empirical diet

An empirical diet involves excluding common food allergens associated with a specific condition when a dietary cause is suspected but cannot be identified. In adults, the common foods and additives excluded include milk, eggs, wheat, peanuts, citrus fruits, fish, tree nuts, preservatives and colours (Lessof *et al.*, 1980b; Nanda *et al.*, 1989; Riordan *et al.*, 1990; Henz & Zuberbier, 1998; Warner, 1999). Similar foods are excluded in childhood, but chicken and soya are also commonly avoided, particularly in food sensitive enteropathy (Walker-Smith, 1994). Examples of empirical diets are given in Table 11.1.

**Table 11.1** Examples of empirical diets used in published studies.

| Age | Symptoms | Foods/ingredients excluded | Author |
|---|---|---|---|
| Adults or children | Atopic eczema | Cows' milk, egg, tomatoes, colours and preservatives | Sloper *et al.* (1991) |
| Young children | Atopic eczema | Cows' milk, wheat, egg | Broberg *et al.* (1992) |
| Young children | Atopic eczema | Natural and artificial food flavourings | Kanny *et al.* (1994) |
| Young children | Atopic eczema | Egg | Lever *et al.* (1998) |
| Adults | Urticaria | Preservatives, food colours, tomatoes | Henz & Zuberbier (1998) |
| Adults | Urticaria, angio-oedema, pruritis, atopic eczema | Nickel salts | Antico & Soana (1999) |
| Adults | Pseudo-allergic dermatopathies | Food additives | Antico & Di Benardino (1995) |
| Children | Autism | Milk | Lucarelli *et al.* (1995) |
| Infants | Colic | Cows' milk – bottle-fed infants. Artificial colours, preservatives, additives; milk, wheat, egg and nuts for breast-feeding mothers | Hill *et al.* (1995) |
| Children | Atopic eczema | Milk and egg | Atherton *et al.* (1978) |

The duration of use of empirical diets before food challenges are tried is variable. In many situations they are continued for at least 6 to 12 weeks. In migraine and urticaria, the duration will depend upon frequency of attacks. If symptoms occur only every week or two, it may take a few months to be certain of success or failure (David, 1993a). In atopic eczema, a minimum of 6 weeks is needed owing to the natural fluctuation in disease state, the time taken for severe eczema to improve and the possibility of chance improvement or placebo response (David, 1993a).

### 11.4.3 Few-foods diet

The few-foods diet is a strict diet, allowing a small selection of low allergen foods to be given for a short period of usually 2 to 3 weeks. It is generally only used when the symptoms are severe, the history is complex and there is some suggestion from the history that foods may be contributing to some of the symptoms. The idea of a few-foods diet is not new; Rowe (1928) first described this type of diet. The diet usually includes one type of meat, one cereal, two fruits and vegetables, a milk substitute and a cooking oil or fat source. There has been a variety of few-foods diets in use (Egger *et al.*, 1985, Littlewood & MacDonald, 1987; Carter, 1994); even the terminology differs from centre to centre. Some workers prefer the term oligoantigenic diet (Egger *et al.*, 1985; Businco *et al.*, 1996), whereas others use the term elimination diet (Broberg *et al.*, 1992; Grazioli *et al.*, 1993; Stefanini *et al.*, 1995; Gaby, 1998) and even the six-food diet (Devlin *et al.*, 1991). Few-foods diets have successfully been used in the diagnosis of food intolerance in atopic eczema (Pike *et al.*, 1989; Devlin *et al.*, 1991), attention deficit syndrome (Egger *et al.*, 1985), migraine (Egger *et al.*, 1983; MacDonald *et al.*, 1989) and even epilepsy (Egger *et al.*, 1989). However, the role of diet in epilepsy is particularly debatable.

It should be noted, however, that because of the prolonged procedures involved in this kind of dietary therapy, it should be considered only if other attempts at identifying contributory factors and more simple methods of treatment have failed. Even in conditions such as eczema, in which food can be a contributory factor (see Chapter 6), dietary management can make demands that the parents of the affected child simply do not value sufficiently to make the exercise worthwhile.

Examples of alternative few-foods diets are given in Table 11.2. The foods permitted in the basic diet can be adapted according to individual food preferences, age of the patient and clinical symptoms. The duration of the basic few-foods diet should not exceed 3 weeks. More prolonged use may result in an inadequate intake of energy and other nutritional deficiencies (Lloyd-Still, 1979). However, in some conditions such as eczema and hyperactivity, it may take the full 3 weeks before there is an improvement in symptoms and, as a result, some advocate the basic diet for longer (Devlin *et al.*, 1991). In general, if symptoms do not improve within 3 weeks, it is probable that foods are not the cause of the symptoms, or alternatively that the patient has failed to comply or that the diet still contains a food to which the patient is intolerant.

**Table 11.2** Examples of few-foods diets.

|  | Diet 1 | Diet 2 |
| --- | --- | --- |
| One meat | Lamb | Chicken |
| One vegetable | Carrots | Cabbage |
| One carbohydrate food | Rice | Potatoes |
| One fruit | Pears | Apples |

*Note:* These foods would be consumed in addition to a milk substitute (or vitamin and mineral supplement), salt, sugar, water and fruit juice.

When symptoms improve, omitted foods are gradually reintroduced into the diet to identify foods associated with the provocation of symptoms. Food reintroduction in few-foods diets should be conducted carefully, slowly and systematically. The rate of food reintroduction varies from one new food every 1 to 2 days to one food every 7 days. The latter approach is better in conditions such as eczema, migraine and hyperactivity, when delayed reactions may occur. Initially, only small portions of a new food should be given and at least one accompanying adult should be present in case of anaphylaxis. However, if there is any suggestion of severe reactions occurring, food challenges should be in a clinical environment under medical supervision.

The order in which foods are reintroduced is flexible, and is influenced by food preferences, food allergenicity and nutritional and culinary properties. For example, it is more useful to introduce foods such as wheat early rather than peas or bananas. Some authors advise introduction of foods by families, *e.g.* Leguminosae family: peanut, soya bean, French bean, carob bean and lentils (American Academy of Allergy and Immunology Committee on Adverse Reactions to Foods & National Institute of Allergy and Infectious Diseases, 1984). This is presumably because, with the exception of animal milks, clinical cross-reactivity between different foods within a family of foods is unusual (David, 1993a).

Throughout the reintroduction phase, accurate records of the foods introduced and the timing and severity of any symptoms should be documented. It can take up to a year to reintroduce all the foods typically consumed, and it requires intensive dietetic supervision and support. Few-foods diets are particularly difficult to follow and reports of non-compliance or diet abandonment are common. Hathaway and Warner (1983) reported, in a group of children with atopic eczema, that 3 out of 14 (21%) children under 3 years of age and 12 out of 26 children (46%) over 3 years gave up their few-foods diet. Devlin *et al.* (1991) reported that 9 out of 63 (14%) children with severe atopic eczema stopped a few-foods diet before 6 weeks. In a study on severe atopic dermatitis in 85 children, 29% (*n* = 25) failed either to adhere to the diet or attend appointments for review (Mabin *et al.*, 1995a,b). Nevertheless, for some, a few-foods diet can lead to identification of food allergens, and their subsequent avoidance can result in a dramatic improvement in symptoms, which far outweighs the trials and tribulations of this difficult diet.

### 11.4.4 Elemental diet

A so-called elemental diet is a chemically defined diet in which the protein source is derived from amino acids, with added carbohydrates in the form of short chain polymers of glucose or disaccharides other than lactose, a small quantity of fat (usually containing a high proportion of medium chain triglycerides), minerals and vitamins. Therefore, these diets contain nutrients in their most easily absorbable form. Elemental diets are generally used only when symptoms are severe and other diagnostic methods have failed. They have provided a diagnostic tool for food intolerance since the mid-1970s (Galant *et al.*, 1977; Hughes, 1978). All food is usually withdrawn and is replaced with a low allergen amino acid based elemental formula, given in liquid form, for a specific time period. This regimen is then used to provide nutritional support whilst foods are formally reintroduced into the diet.

Elemental diets have occasionally been successful in the management of severe atopic eczema in children but not adults (Munkvad *et al.*, 1984; David, 1992), in chronic gastrointestinal symptoms in infancy (de Boissieu *et al.*, 1997), and in paediatric (Cosgrove & Jenkins, 1997) and adult Crohn's disease (Riordan *et al.*, 1993). In paediatric Crohn's disease, an elemental diet aids healing of the mucosa, and downregulation of inflammation (Walker-Smith, 1997). It also improves nutritional status and is as effective as high doses of steroids in inducing remission (Goulet & Ricour, 1995; Beattie *et al.*, 1998). Although it is yet to be shown that, in general, low residue diets have these effects, there is evidence that whole protein (Beattie *et al.*, 1994) and protein hydrolysate (Khoshoo *et al.*, 1996) feeds are equally successful in this condition. It is, therefore, possible that the beneficial effect is derived not from the removal of food allergens from the diet but from the removal of unabsorbed food residues and the rest that this provides for the inflamed bowel (see Chapter 7, Section 7.4.3).

Elemental diets commonly need to be administered by a nasogastric tube but palatability has improved, and some patients drink sufficient volumes orally. Elemental diets are hyperosmolar (*e.g.* 20% weight/volume of unflavoured Elemental 028 Extra (Scientific Hospital Supplies) has an osmolality of 502 mosm/kg), so should be well diluted or taken with extra water. They are best taken as chilled drinks but, for an adult, drinking a potential volume of 2.5 to 3 litres daily for a few weeks means that elemental diets can be tedious and demanding. Daily dietary intake charts should be kept and regular anthropometric measurements made and monitored.

### 11.4.5 Rotation diets

This is a modification of the oligoantigenic or few-foods diet. It can only be used in non-life threatening circumstances and it has not been shown to be effective in any published controlled studies. The diet is based on the belief that the degree of sensitivity to a food is related to the amount of food consumed. It is assumed that increased frequency of intake increases sensitisation; and tolerance to a food will occur after prolonged omission. The diet involves rotating exposure to an individual food or a family of foods, so a food or its family is eaten only once in anything from 3 to 30 days. The aim is to give the body a rest from each food family. Foods are excluded if they are known or suspected of causing symptoms, or are commonly associated with food intolerance reactions (Thomas, 1988). However, once established on this diet and symptom-free, omitted foods can be reintroduced to determine whether symptoms will develop.

Those who recommend rotation diets suggest their use may be temporary or lifelong. Although popular with some practitioners in the USA (Parker *et al.*, 1988), their design is illogical (patients who are genuinely intolerant would not be able to tolerate trigger foods even once a week), potentially dangerous and may be nutritionally imbalanced. Any claims of benefit are anecdotal and recognised food allergy specialists do not advocate this type of diet.

## 11.5 Food challenges

The aim of a food challenge is to study the consequences of food or food additive ingestion (David, 1993a). Food challenges are necessary for several reasons: firstly, to confirm or refute a diagnosis, and secondly, to investigate the development of food tolerance. The food challenge should, ideally, replicate normal food consumption in terms of dose, route and food type (David, 1993a).

### 11.5.1 Open challenges

Initially, in severe cases, minute quantities of challenge food are introduced, because of the risk of anaphylaxis, and the amount is incrementally increased over a period of hours until average portion sizes are being eaten. In clinical paediatric practice, the majority of food challenges are open challenges. These are simple and practical but are disadvantaged by observer bias. The parents, patient and clinical staff know which foods are being given and this may influence the response and the interpretation of any observations made. The challenge may be continued for several days, in cases of reported delayed reactions.

### 11.5.2 Double-blind placebo-controlled food challenge (DBPCFC) tests

The DBPCFC test is considered the 'gold standard' procedure for the diagnosis of food intolerance (see Chapters 4 and 10). A DBPCFC test involves the administration of a challenge substance, which is either the specified food (or food component) or an indistinguishable placebo item. During a DBPCFC, the patient remains unaware of whether a specific food or placebo is being given. A 'neutral' observer such as a doctor or nurse is also unaware of what is being administered and this has the advantage of objectivity. The patient, parent and medical observer each scores responses. During challenge procedures, the patient should remain on a limited diet, eating foods known not to cause symptoms. Suspect foods or food ingredients can either be disguised by mixing with another food, added to opaque capsules or given in a liquid medium. The placebo should always be indistinguishable from the test food.

DBPCFC tests are difficult to do successfully and are time consuming, and as a result they are not commonly used in clinical practice. However, they are necessary when there is doubt about diagnosis and for research purposes. They have helped establish that the population as a whole (Young *et al.*, 1994) and parents (Devlin & David, 1992) mistakenly perceive food or food additives to be responsible for more symptoms than is apparent when the strict protocols of DBPCFC tests are applied (Chapter 4). DBPCFC should not be used if there is a clear history of major allergic symptoms following ingestion of a specific food, because of the risk of anaphylaxis.

There are several practical problems with the administration of DBPCFC tests:

- Ideally the test food should replicate the natural food or food additive that provoked symptoms, *e.g.* whole pasteurised liquid milk should not be substituted for sterilised skimmed milk. How-

ever, practically it is difficult to mask the smell, texture and flavour of certain foods. The challenge mixture should always be palatable and acceptable if given orally.

- Encapsulation of food for challenges is commonly recommended (Bock *et al.*, 1988). However, standard capsules only contain up to 500 mg of food. They, therefore, can contain only a limited quantity of challenge material, and if it is given in a dried format (to increase the quantity), this will probably reduce its allergenicity. Furthermore, patients need to be able to swallow capsules whole, so this type of DBPCFC is unsuitable for young children.

- The amount of allergen needed to provoke a reaction is likely to vary between subjects. Hill *et al.* (1988) demonstrated that 8–10 g of cows' milk powder caused a reaction in some patients, whereas others required up to 10 times this amount before symptoms developed. A negative reaction to the allergen in a blind challenge does not always signify that food intolerance does not exist, as the quantity of food or food ingredient consumed or the length of challenge may have been inadequate. Ideally, before attempting a DBPCFC, the quantity of food needed to cause symptoms should first be established during an open food challenge.

- A reaction may not occur during a DBPCFC test if the challenge is given during a dormant phase of the disease (Carter, 1994), *e.g.* in urticaria, salicylate intolerance may only occur in subjects with active disease. Equally, if symptoms are induced by a combination of food and exercise, which is sometimes reported (Palosuo *et al.*, 1999) (see Chapter 6), exact conditions may be difficult to reproduce with a DBPCFC test.

## 11.6 Milk-free diets

A milk-free diet is usually difficult to follow. It involves the exclusion of not only cows' milk or cows' milk based infant formulas, but also a wide range of other foods that contain cows' milk or components of cows' milk. Cows' milk is used to make foods such as cheese, yogurt, ice cream, milk chocolate, butter and cream. Constituents of milk are also likely to be found in foods such as biscuits, some sweets (*e.g.* whey powder in chewy sweets) and tinned and processed meats. Many spreads (including reduced fat) now include milk components to improve their flavour. Cheese may be added to foods such as tinned spaghetti, the milk component lactose added as a flavour carrier in crisps and delicatessen meats may contain whey/casein in the brine that surrounds meat in pre-packaged products. Cows' milk casein is even added as a stabiliser in some natural latex rubber gloves and can cause contact urticaria (Ylitalo *et al.*, 1999).

A list of milk-containing derivatives is given in Table 11.3, but many people may not be aware that these are associated with cows' milk and may not recognise their significance on food labels. Furthermore, reading the label will not always provide a conclusive answer as UK labelling does not require the constituents of all compound ingredients to be listed (if the compound ingredient forms less than 25% of the final product its individual constituents need not be declared) (Anon, 1984) (Chapter 12). Although many manufacturers choose to provide this information voluntarily, especially for nuts and peanuts, the legislation makes it very difficult for lay individuals to interpret ingredient labels with any certainty. Added to this, there is no legal requirement for all foods to have ingredients listed on labels, *e.g.* chocolate, loose sweets, freshly baked foods or unwrapped meat products are exempt (Chapter 12). Manufacturers produce a range of substitutes for milk containing foods, *e.g.* soya-based spread, soya yoghurt, carob chocolate and soya-based cheese, but sometimes milk derivatives are even added to these. Although rare, David (1993a) reported a 12-year-old boy who died as a result of an anaphylactic reaction after eating a tofu cheese, containing a cows' milk derivative, which was thought to be milk-free.

**Table 11.3** Milk derivatives and possible milk containing derivatives found on food labels.

**Milk products**
Skimmed milk powder
Butter
Cream
Cheese
Cheese powder
Buttermilk
Yoghurt
Fromage frais
Dairy desserts
UHT milk

**Milk components**
Whey
Whey protein, hydrolysed whey protein
Non-fat milk solids
Milk solids
Milk protein
Casein
Caseinates
Hydrolysed casein
Sodium caseinate

**Other milk containing derivatives**
Butterfat
Spreads and low fat spreads
Shortening
Animal fat
Whey syrup sweetener
Artificial cream
Lactose
Flavourings containing lactose for lactose intolerance

### 11.6.1 Milk substitutes

Milk is a cheap, popular and valuable source of nutrition in a young child's diet and its contribution should not be underestimated. Half a litre of cows' milk each day provides 26% of the estimated average requirement for energy, 70% of the vitamin A, and 100% of the calcium and riboflavin dietary reference values for boys aged 1–3 years (Department of Health, 1991). In the absence of milk it is important that those young children who are unable to tolerate cows' milk are provided with a nutritionally adequate low allergenic formula, to provide a source of energy as well as other nutrients. Several factors influence the choice of milk substitute, including nutritional composition, evidence of satisfactory growth and nutritional status in children, palatability of the product, ease of preparation, cost, availability and allergenicity.

There are several choices of milk substitute including:

- soya-based formulas and drinks,
- protein hydrolysates – extensively and partially hydrolysed,
- amino acid formulas,
- meat-based formulas,
- alternative animal milks, *e.g.* goats' milk,
- cereal-based drinks.

### (i) Soya formulas and drinks

Soya beans belong to the leguminosae family, along with lentils, peas and peanuts. The globulin fraction of the soya bean is the major protein component (90%) and is principally composed of the glyco-protein, β-conglycin, and the amino acid glycine. Soya 'milk' was first used to feed babies with cows' milk intolerance as early as 1909 (Ruhrah, 1909). The modern generation of soya bean formulas is based on soya-protein isolate, supplemented with L-methionine, taurine and carnitine. There are now five nutritionally complete infant soya protein isolate formulas sold commercially in the UK (Table 11.4). The infant soya formulas are well accepted, economical and support normal growth, protein status and bone mineralisation. In the literature, the allergenicity of soya has probably been over-estimated. Early reports of secondary soya intolerance to cows' milk protein intolerance varied between 5% and 80% (Gerrard *et al.*, 1973; Kuitunen *et al.*, 1975; Jakobsson & Lindberg, 1979; Kahn *et al.*, 1989), but the results should be viewed with caution because in many of the studies, diagnosis of soya allergy was by clinical evaluation only. In more recent trial reports, including only cases confirmed by DBPCFC tests, soya protein intolerance is lower (Bock & Atkins, 1990; Businco *et al.*, 1992; Bruno *et al.*, 1997; Zeiger *et al.*, 1999). Bock and Atkins (1990) reported that only 7% of 54 children with cows' milk protein intolerance had symptoms of soya protein intolerance following a DBPCFC test. Cantani and Lucenti (1997) did a meta-analysis of 17 different studies of soya formula allergenicity and concluded that, from clinical history based studies with DBPCFC tests, the prevalence of allergy to soya protein formula was only 4% (see Chapter 4 for more information on the prevalence of allergy).

Owing to the possibility of secondary soya intolerance, some experts do not recommend soya formula as the first choice of milk substitute in cows' milk protein intolerance. There is particular concern that soya protein can induce enteropathy in young infants with and without cows' milk protein intolerance, with atrophy of the villi similar to that caused by cows' milk protein intolerance. However, other workers take alternative views (Zeiger *et al.*, 1999) and suggest that soya protein should be the preferred choice for children with cows' milk protein intolerance that is IgE mediated (Businco *et al.*, 1992) and/or associated with skin or lung symptoms.

There are a number of other soya drinks, *e.g.* Granose or Provamel soya drinks, which can be purchased directly from health food stores and supermarkets. None of these are suitable for children under 1 year, but some are enriched with calcium and may be useful for the slightly older child who refuses infant soya formula.

### (ii) Protein hydrolysates

There are a number of hydrolysed protein formulas available internationally, including both exten-

**Table 11.4** ACBS* prescribable infant formulas used for the diagnosis and treatment of cows' milk intolerance.

| Soya formulas | Extensively hydrolysed casein hydrolysates | Extensively hydrolysed whey hydrolysates | Soya and meat hydrolysates | Amino acid formulas |
|---|---|---|---|---|
| Farley's soya (Farley's) | Nutramigen (Mead Johnson) | Alfare (Néstle) | Pepdite 0–2 (Scientific Hospital Supplies) | Neocate (Scientific Hospital Supplies) |
| Infasoy (Cow & Gate) | Pregestimil (Mead Johnson) | Peptijunior (Cow & Gate) | Prejomin (Milupa) | |
| Isomil (Ross) | | | | |
| Prosobee (Mead Johnston) | | | | |
| Wysoy (SMA Nutrition) | | | | |

* Advisory Committee for Borderline Substances.

sively hydrolysed and partially hydrolysed formulas. They are based on whey, casein or a combination of meat and soya protein. Protein hydrolysates are the result of heat treatment and/or enzymic cleavage, which is used in order to produce peptides of minor antigenic activity (Rugo *et al.*, 1992).

Although a number of **partially hydrolysed formulas** are available internationally from a number of manufacturers, only two are available in the UK (Omneo Comfort 1 and Omneo Comfort 2, from Cow & Gate). They are commonly based on whey or a combination of casein and whey protein. They contain a high proportion of non-degraded proteins in the molecular weight range of 800–4000 daltons (Halken *et al.*, 1995). The advantages of partially hydrolysed formulas include cheaper cost, lower osmolality and some improvement in palatability. However, their indications for use remain imprecise. They are designed for allergy prevention rather than treatment, but a study on allergy prevention in 155 infants showed that, when compared to normal infant formula, partially hydrolysed formula had little benefit (Oldaeus *et al.*, 1997). *In vivo* and *in vitro* studies have demonstrated the superior efficacy of extensively hydrolysed compared with partially hydrolysed formulas (Niggemann *et al.*, 1999) and the latter have been shown to cause immunological reactions in children with cows' milk protein intolerance (Oldaeus *et al.*, 1991). A discussion of studies using protein hydrolysates can be found in Chapter 5, Section 5.9.

It should be noted that the partially hydrolysed formulas Omneo Comfort 1 and 2 have not been designed for either the prevention or the treatment of food intolerance. Instead, they have been produced for the treatment of common, minor digestive and feeding problems in infancy, such as colic or posseting. Other features of these formulas are that they have a reduced lactose content, and contain pre-gelatinised potato starch (to increase viscosity) and a mixture of the prebiotic galacto- and fructo-oligosaccharides. They are not currently ACBS (Advisory Committee for Borderline Substances) approved and hence not NHS prescribable in the UK.

**Extensively hydrolysed formulas** usually contain peptides with a molecular weight of less than 1.2 kDa because allergic responses, including anaphylaxis, have been provoked in animals injected with peptides with molecular weights of 1.3 kDa or greater (Knights, 1985).

There is now increasing awareness of clinical symptoms occurring in response to extensively hydrolysed formula (Ammar *et al.*, 1999). The European Society of Paediatric Allergy and Clinical Immunology recommends that, before a protein hydrolysate is given to patients with cows' milk allergy, the allergenicity of the product should be evaluated in each infant prior to treatment. This should be by a skin prick test with a sample of the formula. If the skin prick test is positive, they recommend an open challenge under the supervision of a physician, before the formula is given as the milk substitute (Businco *et al.*, 1993). This is rarely conducted in clinical practice.

Two **casein hydrolysate formulas** have been available in the UK since the early 1940s, Nutramigen and Pregestimil (Mead Johnson). The preparations contain free amino acids and short chain peptides with over 97% of the latter having a molecular weight of less than 1.0 kDa (Hudson, 1995).

Although there is considerable clinical experience with these formulas, most reports of severe reactions to casein hydrolysates (Bock, 1989; Saylor & Bahna, 1991; Rosenthal *et al.*, 1991; Schwartz & Amonette, 1991), including anaphylactic reactions (Lifschitz *et al.*, 1988), are relatively new.

The casein hydrolysate formulas available in the UK are nutritionally complete, contain added selenium, are well tolerated, produce normal growth and are approved by the ACBS, and are therefore NHS prescribable in the UK. However, they have a bitter taste (a result of enzyme hydrolysis), an unpleasant smell and are commonly unacceptable to the young child drinking from a feeding cup. In addition, they are expensive and Nutramigen has been shown to cause frequent watery, green stools (Hyams *et al.*, 1995).

Two lactose-free, extensively hydrolysed and nutritionally complete **whey formulas** are available in the UK. Three per cent of the peptides in Alfare (Nestlé) have a molecular weight greater than 2.0 kDa, compared with 7% in Peptijunior (Cow & Gate). Both formulas have been shown to be clinically effective (Taylor *et al.*, 1988; Siemensma *et al.*, 1993), and to produce adequate growth, although subclinical selenium deficiency was reported with Peptijunior (Taylor *et al.*, 1988).

Severe reactions to extensively hydrolysed whey formulas have been reported (Businco *et al.*, 1989; McLeish *et al.*, 1995). Whey protein trypsin hydrolysates will have epitopes in common with cows' milk protein, including those associated with beta-lactoglobulin, inducing an immunogenic cross-reactivity between hydrolysate and cows' milk proteins (Businco *et al.*, 1989). Practically, the same problems of taste, smell and cost are experienced as with casein hydrolysate formulas.

### (iii) *Soya and meat hydrolysates*

There are few published data and little practical experience to support the use of the two hydrolysed formulas (Prejomin, Milupa; Pepdite 0–2, Scientific Hospital Supplies) based on a mixture of meat and soya hydrolysate. Sixteen per cent of the peptides in Prejomin have a molecular weight greater than 2.0 kDa. No similar data are available for Pepdite 0–2.

### (iv) *Amino acid formulas*

With increasing reports of reactions to protein hydrolysate formulas, use of amino acid based infant formulas is growing (Isolauri, 1995; Ammar *et al.*, 1999; Hill *et al.*, 1999). There is only one amino acid based nutritionally complete formula designed for infants (Neocate, Scientific Hospital Supplies). It consists of L-amino acids, maltodextrin, safflower oil, soya oil, coconut oil, vitamins and minerals. Sampson and co-workers (Sampson *et al.*, 1992b) found that, in 28 children with cows' milk protein intolerance, 5 had positive skin reactions to this amino acid formula, whilst no child reacted to blind or open challenge tests. The product costs twice as much as most protein hydrolysate formulas and poor palatability is a problem.

### (v) *Meat-based formulas*

There is an increasing number of reports of home-made meat-based modular feeds being successfully used as an alternative to protein hydrolysate formulas (Cantani, 1992; Weisselberg *et al.*, 1996). In one study in three infants given a home-made meat-based formula, increased levels of creatinine and blood urea nitrogen, and metabolic acidosis were noted; but these returned to normal after the protein content of the feed was lowered (Weisselberg *et al.*, 1996). In the UK, a commercially available modular feed based on chicken meat is occasionally used for infants with chronic diarrhoea, caused by intolerance to cows' milk, soya or protein hydrolysate. The feed is expensive, unpalatable and allergic reactions to chicken have been noted (Vila *et al.*, 1998). The use of such feeds, therefore, requires close supervision by a paediatric dietitian. The use of meat-based modular feeds has not been evaluated in the management of cows' milk protein intolerance.

### (vi) *Alternative animal milks*

Goats', sheep's and mares' milks have all been used in the management of cows' milk protein intolerance (Egger *et al.*, 1989; Iacono *et al.*, 1992; Bellioni-Businco *et al.*, 1999). They are all nutritionally unsuitable if given in unmodified form to infants under one year, and they contain lactose. A goats' milk formula for infants is now available in the UK (Nanny Goat Infant Nutrition, Vitacare). However, the EC Directive covering infant formulas and follow-on formulas does not recommend goats' milk. There is evidence to demonstrate a strong cross-reactivity between cows', goats' and sheep's milks (Gjesing *et al.*, 1986; Egger *et al.*, 1989; Dean *et al.*, 1993; Bellioni-Businco *et al.*, 1999) and such drinks or formulas should not be used in the management of cows' milk intolerance.

### (vii) *Cereal drinks*

In the UK, there are two cereal-based drinks, one made from oats and one from rice, which can be used as a drink for children with cows' milk protein intolerance. They are of little nutritional value, are unsuitable for infants under one year and should not be used as a main substitute for cows' milk.

## 11.7 Egg-free diets

As with all foods, eggs are not essential in the diet of a child. However, eggs provide good quality protein and are a dietary source of vitamin $B_{12}$, pantothenic acid, folic acid, riboflavin, selenium and biotin, although these nutrients can easily be supplied by other foods. Eggs are used in a wide variety of manufactured products because of their excellent physical properties in food processing (coagulation, stabilisation and emulsification). A list of egg-derived ingredients, which may be found on food labels, is given in Table 11.5. Foods containing egg include cakes, meringues, mayonnaise, salad cream, egg pasta, Quorn and quiche-type flans. Other foods likely to contain egg or egg components include chewy sweets, sauces, biscuits and even malted milk drinks. The food additive lecithin (E322) can be derived from egg, although it is usually extracted from soya. Egg whites may be used as clarifying agents in broths or soups, and this may be a particular problem when eating out. Some baked products with a yellow colour or shiny glaze may have been coated with whole egg or egg white before baking. Some chocolate products may contain egg, but are exempt from the food labelling regulations. In the UK, it is possible to purchase egg replacer and egg white replacer based on potato starch, maize starch or tapioca flour. Egg white replacer is useful for egg-free meringues. The egg replacer acts as a raising agent in cakes and biscuits.

**Table 11.5** Egg-derived ingredients that may be found on food labels.

Fresh egg
Dried egg
Egg white
Egg yolk
Egg lecithin
Ovalbumin
Ovomucin
Ovomucoid
Ovoglobulin
Ovovitellin
Livelin
Vitellin

The measles virus used for the MMR (measles, mumps and rubella) vaccine is grown in chick embryo tissue. The safety of administering the MMR to individuals with egg allergy has been debated for years, but many studies have shown it is safe (Freigang *et al.*, 1994; James *et al.*, 1995). The Royal College of Paediatrics and Child Health (1999) recommends that close medical supervision is only necessary when this vaccine is given to children who have had an anaphylactic reaction to egg. It is not contraindicated in children with other egg intolerance symptoms.

Among children with an allergy to egg, the 80% who develop tolerance, do so by the age of 5 years (Dannaeus & Inganas, 1981). In the first instance, they usually tolerate a small quantity of egg in manufactured foods and cooking. Heat treatment, in particular, helps to denature protein and render it less allergenic.

## 11.8 Peanut-free diet

The peanut is a legume and not a member of the tree nut family. Peanut extracts contain many allergenic proteins (Clarke *et al.*, 1998) and are the most common cause of severe or fatal food-associated anaphylaxis in Europe and North America.

Exposure to peanuts can occur through ingestion, touch or inhalation, and even trace amounts can cause an anaphylactic response (Fries, 1982). Elimination of the following ingredients is necessary for individuals adhering to a peanut-free diet: ground nuts, mixed nuts, peanuts, earth nuts, monkey nuts, peanut butter, peanut flour and cold pressed peanut oil. Foods that may contain peanuts or peanut products include: African, Chinese, Indonesian and Thai dishes; baked goods such as pastries, cakes and biscuits; confectionery; ice cream; cereal bars; vegetarian products; breakfast cereals; satay sauce; curries; hydrolysed plant protein and hydrolysed vegetable protein; and marzipan (can contain a mixture of nuts) (Stoker & Castle, 1996). Minor food ingredients, which may very rarely be of peanut origin, include the food additives E471, E472 (a–e) and lecithin. Ethnic restaurants often use peanuts in a variety of foods, which makes it highly possible for cross-contamination to occur, so these restaurants should be avoided by those allergic to peanuts. Roasting and heat treatment do not alter the allergenicity of peanuts (Keating *et al.*, 1990). Travelling on airlines is a particular problem for peanut sensitive individuals owing to the circulation of peanut dust from opened peanut packets. However, many airlines are now using alternative snack items and airlines may remove peanuts from the plane on receipt of a written request together with a doctor's certificate.

Most UK manufacturers and retailers have voluntarily implemented full disclosure of peanut or nut content (Chapter 12). Packaging often has labels stating 'contains nuts' or similar phrases. Manufacturers may declare 'may contain trace of nuts' if a food item is manufactured to be peanut-free but made in the same area of the factory as a peanut containing food, thus providing the potential for cross-contamination.

The safety of peanut oil has caused debate, although refined peanut oil is probably safe. Cold-pressed peanut oil has been shown to contain protein. In 1981, ten peanut allergic adults were challenged with peanut oil and no adverse reactions were observed (Taylor *et al.*, 1981). Subsequently, Hourihane *et al.* (1997a) challenged 60 subjects, allergic to peanuts, with both refined and crude peanut oil and no subject reacted to refined peanut oil, but 10% reacted in a minor and localised way to crude peanut oil.

There have also been two reported cases of infants reacting to infant formulas that contained peanut oil. The reaction was linked directly to an allergy to peanut oil (Moneret-Vautrin *et al.*, 1991). Labial and oral provocation tests were positive to peanut oil in both children. The infants were calculated to have received 5 to 7 ml of peanut oil daily; its purity was not stated but it was probably refined. Rance and Dutau (1999) found that 17 out of 63 children with peanut hypersensitivity, tested by an oral food challenge, reacted to peanut oil.

Peanut oil is now easier to exclude from the diet as many companies have removed it from their products. Practically, it means exclusion of vegetable oil, arachis oil and ground nut oil. Peanut oil is sometimes used as a carrier for fat soluble vitamins and flavourings in food and (as arachis oil) can be an ingredient of soaps, lotions and toothpaste (McAlister *et al.*, 1997). However, some of the main supermarket chains and other manufacturers produce lists of their peanut-free lines to help with the selection of appropriate products, and ingredient labelling of cosmetics is now a legal requirement.

There is no convincing evidence of clinical cross-reactions between peanuts and tree nuts (Bock & Atkins, 1989), although there is evidence that multiple allergies to peanut and tree nuts appear progressively with age (Ewan, 1998). Ewan demonstrated that out of 62 children with peanut or tree nut allergy, 12 reacted to both peanuts and tree nuts. In addition, Hourihane *et al.* (1996) found a proportion of peanut sensitive individuals cross-reacted with tree nuts, *e.g.* Brazil nuts, hazel nuts

and walnuts, on the basis of skin prick testing. It may, therefore, be appropriate that, if a peanut sensitive individual has not yet been exposed to tree nuts, these are introduced with caution and singly.

## 11.9 Nutritional hazards of diet therapies

There have been several reports in the literature of poor growth and nutritional deficiencies in children on modified diets as a result of allergies, but the diets have usually been self-selected by parents or carers, or have been recommended and supervised by workers with little expertise in the field of nutrition (David, 1989; Labib *et al.*, 1989). Roesler *et al.* (1994) described nine children, who were failing to thrive on limited diets because their parents believed they had allergic reactions to multiple foods. Only two patients reacted during a DBPCFC test. One reacted to milk (one of 14 suspected foods) and the other reacted to eggs and milk (two of 15 suspected foods). David (1987) has described a 10-month-old child with eczema who had been diagnosed by a non-medical allergist as having an allergy to 57 foods. The child was placed on a diet consisting only of mashed potato, pure orange juice and pineapple juice. Not surprisingly, weight loss and failure to thrive accompanied this. In a survey of children between 5 and 11 years, those who were perceived to have food intolerance by their parents and were avoiding three or more foods were, on average, 4.2 cm shorter than children on a normal diet (Price *et al.*, 1988). Furthermore, the existence of scurvy, osteoporosis and megaloblastic anaemia in a patient with alleged food intolerance has been reported (Barratt & Summers, 1996).

Even simple milk-free exclusion diets have been shown to adversely affect nutritional status. Two separate studies have reported young children on milk-free diets to have a lower height for age (Tiainen *et al.*, 1995) and a lower weight for length index (Isolauri, 1998), when compared to healthy age-matched control children. Calcium intakes have been shown to be significantly lower for both adults (McGowan & Gibney, 1993) and children (Stallings *et al.*, 1994) on a milk-free diet. There have been at least two reports identifying rickets in a total of three children on milk-free diets; the rickets probably resulted from inadequate calcium intake (David, 1989; Davidovits *et al.*, 1993).

It is essential that all diet therapy, particularly in

children, is supervised by a state registered dietitian to ensure that the prescribed diet is nutritionally adequate and contains sufficient energy to support normal growth and weight gain. Growth, weight gain and nutritional intake should be regularly monitored throughout dietary trials. Appropriate vitamin and mineral supplementation should be prescribed as necessary.

## 11.10  Other pitfalls and problems of diet therapy

### 11.10.1  Risk of anaphylactic reaction during food challenge

David (1984) reported four patients who suffered an anaphylactic shock following open food challenges. Disturbingly, two of the four reactions occurred at home, following the ingestion of soya-based drink in one case and sweetcorn in the other, as part of the re-introduction phase of a few-foods diet. Where severe reactions are expected, challenges should always be conducted under medical supervision in the clinical setting. Parents or patients should always be informed of the dangers of food challenges.

### 11.10.2  Cost of diet therapies

It is often assumed that the special diets used in food intolerance are more expensive than normal food. This is the case for few-foods diets, which may cost two to three times that of a normal diet (MacDonald & Forsythe, 1986). For other diagnostic diets, *e.g.* milk-free or gluten-free, the cost differences are small, although there may be extra expenditure on special milk substitutes, wheat-free products or non-prescribable vitamin and mineral supplements.

### 11.10.3  Psychosocial effects

It is difficult to measure the true psychosocial effects of diet therapy that limits food choice. Such dietary approaches are likely to take extra effort and time, particularly in shopping and food preparation. Eating socially away from the home may be limited, and suitable foods can be purchased with confidence in only a few restaurants and fast food outlets. Many catering staff may not even understand adequately what is being asked of them when a customer concerned about an allergy enquires about the suitability of items on the menu; this is an issue that needs to be addressed in the training of caterers and chefs, and is covered in the guide *Catering for Health*, developed by the British Nutrition Foundation, for supporting the training in nutrition received by catering students (FSA/DH 2001). The problems associated with eating socially, especially in catering outlets, could cause social isolation. Concerns over potential dietary mistakes may cause anxiety for teachers, school dinner supervisors and other carers, which may restrict some of the activities a child is permitted to do, *e.g.* eat school lunches, or participate in school organised holidays, school visits and in any school activities concerning food.

### 11.10.4  Munchausen's syndrome by proxy

There are occasional reports of parents, mothers in particular, having an obsession with food allergy that results in bizarre diets and life styles. Warner and Hathaway (1984) reported 17 children from 11 families with the allergic form of Munchausen's syndrome by proxy. Most mothers were articulate and middle class. Management proved very difficult and many children remained on a diet despite exclusion of the diagnosis of allergic disease. Gray and Bentovim (1996) also reported a group of children who had illness induced by a parent. Allegation of food allergy and withdrawal of food was a common presentation.

## 11.11  Conclusion

Although the dietary management of food allergy and intolerance is very important there is also evidence that overdiagnosis and unsupervised dietary restriction can not only cause physical harm, but can be socially isolating and very stressful to both parents and child. All diet therapy recommended in the diagnosis and management of food allergy and intolerance should ideally be conducted by experienced health professionals, who have a recognised qualification in nutrition and dietetics.

## 11.12 Key points

- Although a clear history, positive skin tests and IgE-based laboratory tests can be strongly suggestive in some cases, dietary exclusion and challenge is the only reliable tool able to identify food intolerance. In less clear-cut cases, a double-blind placebo-controlled food challenge (DBPCFC) is necessary in order to confirm or refute the diagnosis.

- All diet therapies require dietetic supervision by a state registered dietitian.

- The use and duration of exclusion diets will depend on the diagnosis, severity of symptoms, age of patient and type of food excluded.

- Choice of milk substitute for milk intolerance primarily depends on the type of symptoms, the age of the patient, and the product's nutritional composition, palatability and ACBS (Advisory Committee on Borderline Substances) prescribability.

- Peanuts, the most common cause of fatal food-associated anaphylaxis in the UK, are becoming easier to exclude from the diet owing to full disclosure of peanut or nut content by most UK manufacturers. However, non-packaged food (*e.g.* takeaway and restaurant food) can still pose a major problem.

- Nutritional hazards of inappropriate or unsupervised diet therapy include faltering growth, low calcium intakes and rickets.

# 12
# Food Allergens and the Food Industry

## 12.1 Handling food allergens in manufacturing

Food allergies can be uncomfortable, severe or potentially fatal to those who suffer them, depending on the nature of the reaction (Chapter 6). The most common advice to sufferers is to avoid consumption of the trigger food. Superficially, this seems a relatively simple and straightforward means of avoiding reactions. However, for some individuals recognising, and thus being able to avoid, allergens can be difficult and time consuming as they may react to minute amounts of trigger foods, which are often widespread throughout a variety of foods.

All food manufacturers have an over-riding legal and moral responsibility to ensure that their products are safe and fit for the purpose intended. They must also comply with the relevant labelling legislation. The food manufacturing industry takes the control of food intolerance extremely seriously and has already implemented many initiatives to assist sufferers. This chapter discusses the steps that can be taken during manufacture to reduce the risk of transfer of allergens and the appropriate labelling opportunities that exist to assist sufferers of allergies to select foods with confidence.

In the UK and the USA, the majority of allergic reactions are caused by eight food types (see Table 12.1 and Chapter 6). The list in Table 12.1, which is not ranked in any particular order and is a slight modification of the list generated by Codex, does not include sesame seeds, but these can also cause severe allergic reactions and are mentioned in the leaflet *Be Allergy Aware,* which is now available from the Food Standards Agency (2001). These

**Table 12.1**  The most common causes of allergy.

| |
| --- |
| Peanuts |
| Tree nuts* |
| Eggs |
| Fish |
| Cows' milk |
| Crustacea, molluscs, shellfish |
| Soya beans |
| Cereals containing gluten, especially wheat |

* Tree nuts are listed by the British Retail Consortium (1998) as almond, Brazil, cashew, chestnuts, hazelnut, macadamia, pecan, pine, pistachio, walnut.
*Sources:* ILSI (1998), Codex Alimentarius Commission (1998), Codex Committee on Food Labelling (1999).

are the foods that have been considered in formulating the recommendations in this chapter. Peanuts (strictly a legume) and tree nuts are considered as a special case in manufacturing and retail as currently they are seen to be the major cause of food-induced anaphylaxis in the UK. Peanuts appear to contain one of the most potent allergens and are the main cause of severe reactions in adults (Chapter 6). They seem to initiate reactions in some peanut-sensitised individuals at very low levels. Additional controls at all levels of food production are often introduced to ensure that the presence in a product of even trace amounts of recognised allergens is communicated to consumers.

The main communication tool that the industry has is the ingredients list provided on the majority of products. It is important that ingredients lists are visible, readily accessible, accurate and legible. Food labelling is discussed later in the Chapter (see Sections 12.4 onwards).

## 12.2 Identification of allergens

The first step in identifying a strategy for managing allergens in the food industry is to be aware of the most common allergen-containing foods and food ingredients, so they can be controlled throughout the manufacturing process. Such foods vary from country to country, but certain foods are well established as causing allergy, and these are shown in Table 12.1. Additional foods need to be considered on a case by case basis, for instance celery allergy is seen as an important problem in France.

The eight food types listed in Table 12.1 are the cause of approximately 90% of food allergies in the UK and USA. With the exception of gluten-containing cereals, the other foods listed have the potential to trigger anaphylactic (IgE mediated) reactions. Other foods can cause reactions in a very small number of cases, and in fact the profile of foods causing reactions is in a dynamic state as the food supply and diet changes. For instance, kiwi fruit intolerance has been reported only recently because kiwi fruit are a relatively recent introduction to our diet.

Each product must be assessed by the manufacturer to identify whether recognised allergenic ingredients (listed in Table 12.1) are present. The best practice is to check all steps in the manufacturing process to ascertain whether foods or food ingredients containing allergens are present in the product, or whether there is any chance of cross-contamination with other allergen-containing foods during the manufacturing process. This detailed procedure should always be followed when reviewing products that may contain tree nuts and peanuts, and where the product claims to be free of a common allergen, for example milk-free or gluten-free products.

## 12.3 Good manufacturing practice

Good manufacturing practice (GMP) in the food industry is the series of controls used during production to ensure that all products are consistently manufactured to a quality appropriate to their intended use. GMP aims to produce safe and wholesome food through well-controlled operations that avoid waste and any type of contamination with allergens not normally present in that product. GMP should be applied throughout the whole production and supply chain and covers aspects such as raw material sourcing, hygienic design of buildings and equipment, production processes, food handling, storage and transport conditions, safety procedures, cleaning procedures and personal hygiene. Evidence of the ability to put into practice the principles and measures involved in GMP, and the actions that are taken at a particular manufacturing site, is essential to demonstrate that all reasonable steps have been taken to prevent errors, and indeed offences, from occurring.

The manufacturer of a food product must comply with the relevant legal requirements, including product composition, labelling, safety and hygiene. GMP is an overall system for control and maintenance of quality. In its broadest sense it shows that quality is not only the responsibility of the factory, or group of factories, but also of suppliers, contract manufacturers and all business partners. The principles outlined in GMP have been developed for large scale food industries, but they apply equally well to retail and catering environments, albeit on a smaller scale.

### 12.3.1 Allergens and GMP

The control of allergens in the food industry clearly falls under the remit of GMP. The presence of recognised allergens in products should be labelled since any errors or omissions have the potential to cause serious safety problems for those who are sensitised to allergic reactions. The areas of product composition, labelling and safety are particularly relevant to the control of allergens in the manufacturing process, and these will be discussed in detail throughout this chapter.

To claim a product is free from a particular allergen it must meet the following criteria:

- It must not contain the allergen as an ingredient.
- It must not contain any ingredient that contains the allergen, however small the concentration.
- It must not carry any risk of cross-contamination with the allergen during manufacture or packing.

Ideally, production facilities that handle ingredients containing recognised allergens will be specifically designed and built to enable complete segregation between products containing these ingredients and those that do not contain them. A factory producing foods that contain common allergens should ideally have the following facilities:

- dedicated equipment,
- screened-off manufacturing/packing areas,
- dedicated workwear and washing facilities,
- cleaning regimens and pre-use inspections,
- segregated storage areas,
- air flow management/negative air pressure in nut areas.

However, in practice, many manufacturing plants are used for the production of more than one product, and often one of the products contains a recognised allergen. Therefore, manufacturing plants on large and small scales can be divided into two categories: those that handle particular allergens and those that do not. Where dedicated equipment is not available, additional steps need to be introduced to control the presence of allergens and prevent contamination of other products with allergens.

### 12.3.2  Hazard analysis critical control point studies

Hazard analysis critical control point (HACCP) studies are detailed procedures that are undertaken to evaluate potential safety hazards, to eliminate them where possible or to find ways of keeping them under control. Such studies are an important part of any GMP plan. HACCP studies involve the identification of critical control points (CCPs) in a manufacturing process, by using a systematic and standard approach to hazard analysis.

The presence in a food product of ingredients containing known allergens (Table 12.1) should be declared on the label. CCPs, in relation to allergens, are those specific parts of a manufacturing process where there is a risk of the unintentional presence of allergens occurring through cross-contamination and where a specific control needs to be introduced to minimise the risk. CCPs include critical points in the sourcing and storage of raw materials, in the cleaning of particular parts of the plant following production and in the control of any waste that may be produced. Once CCPs have been identified, the risks need to be detailed and procedures developed to eliminate or control the risks of cross-contamination. Training, reporting and doc-

umentation of the actions taken are also part of any HACCP system to ensure consistency in quality control for every production run (Table 12.2). A practical example of a HACCP assessment is shown in Table 12.3.

**Table 12.2** Systematic approach to HACCP studies, related to allergen control.

| | |
|---|---|
| **Process step details** | What is the nature of the process involved? |
| **Hazard description** | Is there a risk of contamination with allergens? |
| **Control measures** | What procedures will control this risk? |
| **Modifications** | Can changes control the risk – what are they? |

Can the product be regarded as free from the allergen or is extra labelling required?

**Table 12.3** HACCP – Nuts: critical control point No. 8.

| | Disposal of packaging |
|---|---|
| **Hazard** | Contamination of other lines if nut packing materials are used for other purposes, *e.g.* storing other raw materials |
| **Controls** | Prevent use of packaging for other purposes to ensure no cross-contamination to other ingredients |
| **Person responsible** | Mixer operator |
| **Action required** | Dispose of all nut packaging materials once used |
| **Corrective action** | If nut packaging materials are observed being used for other purposes, report this to the LINE MANAGER immediately |

HACCP studies are invaluable in the control of allergens in the manufacturing environment because they give a clear indication of the risk of allergens being present in a specific product, particularly through potential cross-contamination from or to other products. HACCP studies should be undertaken on each production line and are a critical part of any GMP procedures used at a manufacturing site.

### 12.3.3 Cross-contamination

Cross-contamination occurs when small particles of a particular ingredient are transferred from a product, to which the ingredient has been added, to another product, to which addition of the ingredient is not intended. This can happen when two or more products with different ingredients are manufactured or packed on the same line. Cross-contamination of ingredients or products can occur at the level of the raw material supplier (who may process many raw materials), during transport or storage of raw materials or, indeed, during manufacture or packing of the finished product.

It is recommended that HACCP studies (as detailed in Section 12.3.2) should be used to evaluate all aspects of the supply chain, to identify any risks of cross-contamination with the recognised allergens listed in Table 12.1. In most cases, only minute amounts of an allergen are transferred from one product to another. However, it is clear that very sensitive individuals can react to extremely small quantities of allergens, so cross-contamination of any nature must be handled responsibly. Where a risk exists there are two options:

- to control the risk
- to use appropriate labelling on the product.

Peanuts and tree nuts are most often highlighted as potentially being involved in the cross-contamination process, and statements such as 'May contain nut traces' can be seen on a number of products. The use of the 'May contain...' statement is not a substitute for GMP and appropriate controls; it should only be used where a real and demonstrable risk of cross-contamination exists.

Important points:

- *Purchasing raw materials*  A detailed specification will provide information on the suitability of the ingredients for sufferers of particular allergies.
- *Distribution of raw and semi-finished materials*  Controls will minimise any risk of cross-contamination during the distribution of raw materials.
- *Storage of raw materials*  Controls will minimise the risk of cross-contamination whilst ingredients are stored. Clear labelling and correct segrega-

tion of ingredients will be important aspects of these controls.
- *Scheduling of production*  Organising schedules so that products containing allergens, which have the potential to contaminate allergen-free products, are manufactured following production runs of the latter.
- *Manufacturing*  All steps in the manufacturing process must be evaluated with respect to the control of allergens.
- *Reworking product*  Excess product that is reworked, in small amounts, back into production must be strictly controlled to ensure that allergens are not accidentally transferred from one product to another.
- *Air movement*  Emissions from a production area must be controlled to eliminate any risk of transfer of dust, containing allergens, from one area to another.

### 12.3.4 Confirmation of the presence of allergens

Once all the above steps have taken place, food manufacturers are able to make a judgement, based on all evidence obtained, as to whether a product contains or may contain or is free from a particular allergen. This judgement should form the basis of any information provided to allergy sufferers, to enable them to select suitable foods for their needs.

Analytical tests identifying the presence or absence in foods of proteins known to cause allergies are available. These tests can be useful but, in some instances, results need to be interpreted with care. In particular, it is essential that the sample of food analysed is truly representative of the entire food product. The sampling of liquid or fluid foods gives a relatively reliable sample as the food can be further blended to give even distribution of all ingredients. However, the sampling of foods such as breakfast cereals, chocolate bars and other more complex foods poses various difficulties. A random sampling technique could be employed, providing a number of samples from the food, but there is always a chance that the fragment of nut or grain of milk powder containing the allergen will be missed. The results achieved would, therefore, give a false negative, incorrectly suggesting that the product is free from a particular allergen.

Such tests should not be used to give definitive information about the presence or absence of allergens in a product. However, analysis provides a means of monitoring the effectiveness of the HACCP system, which should be undertaken on each product.

### 12.3.5 Labelling and communicating the presence of allergens in food

The food industry has a responsibility to consumers to provide them with certain information on the products that they purchase. The majority of pre-packaged foods have to carry an ingredients list showing all ingredients included in a product, in descending weight order. There are certain exceptions to this rule, for instance food sold loose or through catering outlets is not subject to the same legislation. The ingredients list gives manufacturers the opportunity to provide information that enables sufferers of food allergies to select foods with confidence. In order to provide accurate information, food manufacturers and caterers must understand the ingredients they use and the manufacturing processes involved, and understand in detail which products contain allergens, or are at risk of cross-contamination with allergens during production, packing or serving. The principles involved in GMP are outlined in Section 12.3.1.

The food industry must also consider the impact of other communication and promotional activities, such as product sampling, where allergy issues must be taken into account (Section 12.6).

### 12.3.6 Legislation

Manufacturers also have a responsibility to provide safe food for consumers, and this includes safety from an allergy sufferer's point of view. Responsible food manufacturers know that a number of foods and ingredients can give rise to rapid, life-threatening reactions in a small number of allergic individuals. The adverse publicity that might be received following an incident could be extremely damaging to the reputation of the product concerned and, indeed, the company, and this in itself is a stimulus for self policing. In addition, legislation, covering food safety and food labelling, exists to protect consumers. This includes that which directly relates to food, such as the Food Labelling Regulations, but, in addition, other areas of the law need to be considered, including relevant consumer protection legislation and requirements arising from the European Product Liability and Product Safety Directives.

## 12.4 Food safety legislation

The Food Safety Act 1990 (Anon, 1990) requires that all food manufacturers, caterers and retailers ensure that the food they supply is safe (for the intended use) and is of the nature, substance and quality demanded. The General Product Safety Regulations 1994 (Anon, 1994) apply to food where there is no specific provision under the Food Safety Act or any regulations made thereunder. As a result, information may need to be provided to consumers on any risks that a product might present in relation to a number of factors, such as the potential risk for vulnerable groups, *e.g.* allergic individuals.

A failure to comply with these requirements because of the un-notified, inadvertent presence of a recognised allergen (see Table 12.1) in a product, through manufacture or cross-contamination, is a criminal offence and may result in a prosecution even though no intention to cause harm existed.

There is, however, a due diligence defence available to manufacturers in the event of proceedings under either the Food Safety Act (Anon, 1990) or the General Product Safety Regulations (Anon, 1994), which would require the manufacturer to prove that he had taken all reasonable precautions and exercised all due diligence to prevent inclusion of an allergenic material. Manufacturers can reduce the risk of prosecution and contribute substantially to the establishment of a due diligence defence by implementing good manufacturing practice and documenting all procedures taken as evidence of good manufacturing practice processes, training and results, as detailed in Section 12.3.

### 12.4.1 Food labelling legislation

As indicated in Section 12.3.5, the majority of manufactured and packaged food products have, by law, to carry a full list of the ingredients they contain, in descending order of weight in the finished product (Fig. 12.1). There are currently no specific provisions made under either UK or EU food legislation that require potential allergens to be

---

**Fruit bar example**
Banana, apple juice concentrate, oats, cornflakes (maize, sugar, malt extract), vegetable oil, wafer (wheatflour, potato, starch, water, vegetable oil)

**Chocolate bar example**
Milk chocolate contains cocoa solids 22%, milk solids 20% minimum, vegetable fat, emulsifier (lecithin) and flavourings

---

**Fig. 12.1** Example labels demonstrating full ingredients listings, in descending order of weight in the finished product.

---

labelled. While there is a general requirement that all ingredients added to a food must be declared on the ingredients list, in accordance with the Food Labelling Regulations 1996 (Anon, 1996), there are certain exceptions to this general rule. These relate to compound ingredients (an ingredient that could be sold in its own right and is composed of multiple ingredients) that constitute less than 25% of the finished product. Other exceptions to the Food Labelling Regulations include generic terms (*e.g.* fish can be used for any species of fish); 'carry over' ingredients, such as additives, which do not have any technological function in the end product; additives used as processing aids; solvents/carriers for additives or flavourings; and those products that do not require ingredients lists at all, such as food sold through catering outlets.

A number of product categories are exempt from the general regulations outlined above and these include sugar products, honey, condensed milk, dried milk products, coffee and coffee products, spreadable fats and chocolate. Each of these has its own regulations and needs to be considered individually.

Manufacturers need to consider their legal obligations to inform consumers about the known or adventitious presence of allergens in a product, even where this is not a specific requirement of current food labelling legislation. There are many additional points to consider from a manufacturer's view. For example, it is essential to consider whether it is appropriate to give all relevant information in or adjacent to the ingredients list or whether an alternative location would be preferable. Where the presence of allergens is highlighted on labels,

the prominence of that message is important. Clear responses to these points are not necessarily available in law. However, where an ingredient is knowingly added to a food, the Food Labelling Directive (Anon, 2000) requires that its presence should be declared on the ingredients list. One major exception to this is the '25% rule'.

### 12.4.2 The 25% rule

This rule is contained in European food labelling legislation. It states that compound ingredients, *i.e.* those that themselves contain a number of ingredients (*e.g.* toffee, biscuits, chocolate chips), which are less than 25% of the finished weight of the product, need only be declared as the compound ingredient and not as the constituents that make up the ingredient (other than any additives it contains that perform a technological function in the finished food). For instance, where toffee is an ingredient of an ice cream, and is less than 25% of the weight of the finished product, it could be labelled as 'toffee (contains flavouring)', rather than as the butter and sugar that it contains.

Most manufacturers recognise the importance of providing information on the ingredients list to help sufferers of food allergies to select a suitable diet with confidence. To do this the ingredients list must accurately reflect the ingredients in the product, including those allergens that are present in minute amounts. Consequently, the majority of manufacturers voluntarily ignore the 25% rule and voluntarily label the presence of all allergens via the ingredients list. This includes common allergens (see Table 12.1) that are components of compound ingredients.

### 12.4.3 International trade

The progressive development of international trade is leading to an increasing number of products sold with multi-lingual labels, produced in one, or perhaps two 'European' factories for sale in several countries simultaneously. This situation is no longer confined to large multi-national manufacturers but also applies increasingly to major retailers who, in some cases, are now selling products with European labels. This creates a number of problems from a labelling stance. Firstly, where two factories produce the same product there may be a difference in the other products manufactured at each site and, consequently, a difference in the allergens that could potentially be transferred by cross-contamination. It is essential that the 'worst case' scenario is represented on the label. For instance, where manufacture is split between two factories and one of the production lines also produces nut-containing products with a real risk of cross-contamination, this should be indicated on the labels of both, via appropriate labelling (Sections 12.4.1, 12.4.4). This ensures a consistency of labelling and removes any risk of confusion or any inadvertent consumption of a product that may initiate an anaphylactic reaction.

Secondly, it is known that awareness of, and sensitivities to, allergens vary throughout Europe. The voluntary labelling of particular allergens is specific to some countries whilst for others this additional labelling is not deemed important. Potentially, the presence of an allergen could be mentioned on packaging in one language but not in another, and this is an issue that individual companies need to address. Imported products need to conform to the legislation and the voluntary labelling actions taken in the receiving country that sells the product, which may differ from those in the manufacturing country. This will ensure that consumers have consistent information to enable them to select products with confidence.

### 12.4.4 'May contain' statements

The statement 'may contain *nut* traces' is used to show where there may be small amounts of the allergen (in this case nuts) present in the product, most likely as a result of cross-contamination (Section 12.3.3). Currently it is most commonly used for peanuts and nuts. The statement must only be used where there is a real risk of cross-contamination and not as a catch-all to remove any liability. GMP (Section 12.3.1) and HACCP studies (Section 12.3.2) will identify real areas of risk and the need to use such a statement. Where it is used, it needs to be clearly legible and in a place where consumers would expect to find it. It has become common practice within the UK to place this statement at the end of the ingredients list and, where possible, in a type face slightly larger than that used for the ingredients list and similar to that used for the word 'Ingredients' (Fig. 12.2).

---

**Ingredients**
Wheat flour, sugar, hydrogenated vegetable oils, cocoa powder, modified starch, dried egg, dried skimmed milk powder, raising agents (E500, E450(a)), salt, flavouring, water, chocolate (contains lecithin and vanilla), acetic acid
**May contain nut traces**

---

**Fig. 12.2**　Example of labelling that highlights the potential presence of nuts.

---

The use of 'may contain' advisory labelling in relation to the potential, adventitious presence of a food allergen should be a last resort and it should never be used as a general insurance or a substitute for good manufacturing practice.

## 12.5 Brand extensions

Many brand names are now used across a wide variety of products, for example a chocolate bar brand name may be used for a dessert, ice cream, drink, chocolate spread, Easter egg, and for various shapes and sizes of chocolate bars. It is possible that individuals with a specific food allergy, and for whom the original chocolate bar is acceptable, may assume that the other products sold with the same brand name are also suitable. However, in most cases, different products will contain different ingredients, be manufactured on different production lines, in different factories, using different technologies, and may well contain different allergens to other products under the same brand. Each variant in the product range will have its own ingredients list. It must be stressed that the onus is on the consumer to check the suitability of each product for his or her particular dietary restrictions, using the ingredients list on the label.

## 12.6 Promotional activities

The control of allergens in manufactured products extends beyond production and labelling to all promotional practices linked with the product. Those that need particular attention relate to sampling of the product, *e.g.* in a supermarket. Product sampling can follow a variety of routes, but the most common include:

- Wet sampling – the product is served from a central location in a ready-to-eat or drink format, for immediate consumption.
- Dry sampling – a product that needs preparation is distributed from a central location in a format that needs further preparation.
- Door drop – free samples of products are distributed for trial at home.

It is essential that those using product sampling as a marketing strategy are fully briefed as to the allergenic potential of the product. Wet sampling of products, or the sampling of products intended to be consumed immediately, needs to be undertaken with great care as consumers receive the product without any packaging. Information must be available to advise consumers of the ingredients in the product and notices highlighting the likely presence of common allergens need to be displayed to assist sufferers of allergies in selecting whether or not to sample that product. These procedures apply to dry sampling also, but in these cases the product is often distributed in its outer packaging with a detailed ingredients list. Sampling to children can pose additional difficulties and should only be undertaken with parental consent for the child to take the product. This is particularly relevant with nut and peanut allergies, as the reactions can be severe, even in response to extremely small quantities of the allergen.

Door drop sampling provides an efficient way of inviting a large number of people to try a product. It, too, has difficulties. In households where someone is at risk of suffering an anaphylactic shock on ingestion of a particular ingredient, great care is taken to select foods that are free from the particular allergen to minimise any risk of anaphylaxis occurring. Sometimes, the entire household excludes the problem food, particularly where this is peanuts (or tree nuts), which are relatively easy to exclude compared with foods such as eggs or milk. This is particularly true in households with young children with severe food allergies, who are unable to read labels and unable to be responsible for the foods they choose.

Delivering free samples of foods containing the allergen through the letterbox removes the choice to select suitable foods from the family. A young child could see the food product on the doormat and consume some without parental knowledge.

Consequently, it is recommended that door drop sampling is undertaken with great care and is avoided entirely for products that contain nuts or peanuts. There are alternative options and these include distributing a coupon for the product, which enables sufferers of allergies to choose whether or not to sample that product, or a reply paid card which is returned if the household would like to request a sample of a particular product to be delivered. The latter two mechanisms put the choice directly in the hands of the householders and remove any risk of inadvertent consumption of a product by young children with a food allergy.

## 12.7 Labelling and handling allergens in the catering environment

Most food products sold through retail channels are in packaging that displays an ingredients list, enabling allergy sufferers to check whether or not a product meets their needs. Where products are sold without packaging or the packaging is removed before the product is presented to the consumer, the communication of the suitability of that product for allergy sufferers becomes more difficult. Within both the catering trade and some aspects of retail, communication of the suitability of products for allergy sufferers is extremely difficult because foods are sold without the advantage of labels showing the detail of the ingredients they contain. Allergy sufferers must take it upon themselves to check the suitability of any foods they select. If there is any doubt at all about a particular product or dish, the advice is that it should be avoided.

The Food Standards Agency (2001) has a list of guidelines for catering establishments to raise awareness of the issue of food allergies and to help caterers provide information for sufferers. These guidelines are equally applicable to small retail outlets. An extract from the recommendations is provided in Fig. 12.3.

## 12.8 Additional communication initiatives

The ingredients list on the label of a product is the most accurate way of assessing the suitability of a product for a sufferer of allergies. However, reading labels can be a laborious and time consuming process and can make shopping a lengthy ordeal.

### Advice to Catering Establishments

In case a customer asks you about the ingredients of a meal, aim to make sure that there is always someone on duty who knows or can find out the ingredients of all the foods you provide. If you are not sure whether there is a trace of a life-threatening ingredient in a meal then say so – never guess. If foods contain nuts, make sure this is reflected in the name or the menu description, for example, carrot and nut salad.

### Foods to Watch Out For

Many establishments often use nuts and seeds to decorate cakes, ice creams, speciality breads or savoury dishes. Other less obvious sources of nuts and seeds are:

- Marzipan, which is made from almonds.
- Hummus, which contains sesame seeds.
- Halva, which is made from sesame seeds.
- Sauces, such as satay sauce, which is made from peanuts.
- Products such as Waldorf salad, salad dressings and flavourings.

Customers suffering from severe food allergy will usually know about the foods they must avoid.

### What your staff can do to help customers

If you are asked by a customer, you must:

- Tell them what is in your food – exactly.
- If you don't know don't guess – find out!

### Remember!

- Even tiny traces of these foods can kill.
- Think before using nut and seed oils, salad dressings and seafood sauces.
- Don't let nuts, seeds and shellfish touch food that doesn't contain these ingredients.
- Clean your hands, work surfaces and utensils after handling nuts, shellfish and seeds.
- Think before cooking with oils that have been used to cook other foods.

**Fig. 12.3** An extract from the guidelines *Be Allergy Aware* (Food Standards Agency, 2001).

Most companies and retailers now produce lists of products free from common allergens, which make food selection much quicker and easier. The lists are available from the companies directly and are often on the Internet.

Once again, peanut and tree nut allergies are often handled as a special case as they are the most common food causes of anaphylaxis. 'Free from' lists, in theory, are accurate on the day they are published but out of date after that as product compositions and manufacturing conditions can change. In practice, product modifications are not undertaken frequently and updated lists are generally available every 6 months or so. In the case of anaphylactic reactions, information must always be accurate and up to date. Peanut- and nut-free lists are often controlled closely and carry a 'use by' date after which that list is invalid and recipients are asked to contact the company for an update. During the lifetime of the list, it is recommended that the names and addresses of all recipients are retained. Where changes occur to that list whilst it is 'live', all recipients can be contacted to advise them of the changes, be issued with a new list and asked to discard the old one. The distribution of the lists of individual companies to third parties, such as dietitians and doctors, is often not supported as this removes control of the list from the company. If a change occurred to a list, the company would have to rely on the health professional remembering which patients had received the list from them and passing on the updated information.

These detailed procedures ensure that the company has tight control over the list it has produced at all times and is in a position to do everything it can to help sufferers of allergies to select suitable foods with confidence.

### 12.8.1 Food intolerance databanks

Many countries throughout the European Union have food intolerance databanks managed by a central group, with information provided by companies. They collate information from various food manufacturers and produce comprehensive lists of products 'free from' the common allergens. In many cases, the booklets they produce (milk-free, egg-free, *etc.*) are available to health professionals, especially dietitians, who are then able to work with sufferers of food allergy to help them select suitable

foods and also to meet their nutritional requirements (Chapter 11). In the UK, the Leatherhead Food Research Association manages the UK Food Intolerance Databank, collating information from various food manufacturers and publishing 'free from' lists directed at health professionals.

The lists provide useful compilations of products suitable for particular diets, but are not without their pitfalls. Often they are updated only on an annual basis and risk becoming out of date even whilst they are still being issued. They can, therefore, help the shopper in the search for suitable foods but do not remove the need to check the product label. While these lists have a useful role to play in identification of suitable foods, they are not suitable for provision of information on nuts and peanuts (with which reactions can be very severe), as information can become outdated and could provide a false sense of security.

## 12.9 Manufacturing foods with reduced levels of allergens

A number of foods are available that have been specially developed to assist sufferers of severe allergies in having a balanced and varied diet. These are available both through normal supermarket outlets and/or through specialist outlets such as pharmacies. These can be divided into three categories:

- Foods inherently free of an allergen
- Foods manufactured to be free from an allergen
- Foods specially developed to be hypoallergenic.

### 12.9.1 Foods inherently free of an allergen

Foods inherently free of an allergen are those normal foods that do not contain certain common allergens. For instance, milk is acceptable in an egg-free diet, and fruit, vegetables and eggs are nut-free and acceptable for sufferers of nut allergies. These foods are available through normal retail outlets.

### 12.9.2 Foods manufactured to be free from an allergen

Foods are available that are specially developed for sufferers of allergies to replace specific common and often staple foods in the diet. For instance, gluten-free bread is a valuable staple food for sufferers of coeliac disease (Chapter 9). The current standards for gluten-free bread are described in Fig. 12.4. These foods are now widely available both through retail outlets and pharmacies. In some cases they are more expensive than their normal equivalent, but they do play very important roles in making the overall diet more acceptable and in keeping with the dietary patterns commonly followed by most people. The variety of foods for special diets has increased greatly and this helps to improve compliance.

### 12.9.3 Hypoallergenic foods

Hypoallergenic foods are those foods that, in the original state, contain allergens but which have been specially treated, such that the allergenicity of the protein has been dramatically reduced. The most common application of this type of technology concerns milks for infants and young children, where the protein is treated to reduce its allergenicity (Chapter 11, Section 11.6.1), which is brought about by alteration to the configuration of the molecule.

Very tight controls are essential during the manufacture of such products to ensure that they meet the specification exactly. Release norms are typically applied to each batch of hypoallergenic product that is produced, and these give very strict definitions of the composition that must be achieved before the product can leave the factory. Various tests are undertaken to ensure that the hydrolysis of the protein elements of the products during manufacture was effective and that the product is of the quality demanded to be called hypoallergenic. In the case of milk products, tests using electrophoresis and ELISA techniques allow the detection of intact proteins and other residual allergens.

A variety of very specialist formulas are available for the treatment of severe food allergies and these include hypoallergenic milks, to help reduce the development of allergy in at-risk children, and milks that act as staple foods for children who have severe milk allergy. These are detailed in Chapter 11, Section 11.6.1. Other hypoallergenic foods are manufactured, but infant milks are the most common food type available.

The control procedures identified in the earlier

---

**Gluten-Free Foods**

Claims such as gluten-free are controlled; for instance, Codex has published standards for claims that products are gluten-free and recommends levels below which a product can be classified as gluten-free. The standard for gluten-free foods applies to those processed foods that have been specially prepared to meet the dietary needs of people intolerant to gluten.

Currently, Codex describes a gluten-free food as:

- consisting of or containing as ingredients such cereals as wheat, triticale, rye, barley or oats or their constituents, which have been rendered gluten-free;
- in which any ingredients normally present containing gluten have been substituted by other ingredients not containing gluten.

The standards define three groups of foods, according to the gluten contents of the end product:

- foods from naturally gluten-free ingredients: max level of 20 mg/kg gluten;
- foods from ingredients that have been rendered gluten-free: max 200 mg/kg gluten;
- foods from any mixture of the above two categories: max 200 mg/kg gluten.

These levels cannot currently be monitored because there is as yet no reliable assay method by which to check gluten levels. The situation is being reassessed by Codex through a group of experts, which is particularly discussing the analytical methodology, the limits of detection and also the scientific justification of the levels outlined above. It is likely that a single figure for classifying foods as gluten-free, whether naturally gluten-free or rendered gluten-free, will be agreed.

---

**Fig. 12.4**  Current standards for gluten-free bread (Codex Alimentarius Commission, 2000).

part of this chapter apply equally to these products, especially where a claim is made that a product is free from a major allergen. Additional checks should be undertaken routinely to confirm that the finished product is indeed free from the allergen or contains only minute amounts that are clinically insignificant. There have been incidents where, despite a claim that a product is free from a particular allergen, trace amounts have been present, which have caused uncomfortable reactions in susceptible individuals. In such cases, problems should be reported to the manufacturer and appropriate checks and action taken.

## 12.10 Summary

The management of food allergens in the food industry is a complex and time consuming process, but one that is essential. The main aim of an allergen-handling process is to understand in great detail the ingredients and processes involved and the potential for allergens to be present in the finished product. The procedures outlined are those that should ideally be followed to minimise any risks associated with the presence of allergens in foods; they represent 'best practice'. Most companies take great care in controlling allergens but in practice problems occur on rare occasions, *e.g.* as a result of incorrect classification of an ingredient or cross-contamination during processing. Health professionals can help by reporting incidents to manufacturers, so that they can be investigated in detail, in order to identify the cause and the actions that need to be implemented to prevent any further problems.

The key steps in managing allergens in food manufacture are, firstly, to understand the constituents of all raw materials in detail, secondly to check all procedures used during the manufacture of the product for any risks of cross-contamination with allergens, and finally to provide accurate information to consumers about the allergens the product contains. All steps need to be undertaken thoroughly to ensure that even trace amounts of common allergens are detected. The processes involved in GMP and HACCP studies assist in this process. In all cases, documentation and training ensure that the processes are applied consistently and comprehensively. Controlling food allergens in the food industry is an essential part of GMP.

It is well known that sufferers of anaphylactic shock can react to extremely small quantities of allergens and it is for these people, in particular, that information provided about the product must be accurate and up to date. The labels of packaged food provide the best communication tool. Manufacturers must take responsibility to ensure that the labelling accurately reflects the ingredients in the product, and also any allergens that may be present through cross-contamination during the manufacturing process. But it is the responsibility of the allergy sufferer (or other members of the family or carers) to check the labels of products to ensure suitability.

Communication of the presence of allergens in food sold loose, without ingredients lists, and food sold through catering outlets will continue to be a critical area. Continually raising the awareness of allergen control in these areas of food provision is a key task, which is fundamental in ensuring that those who suffer food allergies are able to select foods and meals with confidence. Another important aspect is the inclusion of information about allergies in the initial training and in-service training received by caterers and chefs of all kinds. A guide, *Catering for Health*, which provides practical information for caterers is available from the Food Standards Agency (FSA/DH, 2001).

For the future, the control of allergens will continue to be an important aspect of quality control for all aspects of food manufacturing, including large scale manufacture, smaller scale operations and catering processes.

In addition, foods are now manufactured that are specifically developed for those who have allergies, *e.g.* protein hydrolysate formula milks for babies and young children unable to tolerate cows' milk. There are also foods manufactured to be free from particular allergens, and the most common class of these is gluten-free foods. These types of foods play very important roles in increasing the dietary variety of allergy sufferers, thus making appropriate diets more accessible and acceptable. Many products are available through normal retail outlets such as supermarkets and chemists, whilst the more specialist products, such as specialised infant milk products, are often prescribable.

## 12.11 Key points

- The food industry has taken steps to control allergens in manufacture and to provide appropriate labelling on packaged food.
- The majority of food intolerance reactions are caused by eight foods (milk, egg, fish, shellfish, peanuts, nuts, soya and wheat gluten). These should always be controlled in manufacture and labelled when present in a product.
- Systems such as good manufacturing practice and HACCP (hazard analysis critical control point) should be employed to control allergens during manufacture. Any controls introduced should be fully documented and included in staff training plans.
- Ingredients lists provide consumers with a list of components of a product and are the key communication method available. The majority of packaged food products have, by law, to carry a full list of the ingredients they contain, in descending order of weight in the finished product.
- Major allergens should always be included in the ingredients list when added to a product.
- There are certain exemptions to some aspects of food labelling legislation. Most manufacturers voluntarily ignore these when they concern allergens, so that information on the deliberate presence of allergens in a food product is made available to the public.
- Where there is a demonstrable risk that traces of an allergen may inadvertently be present, *e.g.* through cross contamination during manufacture, this should be highlighted at the end of the ingredients list, using wording such as 'May contain nut traces'.

- In many companies, the control of allergens extends to distribution of free samples, food provision in staff restaurants and the full control of allergens on factory premises.
- The sale of products without ingredients lists, such as in delicatessens and catering establishments, is an area where it is less easy to communicate the presence of ingredients that are the main causes of food intolerance. Allergy sufferers should be advised to ask for information and, if in doubt, to avoid the food.
- Most manufacturers produce lists of products free from the eight main allergens. Additionally, the Leatherhead Food Research Association has initiated the Food Intolerance Databank, which holds information from various companies. Leatherhead also produces booklets of products, which are free from particular allergens (available to health professionals).
- A number of foods are available that have been manufactured to ensure they are free from certain allergens, *e.g.* gluten-free products. Codex has published standards and recommended levels, below which a product can be classified as gluten-free.
- Where food intolerance is concerned, the main role of food manufacturers is to provide accurate information for consumers, particularly for those ingredients such as gluten and other allergens that produce severe reactions, so consumers are able to choose a suitable diet with confidence.

# 13
# Immunomodulation of Food Allergies

## 13.1 Background

The prevalence of food intolerance is estimated to be 5–8% in children and 1–2% in adults. A proportion of these reactions are considered to be attributable to IgE mediated allergy; the prevalence being 1–2% in children and less than 1% in adults (see Chapter 4). Although some allergic reactions are of late onset and not IgE mediated, it is only the quick onset IgE mediated reactions which have the potential to result in anaphylaxis.

While avoidance of allergenic foods is an essential part of the management of food allergy, this in itself is insufficient. Common allergenic foods such as egg, milk, peanuts and nuts (see Chapter 6) have such widespread use in the food industry that avoidance becomes very difficult. As little as 1 mg of an allergen in a food may suffice to cause a fatal anaphylactic reaction. Children with diagnosed food allergies frequently have repeated allergic exposures despite having received dietary advice. The response by sectors of the food industry has been to use extreme caution in labelling food products with warnings such as 'This food may contain traces of nuts' (see Chapter 12). Consequently, families of allergy sufferers spend much of their time reading ingredients on food packages. Children may be unable to participate in school meals, their social activities may be limited and they may be labelled as being different. Consequently, the quality of life of children with allergic disorders is considerably diminished, even when diagnosis has been made and treatment measures have been introduced (Primeau *et al.*, 2000).

There is, therefore, a real need to provide treatment for individuals with food allergy to enable

them to normalise their lives. Ideally, we would wish to modulate the immune system to 'switch off' the food allergy and enable the individual to resume a normal diet. There have, indeed, historically, been numerous attempts to do this, and the technique has already been successfully applied in other areas. Traditionally the concept of immunotherapy is to expose the allergic subject to sequentially increasing concentrations of allergen, until high dose maintenance therapy is reached. This includes a state of clinical tolerance whereby the process may take many months. This has been used very successfully to treat grass-pollen induced hay fever by injecting allergen subcutaneously (Freeman, 1911, 1927; Noon, 1911). The process can be accelerated using rush immunotherapy whereby the frequency of injection is increased and the maintenance levels of treatment are reached after 1 to 2 weeks (Freeman, 1930). This technique is used to treat hay fever, cat allergy, hymenoptera allergy and certain drug allergies. The effects of immunotherapy are allergen-specific and indeed allergen-specific changes in immunological function have been seen to occur both at the level of B cells and T cells (see below).

There have been isolated reports of attempts to desensitise patients to food by administering increasing amounts of the food by one of different routes until immunological tolerance was achieved. The first report of desensitisation to a food was described in 1908 where a 13-year-old boy with 'a case of egg poisoning' was reported (Schofield, 1908). He was treated by swallowing pills containing egg white and calcium lactate and taking egg in increasing quantities. Whereas before treatment he would develop immediate symptoms of angioedema, after 7 months of treatment he was able to eat four whole eggs. Another case of successful desensitisation to egg has been reported using ovomucoid allergen (Schloss, 1912).

In 1930 Freeman reported successfully using rush immunotherapy to treat a 7-year-old boy with fish allergy (Freeman, 1930). More recently, an attempt at rush desensitisation by subcutaneous injection of peanut was reported in a small double-blind placebo-controlled study (Lack *et al.*, 1996). This study highlighted the danger of traditional desensitisation regimens for food allergy. Although four treated patients in this study demonstrated increased tolerance to peanut on a second challenge, the risk of serious adverse reactions was unacceptably high.

## 13.2 Immunology

In order to desensitise an individual effectively, two immunological goals need to be achieved:

(1) IgE production by B cells should be diminished, and
(2) allergen-specific Th2 responses need to be altered (immunomodulation) or suppressed (tolerance).

There is a fundamental question as to whether it is possible in principle to change the function of IgE-committed B cells and Th2 cells. Changing the function of IgE-committed B cells in principle seems more difficult. During isotype switching from IgM to IgE, genomic rearrangement occurs in the B cell with consequent heavy chain rearrangement (see Chapter 2, Fig. 2.2). Once committed to IgE production, there is no 'going back' for the B cell to make IgE or other isotyopes. Thus, if indeed secondary and subsequent IgE responses to allergen are derived largely from a pool of memory B cells committed to IgE production, it may be too late to intervene and modulate secondary IgE production. If, on the other hand, secondary IgE responses result from IgM-producing memory B cells which must undergo heavy chain rearrangement from $\mu$ to $\epsilon$ (see Chapter 2, Section 2.4.3), there exists a window of opportunity to intervene and modulate secondary IgE production. There is evidence in the mouse that both polyclonal and specific secondary IgE responses are derived mainly from IgM-producing memory B cells. In a mouse model of allergy to ovalbumin it is possible to intervene and

inhibit secondary IgE responses even when nebulised IFN-$\gamma$ is administered to mice after they have developed a primary anti-ovalbumin IgE response (Lack *et al.*, 1996).

In the human there is no direct evidence as to which population of B cells (memory IgE-committed versus IgM-producing B cells) is responsible for secondary and ongoing subsequent IgE production. There is, however, indirect evidence that IgE production by B cells may be altered. Firstly, the majority of children with egg allergy and milk allergies lose their reactivity to these foods before the age of 5 (see Chapter 6, Section 6.5.1). This remission of hypersensitivity responses to food is accompanied by a decline in skin test reactivity and specific IgE to the food allergen.

Secondly, desensitisation to inhalant allergens by subcutaneous injection results in decreased cutaneous reactivity to allergens and a blunting in specific IgE responses to seasonal allergen exposure. Reduction in IgE production is further accompanied by an increase in IgG4 production to allergen, suggesting that this form of immunomodulation has a direct effect on B cell function. There is also evidence that changes in T cell function occur during immunotherapy. Following desensitisation to grass pollen or house dust mite, there is a shift from Th2 like responses to allergen towards Th1 responses (Lack *et al.*, 1997). Other studies looking at bee venom desensitisation show an allergen specific reduction in T cell responses accompanied by an increase in allergen-specific IL-10 production, indicative of a state of 'anergy'. In other systems of desensitisation there is evidence for the induction of regulatory T cell subsets. It seems likely that systems of immunotherapy that use whole allergen and involve extensive antigen processing and presentation will result in IL-12 induction with subsequent Th1 differentiation. Systems of desensitisation based on injecting peptide may lead to tolerance. In the latter, diminished antigenic processing by APCs and the lack of co-stimulatory signals to T cells may result in clonal anergy. In practice, it is likely that a combination of different immunological mechanisms may be involved and determine the success of individual treatment regimens. See Chapter 2 for a summary of the immune system processes referred to in this section.

## 13.3 Novel treatment strategies

### 13.3.1 Exploiting cross-reactivity between allergens

In the 'oral allergy syndrome' (Chapter 6, Section 6.4.5) there is an association between allergic rhinitis to pollens, especially birch pollen, and allergic reactions to cross-reacting proteins in fruits and vegetables (Amlot *et al.*, 1987; Ebner *et al.*, 1995). One of the most common birch pollen associated food allergies reported involves apple. Both B cell epitope and T cell epitope cross-reactivities have been demonstrated between pollen and fruit/vegetable proteins (Fritsch *et al.*, 1998).

Given that the oral allergy syndrome occurs as a result of cross-reacting allergens, one would expect pollen allergen immunotherapy to lead to a resolution not only of allergic rhinitis but also to the resolution of the associated food allergy. There have been a number of trials examining this question. Thus, in one paediatric trial for immunotherapy to birch pollen, 46% of children in the injection immunotherapy group reported an improvement in food allergy compared to 14% in a placebo group (Moller, 1989). Another study showed that 84% of patients with birch pollenosis and oral symptoms after eating apple reported a significant reduction or disappearance of their food allergy symptoms following pollen immunotherapy, whereas not a single patient in the control group reported improvement in oral allergy (Asero, 1998). In this second study, there was a marked reduction in positive skin prick test responses to apple in 88% of the patients receiving immunotherapy; and 69% of skin prick tests to apple became negative. Such studies now need to be replicated using double-blind placebo-controlled food challenges to demonstrate objectively that immunotherapy with birch will decrease oral reactivity to fruits. Clearly, the increasing identification of panallergens or cross-reactive allergens will allow us to exploit the use of immunotherapy with a single allergen to switch off a multiplicity of allergies.

### 13.3.2 Monoclonal antibody to IgE

The binding of allergen-specific IgE to high affinity IgE receptors on mast cells is central to the pathogenesis of food allergy (see Chapter 2, Fig. 2.7). Recently, humanised monoclonal anti-IgE antibodies have been developed that bind to IgE molecules. These antibodies bind to the third domain of the Fc region of IgE which prevents IgE from binding to its receptors (see Chapter 2, Section 2.4.3). This monoclonal antibody is unable to cross link IgE molecules that are already bound to mast cells. IgE receptor expression on mast cells and basophils is regulated by circulating IgE; and monoclonal anti-IgE treatment has the added benefit of downregulating IgE receptor expression (MacGlashan *et al.*, 1997). Clinical trials using this approach have shown success in the treatment of patients with allergic rhinitis (Casale *et al.*, 1997) and asthma (Fahy *et al.*, 1997; Milgrom *et al.*, 1999).

Such an approach might be used successfully to protect patients with peanut or other food allergies, and early trials are underway. This could be particularly beneficial to patients with multiple food allergies who have recurrent anaphylaxis. The drawback of such an approach is that long term antibody injections of anti-IgE will be required. A variation of this approach is where the consideration is to protect allergic patients with anti-IgE treatment during an 'induction phase' and then, while their allergen-specific IgE levels are diminished, inject subcutaneous allergen using a rush protocol. The main limitation in desensitisation trials of peanut has been the severity of side effects which prevented an adequate maintenance dose from being reached. Neutralisation of circulating IgE should in theory decrease these severe reactions and allow allergen desensitisation to proceed uneventfully to a higher and more effective maintenance level.

### 13.3.3 Immunomodulatory cytokines

Clinical trials with recombinant IFN-γ to treat allergic rhinitis and asthma have proved to be disappointing (Li *et al.*, 1990; Boguniewicz *et al.*, 1993). IFN-γ *in vitro* is a potent inhibitor of IgE production by B cells (see Chapter 2, Figure 2.6). *In vivo* treatment failed to reproduce this effect. Subsequent studies in rodents have demonstrated that for IFN-γ to reduce allergen-specific IgE, it needs to be delivered together with allergen, at the site of allergen exposure (Lack *et al.*, 1994, 1996). The reasons are:

(1) IFN-γ has a short half life;
(2) T cells do not constitutively express IFN-γ receptor; and
(3) B cells only show low levels of IFN-γ receptor expression.

Expression of the IFN-γ receptor on T and B cells requires activation through the presentation of allergen. It seems that similar requirements may exist for other potential immunomodulatory cytokines. Studies using a fusion protein comprising the egg protein ovalbumen and IL-12 in a mouse model of OVA sensitisation, found that this fusion protein of allergen and cytokine was most effective at decreasing OVA-specific IgE and increasing IFN-γ synthesis. Ovalbumen and IL-12 given separately were less effective (Kim et al., 1997).

There is, therefore, evidence that immunomodulatory cytokines may be used to decrease IgE production and promote Th1 like responses, but optimal responses require the co-existent delivery of cytokine and allergen. Other approaches have been used in experimental animal models, whereby the injection of the bacterium *Listeria monocytogenes* converted a Th2 response into a Th1 response (Yeung et al., 1998). This approach is now being considered in terms both of the prophylaxis and treatment of allergies, using vaccine products derived from mycobacteria.

### 13.3.4 DNA vaccines

Intradermal or intramuscular injections of plasmid DNA that encode for specific antigens have been shown to elicit prolonged Th1 responses in the host. In this approach, host cells incorporate the injected plasmid and synthesise low levels of the antigen. This has been successfully used in a rodent model with plasmid DNA encoding an allergen (Raz et al., 1996) and has also been used in an oral gene delivery system using the plasmid DNA for a major peanut allergen (Li et al., 1999). Mice immunised orally with plasmid Arah2 monoparticles had subsequently decreased allergic symptoms and specific IgE in response to Arah2, a major peanut allergen. This approach at least in animal models has associated problems. Firstly, it does not necessarily induce Th1 responses, but may augment Th2 responses, depending on the strain of the animal. Secondly, it seems to be less effective at diminishing

allergic responses once sensitisation is already established.

Another form of DNA vaccine is based on the injection of unmethylated cytosine guanine motifs (CpG). These nucleotide sequences, which are highly conserved in certain bacteria and viruses but not found in vertebrates, influence the host immune response and drive a Th1 like response. Approaches in animal models to inject whole allergen bound to these immunostimulatory sequence motifs have shown inhibition of IgE responses and augmented Th1 responses to allergen (Broide et al., 1998).

### 13.3.5 Engineered allergens

Site directed mutagenesis at a specific amino acid in an allergen epitope has the capacity to decrease significantly the ability of the epitope to bind IgE. This has been used to engineer recombinant major house dust mite allergens and recombinant pollen allergens to decrease IgE binding (Ferreira et al., 1998). The strategy is based on injecting engineered allergens which are safe in that they have a decreased IgE binding capacity, but maintain their ability to stimulate T cells. Such an approach is being considered in animal models of peanut allergy (Li et al., 2000). The problem in the case of such food allergies is that there are numerous major and minor allergens, each with several IgE-binding epitopes and it is likely that multiple amino acid substitutions are required. This may lead to alteration in T cell epitopes, which could compromise the efficacy of such vaccines.

### 13.3.6 Peptide vaccines

Defining immunodominant peptides on major allergens has allowed investigators to produce peptides that can be used for desensitisation. This also depends on injecting peptides that do not bind to IgE but have the potential to alter T cell function.

The potential difficulty is that different subjects will respond to different T cell epitopes, given the diverse HLA background of the population. One approach is to use 'peptide cocktails' that include the major epitopes. There is some evidence that even though only one or a few dominant T cell peptides are injected into animal models, bystander suppression is achieved and tolerance is achieved to rebuild peptides on the same antigen. Investigators have recently managed to hydrolyse peanut proteins, producing a diversity of peptides that show reduced IgE binding but nevertheless induce a proliferative T cell response. A different response is to develop a vaccine using overlapping peptide sequences for the major peanut allergens, thus ensuring that all dominant T cell epitopes are covered.

## 13.4  Conclusions

The past few decades have seen an increase in the prevalence of life-threatening food allergies. Although we are able to diagnose specifically such food allergies and in many cases identify the major allergens involved, there nevertheless exists a gap between our diagnostic ability and our ability to treat these allergies effectively. Advances in our understanding of the context of IgE synthesis and the pathophysiology of food allergy will allow us to bridge this gap. Our increased knowledge of the relevant cytokines and identification of target molecules offers a variety of potential therapeutic avenues to treat patients with food allergy. It is likely that modification of traditional allergen immunotherapy will increase its safety and efficacy, and combined approaches that simultaneously target different molecules will allow us to develop vaccines that can successfully treat food allergy.

---

## 13.5  Key points

- A variety of new strategies exist that should allow the development of successful vaccines to treat patients with persistent food allergies. Further experimental data need to be accumulated.

- It is likely that combined approaches, employing monoclonal anti-IgE antibody, immunomodulatory cytokines and altered allergens or peptides will lead to successful treatment regimens.

# 14
# Conclusions of the Task Force

Although adverse reactions to food and food components, in particular food allergy and intolerance, may not in reality be as commonplace as some people believe, they nevertheless have wide ranging public health implications. Not only can food intolerance restrict the food choices of the affected individual and so potentially adversely affect nutritional status, increase the cost of adopting a healthy diet and impact on the lifestyle of family members, it can also be socially isolating, *e.g.* restricting opportunities for children to interact socially with their peers via events such as school lunches, parties and school trips.

Furthermore, there are wider issues in terms of the implications for the food and catering sectors, for the health service (particularly emergency services and specialist clinics), for the training of health professionals and also the training and support of carers of people at risk of anaphylaxis, in particular schools which have pupils who may require administration of adrenaline.

There are also issues for government in terms of ensuring an appropriate legislative framework, including labelling and food safety, to protect the interests of consumers and meet their needs for information. There is also a need for government to ensure an adequate National Health Service in terms of resources to diagnose, treat and manage adverse reactions to food, allergic disease in particular because of the potential for life-threatening symptoms.

The conclusions reached by the Task Force are presented below, in chapter order. The recommendations of the Task Force can be found in Chapter 15.

## 14.1 Chapter 1

- This Task Force Report uses the phrase *Adverse Reactions to Food* to describe a range of different types of responses to food, in particular *food intolerance* (which includes *food allergy*), *food aversion* and *food poisoning*. This classification of terms is consistent with current practice in the UK, although it is acknowledged that other valid classification schemes exist.

- *Food intolerance* is used here to describe a range of reproducible responses including allergic reactions, adverse reactions resulting from enzyme deficiencies, pharmacological effects, and other non-defined idiosyncratic responses, each of which is manifest when the food is given without the subject's knowledge.

- Estimates suggest that no more than 5–8% of children and 1–2% of adults in the general population are affected by food intolerance. Among children, the prevalence of immunoglobulin E (IgE) mediated allergy is thought to be 1–2%, and less than 1% in adults. On the other hand, as many as 20% of people perceive themselves to be intolerant (or 'allergic') to some foods.

- Allergic reactions can either be IgE mediated and rapid (the most severe example being anaphylactic shock) or delayed and involve cell-mediated mechanisms (*e.g.* coeliac disease) or both.

- The most common intolerance linked to an enzyme insufficiency is lactose intolerance, which is widespread in some populations, though not in the UK.

- A number of food components can produce

pharmacological effects, but these are usually insignificant in clinical terms.

- Dislike and subsequent avoidance of various foods (sometimes referred to as 'faddiness') is commonplace and is referred to as *food avoidance*.
- *Food aversion* (dislike and subsequent avoidance of various foods in the absence of organic disease) has been used to describe a response to a food that is associated with sickness, nausea or gastrointestinal discomfort. Sometimes the associated symptoms are similar to those resulting from true food intolerances, which can potentially lead to misdiagnosis.
- *Food poisoning* has been defined as any disease of an infectious or toxic nature caused by, or thought to be caused by, the consumption of contaminated food or water.

## 14.2 Chapter 2

- Many of the adverse reactions described in this report are immunologically mediated, although this mechanism is the underlying factor in the minority of the totality of adverse reactions to foods.
- The immune system is broadly divided into humoral (antibody) and cell mediated immunity. These two processes interact with each other to generate the optimal mechanisms to provide host resistance against microorganisms, this being the primary function of the immune system.
- The immune responses directed against food constituents are no different in principle from those directed against invading microorganisms, it is just that the responses are directed against the 'wrong' target.
- Whereas the elimination of invading microorganisms by the immune system is beneficial to the host, the same immune responses directed against food constituents can result in tissue damage and disease.
- Ingestion of food normally induces a state of immunological unresponsiveness known as oral tolerance. The reasons why, in some children, this does not happen when new foods are introduced to their diet are unclear and warrant further study.
- Allergy is defined as the adverse health effects that may result from a specific immune response.

- Allergic reactions mediated by IgE antibodies are the basis of atopic asthma, atopic eczema, hayfever, IgE mediated food allergy and anaphylactic shock. Interaction between an allergen and IgE antibodies specific for that allergen (located on the surface of mast cells) results in the stimulation of the mast cell to release proinflammatory substances that are responsible for the symptoms experienced during an allergic reaction.
- Non-IgE mediated allergy, which is a delayed reaction featuring T lymphocytes (T cells), is the basis of the reactions associated with gluten sensitivity (coeliac disease), characterised by chronic inflammation and tissue damage.

## 14.3 Chapter 3

- Deficiencies of a wide variety of essential nutrients may impair immune function and increase susceptibility to infectious pathogens. Particular examples of those at most risk include premature infants and in malnutrition, especially in childhood, in old age and in the presence of infections, especially HIV.
- While immune function can be improved when deficient nutrients are replaced, as in institutionalised elderly people, an overcorrection of deficiencies, *e.g.* from zinc or iron, can damage the immune response.
- For some nutrients, the dietary intakes that result in the greatest measurable enhancement of immune function are above currently recommended intakes, but this should not be taken to mean that supplementation is the answer as excess intake of some nutrients can also impair immune function. There is no convincing evidence that the immune systems of non-deficient healthy people on a normal mixed diet benefit from vitamin or other dietary supplements.
- A high fat diet can damage the immune response. Fatty acids are, however, an important substrate for the production of eicosanoids, and fish oils may have beneficial effects which are the subject of on-going investigation.
- A number of nutrients can be shown to influence different components of the immune system in a dose–response fashion. The outcomes of these effects can also interact with one another and also with other substances, such as hormones.

- Relatively little is known about the relationship between nutrient status and function of the gut-associated immune system.
- Despite growing interest in the potential of nutrient supply to influence outcome in diseases involving immune dysregulation, the available evidence is insufficient to support recommendations.

## 14.4  Chapter 4

- The epidemiology of gluten sensitive enteropathy (coeliac disease) is fairly well characterised, with a prevalence of clinically proven disease being 1 to 3 cases per 1000 people. However, screening of the general population suggests there may be a significant number of latent/subclinical cases. The European consensus for the prevalence of all cases of coeliac disease is 3 to 4 cases per 1000 people. Superficially there appears to have been an increase in the prevalence of coeliac disease, but increased awareness and new serological tests probably account for most, if not all, of the increase.
- However, in general, it is very difficult to make meaningful comments on the prevalence of food intolerance and allergy to individual foods, and without further research it is virtually impossible to identify time trends and geographical variation. This is mainly due to the paucity of studies and the lack of consensus regarding standard working definitions, which has resulted in different studies using non-comparable methodologies.
- The limited data available suggest that a significant proportion of people (up to 30% of children and adults) believe they are intolerant of one or more foods. However, estimates suggest that in fact the prevalence of proven food intolerance in children is about 5–8% and in adults 1–2%.
- The prevalence of proven IgE mediated food allergy in children is about 1–2% and in adults less than 1% (typically 0.2–0.5%).
- In children, the prevalence of intolerance to individual foods ranges between 0.5% and 5%, with peanut allergy being present in 0.5%. In adults, the prevalence of peanut allergy is between 0.5% and 1%, depending on the study population.

- The most potent risk factor predisposing to food allergy is a personal or family history of atopy.
- In common with other forms of atopic allergy (*e.g.* atopic asthma), it is highly likely that IgE mediated food allergy has increased in the last 30 years and will probably continue to do so in the foreseeable future. No reliable data on these time trends are yet available.
- Both genetic and environmental factors influence susceptibility. Recent research has demonstrated associations between certain genetic loci and IgE mediated allergy. The relevance of these associations and the potential impact on them of environmental factors, such as changes in the patterns of childhood infection and consumption of dietary constituents, is under active investigation.

## 14.5  Chapter 5

- There is little published evidence to support any benefit of dietary intervention during pregnancy regarding the development of allergic disease in the genetically susceptible child.
- It is generally agreed that exclusive breast feeding should be encouraged for all infants for 3 to 4 months (for a range of reasons, many of which are unrelated to atopy). Exclusive breastfeeding for 4 to 6 months may be particularly important for infants at high risk of atopic disease, although benefits beyond 6 months of age are unclear.
- Early introduction of solids (before 4 months) may predispose high-risk infants (*i.e.* those with a family history) to atopic disease, *e.g.* eczema.
- Protein constituents of foods may be identified in breast milk but there is no consensus that this is harmful, even in infants at high risk of atopic disease.
- There is some evidence to support the exclusive use until 5 to 6 months of hydrolysed infant formulas in bottle-fed infants at high risk of developing atopic diseases. In some studies, the benefit has been similar to that reported with exclusive breast feeding.
- If dietary restriction is advised to reduce the risk of allergy developing in a high risk child, there is little consensus regarding the ideal dietary plan. Prevention programmes are costly and demanding for both families and health professionals.

## 14.6 Chapter 6

- Allergy can be defined as the adverse health effects that may result from the stimulation of a specific immune response. In the context of food allergy, the allergic sensitisation is induced to food proteins, substances that in non-sensitised subjects are tolerated fully.
- Allergy is not the most common result of adverse reactions to food; 2% of infants and young children are affected. In severe cases, allergy can be life threatening. In some cases (for instance peanut allergy), food allergy can persist to later life. Adult onset food allergy is less common.
- Individual susceptibility to a particular food allergy appears to be determined by a number of factors, including genetic makeup and heritable factors; the local environment, and in particular the environment during infancy; the age at which first exposure to the food occurs and the nature, extent and duration of that exposure; and the integrity of the gastrointestinal tract.
- Although an anaphylactic reaction or a strongly positive IgE antibody test is prognostic of food allergy, appropriately conducted challenge tests (preferably double-blind and placebo-controlled) are an important means to diagnose or refute food intolerances. The use of non-validated tests may lead to the neglect of other treatable conditions, and to unnecessary and often harmful dietary restrictions.
- Common foods that can cause food allergic reactions in the UK are hens' eggs, cows' milk, peanuts, various tree nuts, soya beans, fish, shellfish and wheat. Reactions to some fruits and vegetables can also cause problems.
- Allergic cross-reactions occur in some people. For example, people sensitised to birch pollen sometimes also react to apple and hazelnut; people sensitised to rubber latex may also react to bananas, chestnuts, kiwi fruit and avocados. Cross-reactions can also occur in people sensitised to clusters of substances, for example mugwort, parsley, celery and spices; or celery, cucumber, carrot and watermelon.
- Food allergic symptoms can affect all organ systems but often affect the skin, gastrointestinal tract and respiratory tract.
- Treatment of food allergy depends upon the use of a nutritionally balanced diet that nevertheless excludes the offending food, and the availability and proper use of emergency measures for severe cases.

## 14.7 Chapter 7

- In an individual with an apparently strong clinical history of food intolerance, it is important to consider and prove or refute whether specific foods are really triggering factors causing ill health.
- There is good evidence that particular foods and their constituents can affect the well-being of some individuals. While there is reliable evidence in conditions such as food-induced anaphylaxis and food-induced gastrointestinal diseases such as colitis, the evidence in other conditions, such as autism, cot death and rheumatoid arthritis, is far less convincing.
- There are also a number of conditions, including asthma, migraine and irritable bowel syndrome, in which food is merely one of the factors which may be capable of triggering symptoms without necessarily playing a fundamental part in the cause of the disease.
- Well-controlled prospective studies, addressing the question of food-related triggers systematically, are rare but are clearly needed.
- The role of diet and associated factors in the pathogenesis of migraine warrants further study.
- There is no good evidence that foods play a causative role in mental disorders.
- A subgroup of children with ADHD may show signs of food-induced behavioural changes. The size of this group of affected children is unknown.

## 14.8 Chapter 8

- Lactose maldigestion is the most common form of carbohydrate intolerance caused by an enzyme defect, although others do exist. Low levels of the intestinal enzyme lactase prevent the digestion of the disaccharide lactase to its component sugars (glucose and galactose) and hence lactose cannot be absorbed and passes undigested into the colon, causing a range of characteristic symptoms.
- Lactose maldigestion is uncommon in northern

Europe, although it is widespread in most other parts of the world. When milk is consumed, symptoms are typically experienced to varying degrees in people of Asian, African, Jewish and Hispanic descent. Lactose maldigestion can occur after gastroenteritis, but this is also uncommon in the general population. The degree of lactose intolerance, the duration and the symptoms experienced vary widely and treatment should be individualised.

- It is essential that any treatments used for lactose intolerance are safe, nutritionally adequate, closely monitored and have been adequately tested in relevant age groups.
- Lactase levels do not seem to be inducible in those with lactase non-persistence, but there is limited evidence that gradual reintroduction can lead to greater tolerance.
- Complete avoidance of dairy products is not usually necessary. Moderating milk intake, taking milk with meals and, where possible, replacing fresh dairy products with fermented dairy products, which are usually better tolerated, might be enough to keep the intolerance symptoms under control. Hard cheeses, *e.g.* Cheddar, contain only trace amounts of lactose and so are well tolerated even by those who experience symptoms with very small amounts of lactose (2–3 g lactose/100 g food). Such strategies enable calcium intake to be maintained.
- The tolerance of yogurt is, at least in part, thought to occur because the bacteria used in its production contain an enzyme that can aid lactose digestion in the human gut.
- Lactose-reduced milks are now widely available. Commercial lactase preparations also exist, both in a liquid form to be added to milk products before consumption and as tablets to be taken before eating lactose-containing meals.
- People who are very sensitive to lactose should be aware that lactose is widely used as an ingredient in ready-made meals and other food products. Such individuals are advised to check the ingredients labels of foods for lactose and to look for other ingredients that might contain lactose as a component, such as whey powder and dried skimmed milk.

## 14.9  Chapter 9

- It is now recognised that gluten sensitivity may cause a variety of conditions affecting the skin, the gut and possibly in some cases, the nervous system.
- Where the gut is the main organ affected, the condition is known as coeliac disease. This is a permanent condition, requiring a life-long strict gluten-free diet.
- Ingestion of gluten activates T cells in the small bowel, which initiate an immune reaction resulting in release of inflammatory mediators, particularly interferon-$\gamma$. This causes damage to the absorptive surface of the small bowel, which results in malabsorption of nutrients.
- Classically, coeliac disease is characterised by diarrhoea, weight loss and anaemia. However, these may be absent and many individuals may suffer from mild or non-specific symptoms, which may be ignored for many years. Delayed diagnosis can result in osteoporosis, infertility or even cancer.
- Coeliac disease is an heritable condition, with first degree relatives of sufferers having a 10% chance of having the condition.
- The condition is triggered by the ingestion of wheat, rye and barley. Oats are probably safe for consumption by gluten sensitive individuals.
- A strict gluten-free diet, which may include high quality wheat starch, is good protection against the long term complications of gluten sensitivity, particularly cancer.
- Small intestinal biopsy remains the gold standard for diagnosis of coeliac disease. However, use of improved serological tests has aided screening programmes, which indicate that in various countries throughout Europe the prevalence of gluten sensitivity is 1 in 250 to 1 in 300 of the population. There are areas, such as parts of Ireland, where this figure may be as high as 1 in 100.
- The skin can be affected by gluten sensitivity in a condition known as dermatitis herpetiformis. Individuals with this condition almost always have some degree of enteropathy, so a gluten-free diet is recommended.
- Gluten sensitivity may be associated with a number of neurological conditions, such as epilepsy. The nature of the association between

gluten and the nervous system remains obscure.

- Measurement of gluten contamination in foodstuffs is difficult. Legislation to protect the consumer is in place, and will be tightened up when improved methods of measurement of gluten are available.

## 14.10 Chapter 10

- The diagnosis of a food intolerance (including food allergy) depends mainly on taking a careful history, clinical suspicion and a positive response to therapeutic measures. If an IgE antibody mediated disorder is suspected, skin tests and *in vitro* tests of food-specific IgE antibodies are helpful and often diagnostic in patients with immediate reactions.
- The double-blind placebo-controlled food challenge is considered the gold standard for the diagnosis of a (often delayed) food intolerance reaction. This test requires specialist knowledge and clinical supervision.
- Great care needs to be taken when challenging patients suspected to be at risk of anaphylaxis, and tests should be conducted only under supervision in a clinical setting.
- Other specialist tests of proven value and available via hospitals include endoscopic investigations and intestinal permeability tests.
- The value of many other tests offered direct to the public, *e.g.* via the Internet and magazine advertisements, is unproven. The tests quoted have not been validated and advice based on them can be unsafe. Diets based on diagnoses arising from these tests are highly inappropriate and unreliable, and provision of dietary advice by unqualified practitioners is particularly hazardous for children.

## 14.11 Chapter 11

- Although a clear history, positive skin tests and IgE-based laboratory tests can be strongly suggestive in some cases, dietary exclusion and challenge is the only reliable tool able to identify food intolerance. In less clear-cut cases, a double-blind placebo-controlled food challenge (DBPCFC) is necessary in order to confirm or refute the diagnosis.

- All diet therapies require dietetic supervision by a state registered dietitian.
- The use and duration of exclusion diets will depend on the diagnosis, severity of symptoms, age of patient and type of food excluded.
- Choice of milk substitute for milk intolerance primarily depends on the type of symptoms, the age of the patient and the product's nutritional composition, palatability and ACBS (Advisory Committee on Borderline Substances) prescribability.
- Peanuts, the most common cause of fatal food-associated anaphylaxis in the UK, are becoming easier to exclude from the diet owing to full disclosure of peanut or nut content by most UK manufacturers. However, non-packaged food (*e.g.* takeaway and restaurant food) can still pose a major problem.
- Nutritional hazards of inappropriate or unsupervised diet therapy include faltering growth, low calcium intakes and rickets.

## 14.12 Chapter 12

- The food industry has taken steps to control allergens in manufacture and to provide appropriate labelling on packaged food.
- The majority of food intolerance reactions are caused by eight foods (milk, egg, fish, shellfish, peanuts, nuts, soya and wheat gluten). These should always be controlled in manufacture and labelled when present in a product.
- Systems such as good manufacturing practice and HACCP (hazard analysis critical control point) should be employed to control allergens during manufacture. Any controls introduced should be fully documented and included in staff training plans.
- Ingredients lists provide consumers with a list of components of a product and are the key communication method available. The majority of packaged food products have, by law, to carry a full list of the ingredients they contain, in descending order of weight in the finished product.
- Major allergens should always be included in the ingredients list when added to a product.
- There are certain exemptions to some aspects of food labelling legislation. Most manufacturers voluntarily ignore these when they concern allergens, so that information on the deliberate

presence of allergens in a food product is made available to the public.

- Where there is a demonstrable risk that traces of an allergen may inadvertently be present, *e.g.* through cross contamination during manufacture, this should be highlighted at the end of the ingredients list, using wording such as 'May contain nut traces'.
- In many companies, the control of allergens extends to distribution of free samples, food provision in staff restaurants and the full control of allergens on factory premises.
- The sale of products without ingredients lists, such as in delicatessens and catering establishments, is an area where it is less easy to communicate the presence of ingredients that are the main causes of food intolerance. Allergy sufferers should be advised to ask for information and, if in doubt, to avoid the food.
- Most manufacturers produce lists of products free from the eight main allergens. Additionally, the Leatherhead Food Research Association has initiated the Food Intolerance Databank, which holds information from various companies. Leatherhead also produces booklets of products, which are free from particular allergens (available to health professionals).

- A number of foods are available that have been manufactured to ensure they are free from certain allergens, *e.g.* gluten-free products. Codex has published standards and recommended levels, below which a product can be classified as gluten-free.
- Where food intolerance is concerned, the main role of food manufacturers is to provide accurate information for consumers, particularly for those ingredients such as gluten and other allergens that produce severe reactions, so consumers are able to choose a suitable diet with confidence.

## 14.13  Chapter 13

- A variety of new strategies exist that should allow the development of successful vaccines to treat patients with persistent food allergies. Further experimental data need to be accumulated.
- It is likely that combined approaches, employing monoclonal anti-IgE antibody, immunomodulatory cytokines and altered allergens or peptides will lead to successful treatment regimens.

# 15
# Recommendations of the Task Force

## 15.1 General recommendations

- There is a need for better safeguards to protect the public against false diagnostic methods and inappropriate diets (Chapter 10).
- There is a need for an accreditation scheme for laboratories involved in diagnostic tests for adverse reactions to foods, particularly those that offer diagnostic tests direct to the public.
- To protect the public, there is a need to establish an accreditation system for practitioners offering diagnostic tests to the general public. In the first instance, such a scheme could be voluntary.
- There is an urgent need for some sectors of the media to adopt a more responsible attitude to the reporting of information about food allergy and intolerance. Too often the articles on this subject are at best based on anecdote and frequently include or are based on misinterpretations of the available evidence and misuse of the terminology used to describe the various forms of adverse reaction, *e.g.* an overuse of the term 'allergy'.
- There is a need to establish national centres of excellence for the consolidation of clinical research and the diagnosis and treatment of food intolerance (in particular allergy). These would act as hubs and provide the opportunity for district general hospitals to link into the national network. Such a venture would carry with it the need for training specialists in immunology, allergy and other related disciplines.
- There is an urgent need to raise the awareness of all health professionals, both as part of initial training and in continued professional development, of current estimates of the true prevalence of food intolerance, the recommended proce-

dures for diagnosis and management, and of the many myths and half truths that are popularised in the press and through other media channels, including the Internet.
- There is a need for GPs and those in hospital casualty departments to be aware of the diversity of adverse reactions to foods that exist, the typical symptoms and the particular risks associated with severe reactions.
- There is a general need for support for the training and provision of guidance for those whose help might be needed to assist a severely allergic individual. This includes schools, nurseries, child minders and those in charge of after school activities such as brownies and cubs. This need also applies to catering establishments of all types. The guidance should cover how to recognise an anaphylactic reaction and the key trigger foods, the need to contact emergency services immediately and the consequences of any delay in getting appropriate medical help for the person. In some cases, *e.g.* schools, it may be necessary to train individuals in the procedures for administering adrenaline (Chapter 6).
- There is a need to continue to raise awareness of food intolerance, in particular allergy, amongst all manufacturers and caterers (including food service staff, *e.g.* waiters) (Chapter 12). The practice of making up-to-date product information available to consumers and to health professionals should be encouraged.
- Manufacturers have responded to the needs of consumers for on-pack information about the presence (or potential presence) of allergens associated with serious symptoms. However, more can still be done and manufacturers should

177

be encouraged to share information and promote best practice related to the control of allergens and communication about the presence of allergens throughout all areas of the food chain.

- There is also a need to continue to promote the use of practical guidelines, such as the Food and Drink Federation's Advice Notes, the Institute of Grocery Distribution's Food Allergy Guidelines and the Food Standards Agency's *Be Allergy Aware: Advice for Catering Establishments* leaflet and poster (Chapter 12).
- There is a need to work towards an agreed EU list of foods that provoke allergic responses, for which inclusion in the ingredients listing on packaging will always be required. This list should include those foods that are the most common causes of allergic reactions.
- There may be benefits in establishing a system through which health professionals could report adverse reactions to food, *e.g.* a national register of confirmed food allergy.
- Studies conducted in other parts of Europe suggest that there may be a considerable number of cases of coeliac disease that remain undiagnosed. Consideration should be given to the benefits of using new developments in serological testing to screen all children at the age of 18 months.

## 15.2 Recommendations for research priorities

### 15.2.1 Sensitisation to food allergens and understanding food allergy

- There is a need for a more detailed understanding of the mechanisms that result in sensitisation to food allergens (Chapters 2, 5 and 6).
- Associated with the above, a greater understanding of the nature and induction of immunological tolerance to food proteins is required, together with an appreciation of the role of tolerance breakdown in the development of sensitisation (Chapters 2, 5 and 6).
- There is an urgent need to understand whether maternal diet, and exposure to food allergens, during pregnancy and lactation affects the development of sensitisation in infants (Chapter 5).
- In particular, it is important to clarify whether specific modifications to the mother's diet (or

other aspects of lifestyle) during pregnancy and lactation carry any benefits (or risks), and whether there is any specific advantage to the baby of particular infant feeding regimens (Chapters 5 and 11).

- There is a requirement to develop robust methods for identifying and characterising protein allergens. Coupled with this is the need to define the molecular, biochemical and structural features of proteins that confer on them the ability to induce allergic sensitisation (Chapters 2 and 6).
- Associated with the above is a need to understand differences in the nature of food allergic reactions to proteins. For instance, why is it that allergy to some proteins is persistent and severe, while responses to other proteins are often less vigorous and transient (Chapter 6)?
- It is important to try and gauge, particularly with the more common food allergens, the levels of exposure which are required for the induction of sensitisation and those that are required for elicitation of reactions in those who are already sensitised (Chapters 2 and 6).
- Opportunities for reducing (by plant breeding or by appropriate biotechnology) the levels of allergens in some important food sources should be explored (Chapter 13).
- The possibility of developing robust methods for treatment of food allergy by desensitisation or hyposensitisation should be explored (Chapter 13).

### 15.2.2 Epidemiology of food intolerance

The epidemiology of food intolerance is poorly characterised (Chapter 4) and the studies published to date have a number of limitations, which confound their interpretation. Current estimates are based on a limited number of population studies, the results of which are not directly comparable and which have involved different populations. Although there is evidence that the prevalence of allergic disease has increased, there are no comparable time trend data for food intolerance.

- There is a need for better information on the prevalence of food allergy and food intolerance in the UK. Such data should be collected using a large and representative population sample and by applying appropriate objective criteria, such as double-blind placebo-controlled food challenges.

- Also required is a large prospective European collaborative multi-centre study, designed to characterise the prevalence of all forms of food intolerance in defined populations using clear, concise and practical definitions and methodology. In addition to providing high quality data on the prevalence of the various forms of food intolerance to different foods, such a study would also be able to adjust for the effects of confounding and, consequently, might also help in the understanding of geographical variations and aetiological factors.

- The question of whether the prevalence of food allergy is increasing, as seems to be the case for other atopic allergic diseases such as asthma, should be addressed. This will require a series of cross-sectional studies, over a period of time, in age subgroups of the same population (Chapter 4).

- Associated with the above, and relevant to atopic allergic disease in general, is a need to clarify the environmental and heritable factors that influence susceptibility and form the basis of inter-individual differences. Included here should be consideration of the influence of nutritional status and gastrointestinal function (Chapters 3 and 6).

- There is evidence of genetic variation in the predisposition to food intolerance, particularly allergy, and hence the potential existence of subgroups of patients that may benefit from dietary (or other) intervention. There is a need to work towards the identification of markers of risk, using the latest gene technology and studying the effect of genetic variation on protein expression and metabolism.

- There is a need to understand the true underlying prevalence of gluten sensitivity in the UK (studies are underway to address this), and to clarify the impact of environmental factors (including early diet) on the underlying genetic inheritance of a predisposition to the condition (Chapter 9).

### 15.2.3 Coeliac disease

- There are a number of important areas for research in the field of coeliac disease, all of which are receiving attention (Chapter 9). However some of these, particularly the genetic aspects, are extremely expensive and may be held back by financial constraints. Current projects need to be supported further, as well as encouragement given to new initiatives. As in many areas of research, a large amount of money is wasted by duplication of effort. Well co-ordinated collaborative projects should be encouraged. An interface between clinicians, scientists and the food industry is essential.

- Various candidate regions within the genome that are associated with coeliac disease have been identified, and there is a need for further investigation. Identification of predisposing gene(s) may help to illuminate the primary defect that underlies the condition and aid identification of patients.

- There is a need for a better understanding of the primary events that result in an inability to tolerate dietary gluten. These may be events that occur prior to activation of gluten sensitive T cells in the small bowel.

- Further efforts are required to produce a high quality gluten standard for use in laboratories worldwide, such that it is easier to compare the results from various studies.

- A standard method for gluten analysis on-line in the food processing setting is required.

- Large scale double-blind placebo-controlled studies are required to clarify whether there is a relationship between gluten and autism.

### 15.2.4 Other forms of food intolerance

- There is a need for better diagnostic criteria and standardisation of procedures used in the study of the role of food in the aetiology and/or exacerbation of a range of conditions, such as attention deficit hyperactivity disorder, irritable bowel syndrome and migraine (Chapter 7).

- Well-conducted prospective studies, investigating food-related triggers of non-immune food intolerance reactions are needed (Chapter 7).

- Investigation of the role of diet and associated factors in the pathogenesis of migraine is warranted (Chapter 7).

### 15.2.5 Diagnosis

- There is a need for an improved battery of reliable and simple tests that will assist in the diagnosis of adverse reactions to food (Chapters 7 and 10).
- There is a need for improvements in the range of standardised test reagents for RAST and skin prick tests (Chapter 10).
- There is a need for agreed criteria for the objective interpretation of double-blind placebo-controlled food challenges (Chapter 11).
- With regard to the host of non-validated tests proffered for the diagnosis of food intolerance, the onus should be on those offering these tests to provide solid evidence of the efficacy, safety and value of such techniques (Chapter 10). It may be worthwhile establishing standardised protocols for the evaluation of such tests.
- It is important that the contributions of complementary medicine to the prevention and management of allergic reactions are explored and evaluated.

### 15.2.6 Dietary management of food intolerance

- There is a need to investigate the prevalence of milk protein hydrolysate intolerance in cows' milk protein intolerance.
- There is an urgent need for evaluation of the dietary, anthropometric, biochemical and nutritional status of patients on long term dietary restriction (whether self-diagnosed or following the advice of medical experts), compared with the normal healthy population.
- There is a need for evaluation of the psychological and social impact of diet therapy in children with food intolerance. There is also the need for a better understanding of the socio-economic impact on patients and their families of following exclusion diets for long periods of time.
- Although it is recognised that allergic reactions to foods may exacerbate existing atopic allergic disease, often the aetiology of these conditions (*e.g.* asthma) is not understood, and may well have had nothing to do with food. The place of dietary restriction in the management of allergic disease, *e.g.* asthma and atopic eczema, particularly in adults, needs clarification.
- Recent studies have suggested that subjects with lactose maldigestion, resulting from lactase deficiency, can develop a tolerance to lactose-containing foods by starting with a low intake and gradually increasing the amount eaten by modest amounts (Chapter 8). Further work is needed to clarify whether this is a technique that could be applied widely among the 70% of the world's population that is lactase deficient in adult life, hence expanding the dietary variety to which they have access.
- There is also a need to investigate the potential for misdiagnosis of lactase intolerance, *e.g.* being confused with irritable bowel syndrome.

# 16
# Questions on Food Allergy and Intolerance

## Definitions of food allergy and intolerance

### (1) What is the definition of food allergy?

An allergic reaction to a food can be described as an inappropriate reaction by the body's immune system to the ingestion of a food that in the majority of individuals causes no adverse effects. Allergic reactions to foods vary in severity and can be potentially fatal. In food allergy the immune system does not recognise as safe a protein component of the food to which the individual is sensitive (such as some proteins in peanuts). This component is termed the allergen. The immune system then typically produces immunoglobulin E (IgE) antibodies to the allergen, which trigger other cells to release substances that cause inflammation. Allergic reactions are usually localised to a particular part of the body and symptoms may include asthma, eczema, flushing and swelling of tissues (*e.g.* the lips) or difficulty in breathing. A severe reaction may result in anaphylaxis (as with severe peanut allergy) in which there is a rapid fall in blood pressure and severe shock. Food allergy is relatively rare, affecting an estimated 1–2% of children and less than 1% of adults (see Question 7), and is often wrongly used as a general term for adverse reactions to food (Chapter 1) (and for food aversion, see Question 5).

### (2) Are there different types of allergy?

There are two well-defined mechanisms via which allergic reactions to food (*i.e.* reactions that involve the immune system) can occur (Chapter 2). Most cases of food allergy involve the production of immunoglobulin E (IgE) and are known as IgE mediated allergies. Symptoms develop quickly and can vary in severity, but the severest form of this type of reaction is anaphylactic shock. The other recognised mechanism is a delayed response (taking hours or even days to develop), which involves a different immune system component, T lymphocytes (T cells). The best defined example of this type of reaction is coeliac disease (sensitivity to the protein, gluten, found in wheat and other cereals), but delayed reactions can also on occasion occur in response to a range of other foods, including milk and soya.

### (3) What causes an allergic reaction?

Most allergic reactions, whether to food or to other allergens, *e.g.* pollen and animal fur, are IgE mediated and such immune responses are also the basis of atopic asthma, atopic eczema, hayfever and anaphylactic shock (Chapter 2). In an allergic reaction, an allergen, to which the individual is already sensitised, interacts with IgE antibodies that are specific to the antigen, which are attached to the surface of cells (mast cells). This interaction triggers an explosive reaction characterised by the release from mast cells of lots of substances which directly cause the inflammatory response that is characteristic of an allergic reaction.

The nature and the extent of the symptoms resulting from this process are dependent on the site, dose of antigen and the levels of IgG antibodies present. IgG antibodies are thought to provide a mechanism to 'mop up' any antigen that is inadvertently absorbed into the bloodstream. For example, the allergen can cause localised effects in the gastrointestinal tract, but it can also cause symptoms in other parts of the body, ranging from a skin rash to a dangerous systemic effect (anaphylactic shock). IgE mediated reactions are usually immediate and are usually localised in one or two organs of the body, such as the nose, eyes and respiratory tract. Inflammatory reactions occur in the membrane lining of these organs causing symptoms such as flushing and swelling, or a runny nose. But these symptoms can be mimicked (or even exacerbated) in response to substances other than allergens (Chapters 1 and 6).

### (4) Why don't all people develop allergies?

Under normal circumstances, a baby rapidly becomes tolerant (non-responsive) to the many proteins that it encounters in the early days and months of its life (Chapters 5 and 6). This process is known as the development of tolerance. The mechanisms that underpin this process are not fully understood. Similarly, it remains unclear exactly why some babies fail to develop tolerance to certain foods and other sources of allergens in their environment. The immune system has evolved to fight infection and one theory is that if a baby's environment is so clean that it does not encounter infections, the sensitivity of the response of the system will be inappropriately set and responses will be triggered by tiny amounts of food protein. This theory is supported by the fact that allergy tends to be more common in first and single children who from the outset may have less contact with other children, and hence childhood infections (Chapter 5).

It is also unclear why some childhood allergies disappear after 12 to 24 months (*e.g.* milk allergy) whilst others are present for life (*e.g.* peanut allergy). Another aspect that is poorly understood is the relative importance of diet in the development of allergic diseases, although it is recognised that diet can aggravate existing conditions such as asthma and atopic dermatitis (many other factors may also be involved). Similarly, the benefit of dietary restriction in the treatment for these conditions is uncertain, particularly among adults.

### (5) What is the definition of food intolerance?

Food intolerance is the general term used to describe a range of adverse responses to food, including allergic reactions (*e.g.* peanut allergy or coeliac disease), adverse reactions resulting from enzyme deficiencies (*e.g.* lactose intolerance or hereditary fructose intolerance), pharmacological reactions (*e.g.* caffeine sensitivity) and other non-defined responses (Chapter 1). Food intolerance does not include food poisoning from bacteria and viruses, moulds, chemicals, toxins and irritants in foods, nor does it include food aversion (dislike and subsequent avoidance of various foods). Food intolerance reactions are usually reproducible adverse responses to a specific food or food ingredient, which can occur whether or not the person realises they have eaten the food.

### (6) How do the symptoms and severity of food allergy and other forms of food intolerance compare?

Food intolerance reactions vary considerably in the severity of the associated symptoms and the length of time for which they persist. For example, peanut allergy is often a life-long affliction and can cause severe, even life-threatening, anaphylactic reactions to tiny amounts of peanut protein (Chapter 6). Cows' milk intolerance may be severe in early life, but typically disappears as the child grows older. The majority (about 90%) have outgrown the intolerance by the time they go to school (typically by the age of 3 years) (Chapter 6). Similarly, egg intolerance is usually a temporary phenomenon associated with early childhood. Coeliac disease (gluten sensitivity) is normally life-long and requires adherence to a diet that excludes all gluten (Chapter 9), but in some the disease is mild and goes undiagnosed as the individual is not aware of any symptoms. Lactose intolerance results in abdominal symptoms such as bloating and diarrhoea in response to test doses of lactose (Chapter 8). The severity of symptoms varies between individuals and most people with this condition can consume moderate amounts of milk and milk products, particularly with meals (see Question 24).

## Prevalence of food allergy and intolerance

### (7) How common is food allergy and food intolerance?

In general, food allergy and food intolerance are more common in children than in adults. It is estimated that true food intolerance affects no more than 5–8% of children and less than 1–2% of adults (Chapter 4). This is much lower than the 20% of people who perceive themselves to have an intolerance or an allergy to food. Food allergy, which specifically involves an adverse response of the immune system, is estimated to affect 1–2% of children and less than 1% of adults (typically 0.2–0.5% depending on the group studied). These estimates of food allergy and intolerance are derived from the results of a few (mostly European) epidemiological studies conducted in children and adults. The studies have measured reactions to the most common food allergens (such as those present in peanuts, hens' eggs and cows' milk).

### (8) How common is gluten sensitivity (coeliac disease)?

The prevalence of clinically proven coeliac disease is 1 to 3 cases per 1000 people. However, recent advances in the methods for diagnosing gluten sensitivity, based on blood measurements rather than an intestinal biopsy, have enabled screening of the general population and the identification of unrecognised cases. As a result, the European consensus is a total prevalence of 3 to 4 cases per 1000 people. Superficially there appears to have been an increase in the prevalence of coeliac disease, but increased awareness and these new blood tests probably account for most, if not all, of the increase. (See Chapter 9 and Question 25.)

### (9) What causes lactose intolerance and how common is it?

Lactose intolerance occurs in individuals who lack or have low levels of the enzyme lactase, which is needed to digest the sugar lactose (found in milk) to its constituent sugars (glucose and galactose) in readiness for absorption in the small intestine. In the absence of lactase, undigested lactose passes into the large intestine causing the characteristic symptoms of diarrhoea, wind and general discomfort. In about 70% of the world's population, a reduction in lactase production after early childhood is the norm. When milk is consumed, symptoms are typically experienced to varying degrees in people of Asian, African, Jewish and Hispanic descent. Nevertheless, the majority of affected individuals can still tolerate moderate amounts of dairy products (*e.g.* a glass of milk), particularly if these are consumed as part of a meal. People of northern European descent, on the other hand, usually retain the ability to produce lactase throughout their life, presumably as a result of genetic inheritance. As a direct result, the prevalence of lactose intolerance in the UK is relatively very low, affecting an estimated 2% of older children and adults (Chapter 8 and Question 24.)

### (10) How strong is the evidence supporting the estimates of the prevalence of food intolerance?

Although population studies in Europe and the USA are reasonably consistent in the estimates they provide of the prevalence of food intolerance and food allergy (Chapter 4), it is virtually impossible to identify time trends and geographical variation. This is mainly because of the small number of population studies (much of the work has been done in small groups of patients with severe allergic reactions) and lack of consistency between the methods employed in the studies. There is an urgent need for a large prospective European collaborative multi-centre study, designed to characterise the prevalence of all forms of food intolerance in defined population groups. The methodology should be consistent and clearly defined. Such a study would also be able to provide much needed data to identify geographical variation, time trends and aetiological factors.

### (11) Are allergy or intolerance becoming more common, or more diagnosed, or both?

There is good evidence that the prevalence of atopic allergic diseases such as asthma, eczema and hayfever has increased in the past 30 years (Chapter 4). This has caused speculation that the prevalence of food allergy has increased in a similar manner over the same time period. However, the evidence to support this conclusion is lacking as there have been no repeated cross-sectional or longitudinal studies specifically designed to investigate time trends in food allergy. The exception is with coeliac disease. Superficially there appears to have been an increase in the prevalence of coeliac disease, but increased awareness and new blood tests may account for most, if not all, of the reported increase (Question 8).

### (12) How does the estimated frequency of food allergy and intolerance in the UK compare with other industrialised countries?

Comparison of prevalence rates between countries is difficult owing to the lack of published scientific data. A general impression is that there is geographic variation in the prevalence of specific conditions, influenced by habitual dietary practices (Chapter 4). For example, allergy to fish is more common in children who live in a country with a high fish consumption, rice allergy is more common in the Far East, and peanut allergy is rare in countries with a low peanut consumption. Paradoxically, reports of peanut allergy are also rare in high peanut consumption countries (*e.g.* parts of Africa and Indonesia), although it is possible that this may reflect failure to diagnose cases in the face of many other health problems. There is a general consensus that allergy in general is more prevalent in affluent westernised countries and that the allergens to which children become sensitised reflect early exposure to commonly ingested allergens in the local diet and the environment. The reasons for this are unclear but are likely to include genetic predisposition and may also be linked to environmental factors such as lower exposure to infection in early life (Chapter 5 and Question 4).

## Common causes of food allergy and food intolerance

### (13) Which foods are the most common causes of allergic reactions and food intolerance?

The majority of allergic reactions to dietary components are caused by a small number of foods, namely cows' milk, hens' eggs, peanuts, tree nuts, soya beans and soya products, fish, shellfish and gluten-containing cereals, *e.g.* wheat. Citrus fruits

can also be a cause (Chapter 6). In children it has been estimated that 9 out of 10 reactions are in response to milk, eggs, soya, peanuts, tree nuts or wheat. Many of these reactions are outgrown in early childhood, and the majority of allergic reactions in adults result from sensitisation to shellfish, fish, peanuts and tree nuts. It is unusual for food allergy to begin in adulthood. The most common food component that causes a non-IgE mediated allergic response is gluten (in wheat and some other cereals) in coeliac disease (Chapter 9). The most common food component that causes a non-immune intolerance is lactose (in cows' milk and other dairy products) in lactose intolerance (Chapter 8). Occasionally, a wide range of other foods can trigger responses (Chapter 6 and Question 17).

### (14) How common is peanut allergy and what is the current advice for pregnant women?

As peanut allergy is one of the few allergies that is typically life-long, its prevalence is estimated to be greater in adults (0.5–1.0% of the population) than in children (0.5%). These figures are based on a limited number of studies, for example one on the Isle of Wight and another in the USA (Chapter 4). It remains unclear whether sensitisation to peanuts can occur prior to birth, but as a precaution, the government's advisory committee, COT (Committee on Toxicity of Chemicals in Food, Consumer Products and the Environment), has recommended that pregnant women who are atopic (predisposed to allergic reactions), or for whom the father or any sibling of the unborn child has an atopic disease (*e.g.* allergic asthma or eczema), may wish to avoid eating peanuts and peanut products during pregnancy. There is no justification for the avoidance of peanuts if there is no history of allergy in the parents or brothers and sisters of the new baby. All people who are known to be sensitive to peanuts should carry preloaded adrenaline syringes and (with the exception of very young children) be trained in their use. Those caring for children at risk of anaphylaxis, including schools, must be trained in the use of adrenaline and have access to supplies. Even a slight delay in the administration of adrenaline can be fatal.

### (15) Is migraine caused by food allergy?

It is likely that some of the headaches and migraines experienced by some people are provoked by food. However, there is unlikely to be a common cause. Various mechanisms may be involved, but allergy is not a likely candidate. Coffee, chocolate and alcoholic drinks are possible triggers for some people, but will be without effect in others. Progress in this field requires a better understanding of the different types of headache syndrome.

### (16) Is it possible to grow out of a food allergy?

Some allergies are characteristically present in young children and normally disappear as the child gets older, *e.g.* allergies to egg and milk (see Chapter 6). On the other hand, allergy to peanuts tends to be life-long, as does gluten sensitivity. The exclusion diets used in the management of allergy are difficult to follow and can lead to social exclusion, even for children once they start to go to parties. So, it is important that allergic children are checked periodically, under medical supervision particularly when the symptoms have been severe, to see whether their allergy has resolved. Sometimes foods may be eaten accidentally, and if found to be well tolerated may no longer need to be excluded from the diet.

### (17) Can allergies exist singly?

Cases of allergic reactions to single foods can occur. Equally, patients can react to more than one allergen (*i.e.* more than one food) and cross-reactions to clusters of foods and non-food items are also recognised. Interestingly, within these clusters the foods and non-food allergens are not always directly related. For example, cross-reactions involving sensitivity to latex (as used in rubber gloves, for example) and to various fruits (*e.g.* banana, kiwi fruit and avocado) have been reported. People sensitised to birch pollen also sometimes react to apple and hazelnut (Chapter 6).

### (18) If a parent suffers from a food allergy, is their child likely to be affected too? If so, what measures can be taken to prevent this?

Of all the factors that influence sensitisation to foods in the neonatal period, the inherited susceptibility to allergic disease is usually the most powerful. Current thinking is that allergy is more likely to be inherited from the mother than the father, although a predisposition to allergy in both parents dramatically increases the likelihood of allergy in their child (Chapter 5). But the specific triggers of the allergic reactions, *e.g.* pollen, animal fur or food, are not thought to be inherited.

As to what can be done, there is little evidence to support the use of any particular dietary modifications during pregnancy as a guarantee that allergy in the child will be prevented. Exclusive breast-feeding for 4 to 6 months may be of value in babies at high risk of inheriting a predisposition to allergy, and not introducing solids before 4 months is also likely to be helpful. But there is little scientific support for modifications of the mother's diet whilst she is breastfeeding. Although many protein constituents of foods can be identified in breast milk, there is no evidence that this is detrimental and it may in fact be part of the important process by which the baby develops tolerance to the many foods that will constitute the diet it is about to encounter. Furthermore, restriction of the mother's diet during pregnancy and breastfeeding may well be harmful to both her and her baby if intake of essential nutrients is compromised.

## Diagnosis and treatment

### (19) What are the best methods to use to diagnose food allergy and other forms of food intolerance?

Although an anaphylactic reaction or a strongly positive IgE antibody test is almost diagnostic of food allergy, most adverse reactions to foods are not IgE mediated and so properly conducted challenge tests (preferably double-blind and placebo-controlled) are important. Double-blind means that neither the patient nor the practitioner (*e.g.* the doctor) knows whether it is the suspect food or a placebo that is being given to the patient. To conduct these challenges properly, specialist knowledge is required and, as a precaution, they should be conducted in a setting where medical support is available, particularly if there is any suspicion that the patient might be at risk of suffering an anaphylactic shock (Chapters 10 and 11). Indeed, rather than take this risk, hospital specialists in this area often prefer to base their diagnosis on skin and blood antibody tests if they suspect that a patient is suffering an antibody-mediated allergic reaction. Such tests, that measure IgE antibodies, are of no use for diagnosis of other forms of food intolerance.

In practice, the diagnosis of a food intolerance (including food allergy) depends mainly on taking a careful patient history, the clinical experience of the doctor and a positive response to therapeutic measures. Such measures are typically the removal of the suspect food from the diet, a positive response being disappearance of the symptoms on removal of the suspect food, followed by their return when it is reintroduced (Chapter 11 and Question 21).

### (20) What evidence is there that alternative methods of allergy detection are effective or, on the other hand, can be harmful?

The vast majority of so-called methods of allergy diagnosis advocated in magazines and via the Internet are without scientific basis and have not been independently validated (Chapter 10). Such tests include hair and nail assessment, VEGA testing and kinesiology. At best the patient is likely just to have wasted money, at worst these tests can result in misdiagnosis and the unnecessary treatment of a disease that does not exist, by the use of an inappropriate and potentially dangerous diet. Misdiagnoses through these routes can also result in the delayed treatment of a real health problem. Because of the impact an inappropriate diet can have on a child's growth, development and social integration, it is particularly important that parents seek advice from appropriately qualified and trained staff. Referral via a GP is recognised as an important first step in this process.

### (21) Which treatments are best supported by research?

Diet is the cornerstone of the treatment and management of food intolerance (Chapter 11). Food(s)

or food constituents that are suspected of causing symptoms are removed from the diet for a specified period to see if symptoms improve. This is followed by a series of open or double-blind, placebo-controlled food challenges (DBPCFC) in an attempt to reproduce the original reaction and prove the diagnosis. It is important that such tests are conducted under medical supervision in case of anaphylaxis. Once diagnosed the patient should receive dietary advice from a state registered dietitian to ensure that excluded foods are replaced by alternative palatable, readily accessible, affordable substitutes, which provide a beneficial nutrient profile, and to ensure that overall the diet is nutritionally adequate. The dietitian will also be able to provide practical advice on issues such as shopping, eating out and interpreting food labels. The involvement of a dietitian is especially important if the patient is a child as an inadequate diet can adversely affect growth and development.

### (22) When a GP thinks a patient may have a food allergy, what is the recommended route for him or her to follow?

Usually the GP should refer the patient to a specialist team, who will confirm diagnosis through a step-by-step process, which takes account of the patient's medical history and may involve a clinical assessment; clinical and laboratory tests; a diagnostic exclusion diet; open food challenges; or double-blind, placebo-controlled food challenges (Chapters 10 and 11). While sufficient centres exist for paediatric treatment, the Task Force believes that there is a gross underprovision of services for adults, and as a result people with a genuine concern about their health feel forced to seek advice from alternative sources, some of which may not be appropriately qualified to advise on these matters.

### (23) If a patient faces several months of waiting for a referral for allergy tests, what interim measures can be taken?

Keeping a diary of food and drink consumed and symptoms experienced can be extremely useful, not only for the patient but also for the practitioner, in helping to identify the problematic food or food constituents. If the patient suspects a specific food, there may be no harm in eliminating this food from his diet until he can be seen by a specialist team. An exception to this is if there is a suspicion that the patient may be suffering from gluten sensitivity (coeliac disease), the diagnosis of which can be severely hampered if the patient has embarked on a gluten-free diet prior to investigation by a gastroenterologist. However, people should be discouraged from eliminating a number of foods simultaneously or following a restrictive diet in an attempt at self-help to reduce symptoms, as the diet may become unbalanced and lead to nutritional deficiencies. It is particularly important to avoid this sort of action with children. Once diagnosed, consultation with a state registered dietitian will ensure that the diet used in management is nutritionally balanced.

### (24) What type of diet do people diagnosed as lactose intolerant have to follow?

Complete avoidance of milk and milk products is rarely necessary as most people still produce some lactase enzyme. Yogurt is usually better tolerated than ordinary milk. This is thought to be due in part to the fact that an enzyme very similar to human lactase is present in the bacteria used in the manufacture of yogurt (the bacterial culture), although other factors are likely to be of relevance too (Chapter 8). Hard cheeses such as Cheddar contain only trace amounts of lactose and so are well tolerated. Having milk as part of a meal is also more likely to be tolerated and most people can consume 200 ml without adverse effects, and so can benefit from the nutrients, particularly calcium, provided by these foods. For people who are very sensitive, lactose reduced milks are now widely available. Although it is not possible to induce the enzyme once levels have fallen, there is some limited evidence that it is possible to develop a tolerance to lactose by gradually modifying the profile of bacteria that reside in the large bowel in favour of ones that cope with the lactose without causing symptoms (Chapter 8).

### (25) What type of diet do people diagnosed as coeliac have to follow?

Coeliac disease is usually a life-long condition requiring a life-long and strict gluten-free diet, and the main organ affected is the small intestine.

Ingestion of gluten activates immune cells in the small intestine, which trigger inflammation and local damage, which disrupts the normal processes used to digest and absorb foods. As a result, untreated coeliac patients lose weight, develop deficiency syndromes such as anaemia, and experience symptoms such as diarrhoea. Gluten is found in wheat, barley and rye, which means that many dietary staples such as bread, many breakfast cereals and foods such as pizza and pasta are no longer acceptable. Oats were thought to trigger reactions, though this is looking less and less likely. The gold standard for diagnosis is the intestinal biopsy, but the availability of improved blood tests is a help in screening larger numbers, *e.g.* the relatives of patients (Chapter 9).

### (26) What should consumers look for on labels?

By law, the majority of packaged food products have to carry a full list of the ingredients they contain, in descending order of weight in the final product. Manufacturers are increasingly deciding, voluntarily, to include information on the presence of small quantities of allergens associated with severe reactions, even when it is not required by law (Chapter 12). This information can help consumers identify whether or not a food contains an ingredient that they need to avoid. In addition, where there is a demonstrable risk that traces of an allergen, such as nut protein, may be present as a result of cross-contamination during manufacture, this is generally highlighted at the end of the ingredients list.

### (27) What does the future hold with regard to desensitisation and food allergy?

Research in this area is being pursued. A variety of new strategies exist that, in the future, should allow the development of successful vaccines to treat patients with persistent food allergies. However, it is early days and much more work is needed before effective new treatments are available. Nevertheless, it is likely that, in the future, combined approaches employing various different techniques coupled with moves to modify the allergenicity of, or remove, particular protein allergens present in foods, will lead to the basis of a successful desensitisation programme (Chapter 13).

### (28) Can we boost the immune system through nutrition?

Deficiencies of a wide variety of essential nutrients impair immune function and increase susceptibility to infectious pathogens. Provision of these nutrients to deficient individuals restores immune function and improves resistance to infection. This has been shown to be important in elderly people and people who are undernourished, for example. For some nutrients, the dietary intakes that result in the greatest enhancement of immune function in experimental studies are above currently recommended intakes; however, this should not be taken to mean that supplementation is the answer, as excess intake of some nutrients also impairs immune function. On the basis of the available evidence, the immuno-enhancing effect of supplementation of healthy individuals is unproven and, as far as micronutrients are concerned, may even be harmful (Chapter 3).

# Appendix 1
# Food Additives

A food additive is defined as:

'any substance not normally consumed as a food in itself and not normally used as a characteristic ingredient of food, whether or not it has a nutritive value, the intentional addition of which to food for a technological purpose in the manufacture, processing, preparation, treatment, packaging, transport or storage of such food results, or may reasonably, be expected to result, in it or its by-products becoming directly or indirectly a component of such foods' (Regulation 2 (1) (a) of the Miscellaneous Food Additives Regulations 1995)

There are over 300 substances (colours, sweeteners and 'miscellaneous' additives) listed in legislation as permitted additives for use in food under EC/UK legislation (Saltmarsh, 2000). The permitted list is continually being updated as new additives receive safety endorsements. Others, which are not listed, may be used for functions that fall outside the control of the legislation, *e.g.* the use of enzymes as processing aids.

Food additives can be categorised in three groups (Food Standards Agency, 2000):

- **natural:** such as the red colouring, beetroot red, derived from beetroot juice,
- **nature-identical:** man-made chemicals, which are identical to something found in nature, such as the flavouring vanillin, and
- **artificial:** man-made and not found in nature, such as saccharin, a low calorie sweetener used to replace sugar.

All additives, regardless of whether they are natural, nature-identical or artificial, are controlled by means of the same legislation, and all undergo the same stringent approval procedures. They are only permitted for use if they are considered both necessary and safe, following scrutiny of the evidence by independent experts. Specific procedures are in place for this process.

The use of food additives is prohibited or severely restricted in some categories of foods, *e.g.* unprocessed foods, and those specially prepared for infants and young children under 36 months of age.

Food additives are often blamed for food intolerance and behavioural problems, especially in young children, but as described in Chapter 4 the actual prevalence of food additive induced reactions is very low. The mechanism is unknown but seldom seems to involve IgE. This subject is discussed in detail in a report from the government's advisory Committee on Toxicity of Chemicals in Food, Consumer Products and the Environment (COT) (Food Standards Agency, 2000). Those additives most frequently mentioned are benzoic acid and benzoates, sulphites, food colours such as tartrazine, and monosodium glutamate.

Benzoic acid and benzoates are used as food preservatives to retard the growth of bacteria and yeasts. Small amounts occur naturally in some berries, such as cranberries, and in some types of honey. Sound published evidence of intolerance to ingested benzoates in childhood is scanty and there is no evidence that benzoates can provoke behavioural problems in otherwise normal children (David, 1993a). However, in children with co-existing atopic disease, *e.g.* asthma and eczema, symptoms may be aggravated as an indirect effect.

Sulphites are widely used as preservatives (Saltmarsh, 2000). They are formed naturally during the production of wine and beer, and are also sometimes added to inhibit the growth of undesirable yeast species and to prevent secondary fermentation. Virtually all asthmatics respond with bronchoconstriction when exposed to sulphur dioxide by inhalation and many respond in a similar way to the ingestion of acidic solutions of sulphites. In a minority of asthmatics, the reaction can be very severe (Taylor *et al.*, 1997). Apart from initiating an asthma attack, other symptoms include flushing, and itching of the mouth and skin.

Tartrazine (E102) is a yellow colour used in foods such as soft drinks, desserts, confectionery, pickles and sauces, and in some drugs. The evidence concerning tartrazine has been reviewed by David (1993a). He concluded that tartrazine can provoke urticaria, asthma or rhinitis in a small number of subjects, but the mechanism for these effects is unknown and there is no evidence that it can result in a worsening of atopic eczema. Tartrazine has been linked anecdotally with attention deficit disorder hyperactivity (ADHD). There is no evidence from double-blind challenge studies that tartrazine can provoke behavioural problems in otherwise normal children but, again, in children with coexisting eczema or asthma, symptoms may be aggravated as an indirect effect (David 1993a). It is important to recognise that hyperactive behaviour has many causes, which are often neglected when undue attention is focused on diet: blind challenge

tests are therefore an essential part of management (Lessof, 1995). The limitations of the evidence concerning diet with ADHD have been reviewed recently (Food Standards Agency, 2000).

Monosodium glutamate (MSG) was linked with 'Chinese restaurant syndrome' in the late 1960s. Although this link is still widely cited, the notion of a specific pattern of gastrointestinal and systemic disorders after ingestion of MSG has not been confirmed in a variety of trials (Food Standards Agency, 2000). (See Chapter 7, Section 7.6.5.)

In conclusion, although asthmatics have been reported to have had severe reactions provoked by sulphites, major reactions to food additives are rare. Indeed, if those additives that improve the keeping qualities of foods were to be removed, this would add to the risk of food-transmitted infection, which already affects many more people than all types of food additive combined (Chapter 1). It remains a concern that many vulnerable people with vague symptoms have been led to adopt inadequate and restricted diets in the misguided belief that food, or food additives, has caused their illness (Lessof, 1995). The same can apply to parents who are worried about behavioural problems in their child and impose a strict dietary regimen on an already disturbed child. While food restriction can sometimes help, it can only be justified in a growing child if its relevance can be objectively confirmed.

# Glossary

**Adrenaline:** A catecholamine that occurs naturally in the body and is also used for the treatment of anaphylaxis.

**Allergen:** Substance, usually a protein or glycoprotein, capable of inducing an allergic response.

**Allergy:** Adverse health effects resulting from a specific immune response.

**Anaphylaxis:** An immediate (IgE mediated) reaction to a foreign substance, which in severe cases can be generalised and life-threatening.

**Angioedema:** Presence of fluid in subcutaneous tissues or submucosa, particularly of the face, eyes, lips and sometimes tongue and throat; may occur during an anaphylactic reaction.

**Antibody:** Immunoglobulin which is specific for an antigen or allergen.

**Antigen:** Substance recognised by the immune system.

**Arachis oil:** Peanut oil.

**Asthma:** Chronic inflammatory disease of the airways which renders them prone to narrowing. The symptoms include paroxysmal coughing, wheezing, tightness and breathlessness. Asthma may be caused by an allergic response or may be induced by non-immunological mechanisms.

**Atopic dermatitis:** Disease of the skin characterised by itching and dry and lined skin.

**Atopy:** Predisposition to IgE production associated with allergy to several common allergens.

**Attention deficit hyperactivity disorders:** Condition characterised by inattentiveness, overactivity and/or impulsiveness.

**B lymphocyte (B cells):** Bursa-equivalent lymphocytes. After maturation into plasma cells they produce antibodies (immunoglobulins) during humoral immune responses. (They were first discovered in the Bursa of Fabricius in the chicken; hence the name.)

**Basophils:** Type of white blood cell, classed as a granulocyte.

**Cell mediated immunity:** Specific immunity dependent upon T lymphocytes.

**Coeliac disease:** Disease characterised by damage to the small intestinal wall due to intolerance of gluten, a protein present in wheat flour.

**Complement:** An enzyme system which is activated characteristically, but not invariably, by the combination of antibody and antigen, and which triggers the changes associated with inflammation and other biological reactions.

**Committee on Toxicity of Chemicals in Food, Consumer Products and the Environment (COT):** A committee composed of independent experts, which advises government on the human health risk of chemicals in food, consumer products and the environment.

**Crude oil:** Unrefined edible oil that may contain sufficient quantities of protein to induce an allergic reaction. Also known as 'gourmet oil'.

**Cystitis:** Inflammation of the urinary bladder, usually characterised by painful urination.

**Cytochrome:** A class of oxidation-reduction enzymes that are principally concerned with the transfer of electrons from flavoproteins to oxygen or other electron acceptors and which employ haem as co-enzyme.

**Cytokine:** Mediators produced by a variety of cell types, and which influence immune and inflammatory responses in a variety of ways.

**Cytotoxic:** Harmful to cells.

**Cytotoxic T cell:** A type of T lymphocyte that interacts directly in an antigen-specific manner with virus-infected, parasite-infected, or otherwise antigenically altered or abnormal cells, and destroys them.

**Dermatitis:** Inflammation of the skin.

**Dermatitis herpetiformis:** Skin disease often associated with gluten-sensitive enteropathy.

**Double-blind placebo-controlled food challenge:** An *in vivo* test in which the patient and doctor do not know which food is being tested until after the tests and the recording of responses have been completed. Often regarded as the 'gold standard' for testing for allergenicity.

**Dysuria:** Painful and difficult urination.

**Elimination diet:** A diet in which a suspect food is eliminated from the diet until all the symptoms have disappeared; it is then reintroduced to see if the symptoms recur. The diet must be strictly supervised by a state registered dietitian.

**Endorphins:** Proteins, which occur naturally in the brain and have analgesic properties

**Enzymes:** Proteins which catalyse chemical reactions in the body.

**Enzyme linked immunosorbent assay:** A sensitive technique for the detection and measurement of compounds, especially proteins.

**Eosinophils:** Type of white blood cell, classed as a granulocyte.

**Epitope:** Peptide sequence within an antigenic molecule which is recognised by the immune system (either lymphocytes or antibodies).

**Food additive:** Substance added to food to facilitate some part of the processing or manufacture of the foodstuff or to impart a particular characteristic; they can be classified according to the purpose for which they are used, *e.g.* food colours, antioxidants, acidity regulators.

**Food allergy:** Adverse reaction to food, mediated by immunological mechanisms.

**Food intolerance:** General term for adverse reaction to food and food ingredients. In this report, the term embraces both allergic and non-allergic reactions.

**Gluten:** Protein present in wheat, intolerance to a component of which is a characteristic of coeliac disease.

**Gluten-sensitive enteropathy:** *see* **Coeliac disease**.

**Glycoproteins** Proteins conjugated with carbohydrate groups.

**Granulocyte:** Class of white blood cells including basophils, eosinophils and neutrophils.

**Histamine:** Decarboxylation product of the amino acid histidine. It is an important inflammatory mediator.

**Human leukocyte antigens:** Gene products of the major human histocompatability complex. They are complex glycoproteins on the surface of cells that provide individual immunological identity.

**Hypersensitivity:** Heightened responsiveness induced by allergic sensitisation.

**Immunoglobulin (Ig):** A member of a family of proteins from which antibodies are derived. There are five main classes in humans known as IgM, IgG, IgA, IgD and IgE.

**IgE:** One of the five main classes of immunoglobulin. IgE is involved in allergy and anaphylaxis as well as protecting against intestinal parasites. IgE mediated hypersensitivity is characterised by the rapid release of mediators such as histamine.

**IgG:** One of the five main classes of human immunoglobulin. The most abundant.

**Incidence:** The number of new cases of a disease that occur during a particular period of time in a defined population.

**Interferon:** Any one of a group of small proteins produced by vertebrate cells in response to viral infection and other stimuli, inhibiting viral multiplication and also having an effect on cell growth and the immune system.

**Interferon gamma:** A substance produced by various cells (including Th1 cells), which antagonises IgE antibody production.

**Interleukins:** Soluble polypeptide mediators, produced by activated lymphocytes and other cells during immune and inflammatory response.

**Lactase:** The enzyme that breaks down lactose (milk sugar) in the small intestine.

**Lactose intolerance:** The inability or reduced ability to break down lactose (milk sugar).

**Lymphoblast:** Precursor cell in lymphoid tissue that divides to form mature lymphocytes.

**Lymphocyte:** A specialised white cell with a variety of immunological functions, including antibody production (B lymphocytes) and cell mediated reactions (T lymphocytes). T lymphocytes also have a regulatory effect on antibody production.

**Lymphoid tissue:** All tissues in which the predominant active cells are lymphocytes – lymph nodes, Peyer's patches, tonsils, adenoids, spleen and thymus.

**Macrophages:** A mobile cell which can ingest

foreign particles, process antigen and release a number of enzymes.

**Major histocompatibility complex:** A cluster of genes encoding the major histocompatibilty antigens, some complement proteins, and other surface proteins of immune system cells. A synonymous term is human leukocyt antigen (HLA).

**Mast cells:** Cells found predominantly in connective tissue, although a specialised population of mast cells is found in mucosal sites (*e.g.* the gut). Following degranulation, mast cells release preformed and newly synthesised mediators of inflammation, including histamine.

**Migraine:** Type of headache, characterised by usually being unilateral and/or accompanied by visual disturbance.

**Monocytes:** A large phagocytic white blood cell found in blood that develops into a macrophage.

**Monosodium glutamate:** Monosodium salt of glutamic acid, an amino acid. Monosodium glutamate is used as a flavour enhancer.

**Natural killer cells:** Class of large granular lymphocytes that recognise and kill cells, especially tumour cells.

**Neutrophils:** Type of white blood cell, classed as a granulocyte.

**Open challenge:** In the context of adverse reactions to food, challenging the patient with the food suspected to cause the adverse reaction, without any attempt to hide the nature of the challenge from the observer or the patient.

**Peanut:** Nut from a herbaceous plant. It is also known as the groundnut or monkey nut, botanical name *Arachis hypogaea*. It is a member of the Leguminosae family and thus related botanically to peas and beans, rather than tree nuts such as brazil, hazel or almond. Used in a number of foodstuffs and also used to produce peanut oil.

**Peanut oil:** Also known as arachis oil. Used in foods and other products such as skin creams.

**Phagocyte:** A cell which ingests and deactivates foreign particles or the body's breakdown products (monocytes, macrophages and neutrophil granulocytes).

**Pharmacological:** Concerned with the action of drugs.

**Prevalence:** Total number of cases of a disease in existence at a certain time in a designated population (including new and old cases).

**Radioallergosorbent test:** A method for measurement of specific IgE antibodies in the blood.

**Refined oil:** Oils containing no detectable protein and therefore unlikely to cause an allergic reaction.

**Rhinitis:** Inflammation of the nasal passages, resulting in runny nose.

**Serotonin:** Vasoactive decarboxylation product of the amino acid tryptophan, also known as 5-hydroxytryptamine.

**Skin prick test:** A clinical test of allergic reactivity, commonly used in allergy clinics.

**State registered dietitian:** An appropriately qualified practitioner able to offer clinical nutritional advice on an individual basis, often working within the NHS

**T cell receptor (TCR):** A highly variable glycoprotein on the surface of T lymphocytes, which specifically recognises and binds a particular antigen, leading to the activation and proliferation of T lymphocytes.

**T helper cells:** T cells which help B lymphocytes to produce antibodies. Two main subtypes exist. Th1 cells produce IFN-$\gamma$ amongst other cytokines and antagonise the IgE response. Th2 type cells produce interleukins that promote IgE production and allergic sensitisation.

**Th1 cells:** T helper lymphocytes of the type 1 subgroup which produce cytokines such as IFN-$\gamma$. In general, their actions antagonise the IgE and allergic responses.

**Th2 cells:** T helper lymphocytes of the type 2 subgroup which produce cytokines e.g. interleukins that promote IgE production and allergic responses.

**T lymphocytes (T cells):** Thymus-dependent lymphocytes which, amongst other functions, help B lymphocytes (B cells) during immunological responses and provide protection from intracellular microbial infection. Distinct subpopulations have been characterised (see T helper cells).

**Tumour necrosis factors $\gamma$ and $\beta$:** Two cytokines produced by monocytes, macrophages and other cells (TNF-$\alpha$) or lymphocytes (TNF-$\beta$).

**Urticaria:** An itchy rash which results from inflammation and leakage of fluid from the blood into the superficial layers of the skin in response to various mediators. Synonyms are 'hives' or 'nettle rash'.

**Vasoactive amines:** Nitrogen containing substances that affect the tone of blood vessel walls.

# Abbreviations

| | | | |
|---|---|---|---|
| CD | Cluster of differentiation T cell antigens | IL | Interleukin |
| COT | Committee on Toxicity of Chemicals in Food, Consumer Products and the Environment | MHC | Major histocompatibility complex |
| | | RAST | Radioallergosorbent test |
| | | SRD | State registered dietitian |
| ELISA | Enzyme linked immunosorbent assay | TCR | T cell receptor |
| HLA | Human leukocyte antigen, synonymous with MHC | TGF-β | Transforming growth factor β |
| | | Th | T helper lymphocytes |
| IFN-γ | Interferon gamma | TNF-α/β | Tumour necrosis factors α and β |
| Ig | Immunoglobulin | | |

# References

Aalberse RC (2000) Structural biology of allergens. *Journal of Allergy and Clinical Immunology*, **106**, 228–38.

Aalberse RC, van der Gaag R, van Leeuwen J (1983) Serologic aspects of IgG4 antibodies. I. Prolonged immunization results in an IgG4-restricted response. *Journal of Immunology*, **130**, 722–6.

Aalberse RC, van Ree R (1997) Crossreactive carbohydrate determinants. *Clinical Reviews of Allergy and Immunology*, **15**, 375–87.

Abbas AK, Murphy KM, Sher, A (1996) Functional diversity of helper T lymphocytes. *Nature*, **383**, 787–93.

Aberg N (1989) Asthma and allergic rhinitis in Swedish conscripts. *Clinical and Experimental Allergy*, **19**, 59–63.

Advisory Committee on the Microbiological Safety of Food (1993) *Report of Progress 1990–1992*, p. 5. London: HMSO.

Allen JE, Maizels RM (1997) Th1–Th2: reliable paradigm or dangerous dogma? *Immunology Today*, **18**, 387–91.

Alun Jones VA (1985) Irritable bowel syndrome. In: *Food and the Gut* (eds JO Hunter, VA Alun Jones). London: Bailliere Tindall.

American Academy of Allergy and Immunology Committee on Adverse Reactions to Foods and National Institute of Allergy and Infectious Diseases (1984) *Adverse reactions to foods*. US Department of Health and Human Services. NIH Publications No. 84–242.

American Academy of Pediatrics ad hoc Committee on Anaphylaxis in school (1993) Anaphylaxis at school: etiological factors, prevalence, and treatment. *Pediatrics*, **91**, 316.

American Psychiatric Association (1996) *Diagnostic and Statistical Manual of Mental Disorders*, 4th edn. Washington DC.

Amlot PL, Kemeny DM, Zachary C, Parkes P, Lessof MH (1987) The oral allergy syndrome (OAS): symptoms of IgE mediated hypersensitivity to foods. *Clinical Allergy*, **17**, 33–42.

Ammar F, de Boissieu D, Dupont C (1999) Allergy to protein hydrolysates. Report of 30 cases. *Archives of Pediatrics*, **6**, 837–43.

Anderson CM (1992) The evolution of a successful treatment for coeliac disease. In: *Coeliac Disease* (ed. MN Marsh). Oxford: Blackwell Science.

Anderson J, Sogn D (eds) (1984) *Adverse reactions to foods*. Bethesda, Maryland: National Institute of Allergy and Infectious Disease, NIH Publication No. 84–2442.

Angold A, Erkanli A, Egger HL, Costello FJ (2000) Stimulant treatment for children: a community perspective [see comments]. *Journal of the American Academy of Child and Adolescent Psychiatry*, **39**, 975–84; discussion 84–94.

Anon (1984) The Food Labelling Regulation (1984) No 1305. London: HMSO.

Anon (1990) Food Safety Act 1990. London: HMSO.

Anon (1994) General Product Safety Regulations 1994, SI 2328. London: HMSO.

Anon (1996) Food Labelling Regulations 1996, SI 1499. London: HMSO.

Anon (2000) Food Labelling Directive 2000/13/EC. *Official Journal of the European Communities*, L109/29 (6.5.2000).

Antico A, Di Benardino L (1995) The role of additives in chronic pseudo-allergic dermatopathies from food intolerance. *Allergy and Immunology*, **27**, 157–60.

Antico A, Soana R (1999) Chronic allergic-like dermatopathies in nickel-sensitive patients. Results of dietary restrictions and challenge with nickel salts. *Allergy and Asthma Proceedings*, **20**, 235–42.

Arentz-Hansen H, Körner R, Molberg Ø et al. (2000) The intestinal T-cell response to α-gliadin in adult coeliac disease is focused on a single deaminated glutamine targeted by tissue transglutaminase. *Journal of Experimental Medicine*, **191**, 603–12.

Arm JP, Lee TH (1992) The pathophysiology of bronchial asthma. *Advanced Immunology*, **51**, 323–82.

Arrigoni E, Marteau P, Briet F *et al.* (1994) Tolerance and absorption of lactose from milk and yogurt during short bowel syndrome in humans. *American Journal of Clinical Nutrition*, **60**, 926–9.

Arshad SH, Matthews S, Gant C, Hide DW (1992) Effect of allergen avoidance on development of allergic disorders in infancy. *Lancet*, **339**, 1493–7.

Ascher H (1996) The role of quantity and quality of gluten containing cereals in the epidemiology of coeliac disease. In: *Coeliac Disease: Proceedings of the Seventh International Symposium on Coeliac Disease* (eds M Maki, P Collin, JK Visakorpi) Finland: Tampere.

Asero R (1998) Effects of birch pollen-specific immunotherapy on apple allergy in birch pollen-hypersensitive patients. *Clinical and Experimental Allergy*, **28**, 1368–73.

Astwood JD, Fuchs RL, Lavrik PB (1997) Food biotechnology and genetic engineering. In: *Food Allergy: Adverse Reactions to Foods and Food Additives* 2nd edn (eds DD Metcalfe, HA Sampson, & RA Simon). Cambridge, Mass: Blackwell Science.

Astwood JD, Leach JN, Fuchs RL (1996) Stability of food allergens to digestion in vitro. *Nature Biotechnology*, **14**, 1269–73.

Atherton DJ (1984) Diagnosis and management of skin disorders caused by food allergy. *Annals of Allergy*, **53**, 623–8.

Atherton DJ, Sewell M, Soothill JF, Wells RS, Chilvers CE (1978) A double-blind controlled crossover trial of an antigen-avoidance diet in atopic eczema. *Lancet*, **25**, 401–3.

Atkins FM, Steinberg SS, Metcalfe DD (1985a) Evaluation of immediate adverse reactions to food in adults. I. Correlation of demographic, laboratory, and prick test data with response to controlled oral food challenge. *Journal of Allergy and Clinical Immunology*, **75**, 348.

Atkins FM, Steinberg SS, Metcalfe DD (1985b) Evaluation of immediate adverse reactions to food in adults. II. A detailed analysis of reaction patterns during oral food challenge. *Journal of Allergy and Clinical Immunology*, **75**, 356.

Auranen M, Nieminen F, Majuri S *et al.* (2000) Analysis of autism susceptibility gene loci on chromosomes lp, 4p, 6q, 7q, 13q, 15q, 16p, 17q, 19q and 22q in Finnish multiplex families. *Molecular Psychiatry*, **5**, 320–2.

Baldwin JL (1997) Pharmacological Food Reactions. In: *Food Allergy: Adverse Reactions to Food and Food Additives* 2nd edn (eds. DD Metacalfe, HA Sampson, RA Simon). Cambridge, Mass: Blackwell Science.

Banchereau J, Steinman RM (1998) Dendritic cells and the control of immunity. *Nature*, **392**, 245–52.

Barbul A, Lazarou SA, Efron DT, Wasserkrug HL, Efron G (1990) Arginine enhances wound healing and lymphocyte immune responses in humans. *Surgery*, **108**, 331–7.

Barbul A, Sisto DA, Wasserkrug HL, Efron G (1981) Arginine stimulates lymphocyte immune response in healthy human beings. *Surgery*, **90**, 244–51.

Barnes RM, Johnson PM, Harvey MM, Blears J, Finn R (1988) Human serum antibodies reactive with dietary proteins. IgG subclass distribution. *International Archives of Allergy and Applied Immunology*, **87**, 184–8.

Barnes RM (1995) IgG and IgA antibodies to dietary antigens in food allergy and intolerance. *Clinical and Experimental Allergy*, **25**, S7–S9.

Barone J, Hebert JR, Reddy MM (1989) Dietary fat and natural killer cell activity. *American Journal of Clinical Nutrition*, **50**, 861–7.

Barratt JA, Summers GD (1996) Scurvy, osteoporosis and megaloblastic anaemia due to alleged food intolerance. *British Journal of Rheumatology*, **35**, 701–702.

Bateson MC, Hopwood D, MacGillivray JB (1979) Jejunal morphology in multiple sclerosis. *Lancet*, **i**, 1108–10.

Battaglia G, Morselli-Labate AM, Camarri E *et al.* (1998) Otilonium bromide in irritable bowel syndrome: a double-blind, placebo-controlled, 15-week study. *Aliments and Pharmacological Therapy*, **12**, 1003–10.

Beattie RM, Bentsen BS, MacDonald TT (1998) Childhood Crohn's disease and the efficacy of enteral diets. *Nutrition*, **14**, 345–50.

Beattie RM, Schiffrin EJ, Donnet-Hughes A *et al.* (1994) Polymeric nutrition as the primary therapy in children with small bowel Crohn's disease. *Aliments in Pharmacological Therapy*, **8**, 609–15.

Beck FW, Prasad AS, Kaplan J, Fitzgeral JT, Brewer GJ (1997) Changes in cytokine production and T cell subpopulations in experimentally induced zinc deficient humans. *American Journal of Physiology*, **272**, E1002–E1007.

Beezhold DH, Sussman GL, Liss GM, Chang NS (1996) Latex allergy can induce clinical reactions to specific foods. *Clinical and Experimental Allergy*, **26**, 416–22.

Bellioni-Businco B, Paganelli R, Lucenti P *et al.* (1999). Allergenicity to goat's milk in children with cow's milk allergy. *Journal of Allergy and Clinical Immunology*, **103**, 1191–4.

Belluzzi A, Miglio F (1998) *n*-3 Fatty acids in the treatment of Crohn's disease. In: *Medicinal Fatty Acids in Inflammation* (ed. J Kremer). Basel: Birkhauser Verlag.

Bendich A (1993) Vitamin E and human immune functions. In: *Nutrition and Immunology* (ed. DM Klurfeld). New York and London: Plenum Press.

Bentley SJ, Pearson DJ, Rix KJ (1983) Food hypersensitivity in irritable bowel syndrome. *Lancet*, **2**, 295–7.

Berney TP (2000) Autism – an evolving concept. *British Journal of Psychiatry*, **176**, 20–25.

Bernstein IL (1994) Development of food aversions during illness. *Proceedings of the Nutrition Society*, **53**, 131–7.

Bernstein JM (1992) The role of IgE-mediated hypersensitivity in the development of otitis media with effusion. *Otolaryngologic Clinics North of America*, **25**, 197–211.

Bernt KM, Walker WA (1999) Human milk as a carrier of biochemical messengers. *Acta Pediatrica*, **88**, 27–41.

Beyer K, Niggemann B, Nasert S, Renz H, Wahn U (1997) Severe allergic reactions to foods are predicted by increases of CD4 + CD45RO + T cells and loss of L-selectin expression. *Journal of Allergy and Clinical Immunology*, **99**, 522–9.

Biagi F, Parnell ND, Ellis HJ, Ciclitira PJ (2000) Endomysial antibody production is not related to histological damage after in-vitro challenge. *European Journal of Gastroenterology and Hepatology*, **12**, 57–60.

Biagi F, Zimmer KP, Thomas PD, Ellis HJ & Ciclitira PJ (1999) Is gliadin misrepresented to the immune system in coeliac disease. Quarterly Journal of Medicine 92, 119–22.

Bielory L & Gandhi R (1994) Asthma and vitamin C. *Annals of Allergy*, **73**, 89–96.

Bindsley-Jensen C, Poulsen LK (1997) In vitro diagnostic methods in the evaluation of food hypersensitivity. In: *Food Allergy: Adverse Reactions to Foods and Food Additives* 2nd edn (eds DD Metcalfe, HA Sampson, RA Simon). Cambridge, Mass: Blackwell Science.

Bischoff SC, Herrmann A, Manns MP (1996) Prevalence of adverse reactions to food in patients with gastrointestinal disease. *Allergy*, **51**, 811–8.

Bishop JM, Hill DJ, Hosking CS (1990) Natural history of cows' milk allergy: clinical outcome. *Journal of Pediatrics* **116**, 862–7.

Bjornsson E, Janson C, Plaschke P, Norrman E, Sjoberg (1996) Prevalence of sensitization to food allergens in adult Swedes. *Annals of Allergy, Asthma and Immunology*, **77**, 327–32.

Black PN, Sharpe S (1997) Dietary fat and asthma: is there a connection? *European Respiratory Journal*, **10**, 6–12.

Bock SA (1987) Prospective appraisal of complaints of adverse reactions to foods in children during the first 3 years of life. *Pediatrics*, **79**, 683–8.

Bock SA (1989) Probable allergic reaction to casein hydrolysate formula. *Journal of Allergy and Clinical Immunology*, **84**, 272.

Bock SA (1992) Respiratory reactions induced by food challenges in children with pulmonary disease. *Pediatric Allergy and Immunology*, **3**, 188–92.

Bock SA, Atkins FM (1989) The natural history of peanut allergy. *Journal of Allergy and Clinical Immunology*, **83**, 900–4.

Bock SA, Atkins FM (1990) Patterns of food hypersensitivity during sixteen years of double-blind, placebo-controlled food challenges. *Journal of Pediatrics*, **117**, 561–7.

Bock SA, Dorion B (1992) Incidence of severe food reactions in Colarado. *Journal of Allergy and Clinical Immunology*, **89**, 192 (abstract).

Bock SA, Sampson HA, Atkins FM *et al.* (1988). Double-blind, placebo-controlled food challenge (DBPCFC) as an office procedure: a manual. *Journal of Allergy and Clinical Immunology*, **82**, 986–97.

Bodmer S, Imark C, Kneubuhl M (1999) Biogenic amines in foods: histamine and food processing. *Inflammation research*, **48**, 296–300.

Boguniewicz M, Schneider LC, Milgrom H *et al.* (1993) Treatment of steroid-dependent asthma with recombinant interferon-gamma. *Clinical and Experimental Allergy*, **23**, 785–90.

de Boissieu D, Dupont C, Badoual J (1994) Allergy to nondairy proteins in mother's milk as assessed by intestinal permeability tests. *Allergy*, **49**, 882–4

de Boissieu D, Matarazzo P, Dupont C (1997) Allergy to extensively hydrolyzed cow milk proteins in infants: identification and treatment with an amino acid-based formula. *Journal of Pediatrics*, **131**, 744–7.

Bonamico M, Ballati G, Mariani P *et al.* (1997) Screening for coeliac disease: the meaning of low titers of anti-gliadin antibodies (AGA) in non-coeliac children. *European Journal of Epidemiology*, **13**, 55–9.

Booth IW (1997) Gastroenterology. In: *Illustrated Textbook of Paediatrics* (eds T Lissauer, G Clayden). London: Mosby.

Boris M, Mandel FS (1994) Foods and additives are common causes of the attention deficit hyperactive disorder in children. *Annals of Allergy*, **72**, 462–8.

Borish L (1999) Genetics of allergy and asthma. *Annals of Allergy, Asthma and Immunology*, **82**, 413–24.

Bousquet J, Neukirch F, Noyola A, Michel F-B (1992) Prevalence of food allergy in asthma. *Pediatric Allergy and Immunology*, **3**, 206–13.

Bresser H, Sandner C, Rakoski J (1995) Anaphylactic emergencies in Munich in 1992. *Journal of Allergy and Clinical Immunology*, **96**, 368 (abstract).

Brett PM, Yiannakou JY, Morris M-A *et al.* (1999) Common HLA alleles, rather than rare mutants, confer susceptibly to coeliac disease. *Annals of Human Genetics*, **63**, 217–25.

Briet F, Pochart P, Marteau P *et al.* (1997) Improved clinical tolerance to chronic lactose ingestion in subjects with lactose intolerance. A placebo effect? *Gut*, **41**, 632–5.

British Nutrition Foundation (1992) *Report of the Task Force on Unsaturated Fatty Acids*. Chapman & Hall, London.

British Nutrition Foundation (1999) *Briefing Paper:* n-*3 Fatty Acids and Health*. British Nutrition Foundation, London.

British Retail Consortium (1998) *Guidelines for the Handling of Nuts and the BRC Nut Classification*. London: British Retail Consortium. (Available from BRC, 5 Grafton Street, London W1X 3LB; Tel: 020 7647 1500, Fax: 020 7647 1582.)

British Society of Gastroenterology (1996) *Guidelines in Gastroenterology: Guidelines for the Management of Patients with Coeliac Disease*. London, British Society of Gastroenterology.

Broberg A, Engstrom I, Kalimo K, Reimers L (1992) Elimination diet in young children with atopic dermatitis. *Acta Dermato Venereologica (Stockholm)*, **72**, 365–9.

Broide D, Schwarze J, Tighe H *et al.* (1998) Immunostimulatory DNA sequences inhibit IL-5, eosinophilic inflammation, and airway hyperresponsiveness in mice. *Journal of Immunology*, **161**, 7054–62.

Broughton KS, Johnson CS, Pace BK, Liebman M, Kleppinger KM (1997) Reduced asthma symptoms with n-3 fatty acid ingestion are related to 5-series leukotriene production. *American Journal of Clinical Nutrition*, **65**, 1011–7.

Brown KH, Black RE, Lopez de Romana G, Creed de Kanashiro H (1989) Infant feeding practices and their relationship with diarrheal and other diseases. *Pediatrics*, **83**, 31–40.

Brown KH, Peerson JM, Fontaine O (1994) Use of non-human milks in the dietary management of young children with acute diarrhoea: a meta-analysis of clinical trials. *Paediatrics*, **93**, 17–27.

Brown P, Gadjusek DC (1978) Acute and chronic pulmonary airway disease in pacific micronesians. *American Journal of Epidemiology*, **108**, 226–33.

Bruijnzeel-Koomen C, Ortolani C, Aas K *et al.* (1995) Adverse reactions to food. *Allergy*, **50**, 623–35.

Bruno G, Giampietro PG, Del Guercio MJ *et al.* (1997) Soy allergy is not common in atopic children: a multicenter study. *Pediatric Allergy and Immunology*, **8**, 190–3.

Burkitt DP, Walker AR, Painter NS (1972) Effect of dietary fibre on stools and transit times, and its role in the causation of disease. *Lancet*, **2**, 1408–11.

Burks AW, James JM, Hiegel A *et al.* (1998) Atopic dermatitis and food hypersensitivity reactions. *Journal of Pediatrics*, **132**, 132–6.

Burks AW, Mallory SB, Williams LW, Shirrell MA (1988) Atopic dermatitis: clinical relevance of food hypersensitivity reactions. *Journal of Pediatrics*, **113**, 327–34.

Burr ML, Butland BK, King S, Vaughan-Williams E (1989) Changes in asthma prevalence: two surveys 15 years apart [see comments]. *Archives of Diseases in Childhood*, **64**, 1452–6.

Businco L, Bruno G, Giampietro PG, Cantani A (1992) Allergenicity and nutritional adequacy of soy protein formulas. *Journal of Pediatrics*, **121**, S21–28.

Businco L, Cantani A, Longhi MA, Giampietro PG (1989) Anaphylactic reactions to a cow's milk whey protein hydrolysate (Alfa-Re, Nestle) in infants with cow's milk allergy. *Annals of Allergy*, **62**, 333–5.

Businco L, Dreborg S, Einarsson R *et al.* (1993) Hydrolysed cow's milk formulae. Allergenicity and use in treatment and prevention. An ESPACI position paper. European Society of Pediatric Allergy and Clinical Immunology. *Pediatric Allergy and Immunology*, **4**, 101–11.

Businco L, Megho P, Amato G *et al.* (1996) Evaluation of the efficacy of oral cromolyn sodium or an oligoantigenic diet in children with atopic dermatitis: a multicenter study of 1085 patients. *Journal of Investigation in Allergy and Clinical Immunology*, **6**, 103–9.

Calder PC (1997) n-3 polyunsaturated fatty acids and cytokine production in health and disease. *Annals of Nutrition and Metabolism*, **41**, 203–34.

Calder PC (1998a) Dietary fatty acids and the immune system. *Nutrition Reviews*, **56**, S70–83.

Calder PC (1998b) Dietary fatty acids and lymphocyte functions. *Proceedings of the Nutrition Society*, **57**, 487–502.

Calder PC (1998c) n-3 Polyunsaturated fatty acids and mononuclear phagocyte function. In: *Medicinal Fatty Acids in Inflammation* (ed. J. Kremer). Basel: Birkhauser Verlag.

Calder PC, Jackson AA (2000) Undernutrition, infection and immune function. *Nutrition Research Reviews*, **13**, 3–29.

Calder PC, Miles EA (2000) Fatty acids and atopic disease. *Pediatric Allergy and Immunology*, **11**, 529–36.

Calder PC, Yaqoob P (1999) Glutamine and the immune system. *Amino Acids*, **17**, 227–41.

Cant AJ, Gibson P, Dancy M (1984) Food hypersensitivity made life threatening by ingestion of aspirin. *British Medical Journal*, **288**, 755–6.

Cantani A (1992) Home-prepared meat diet for feeding the allergic child. *Revue Europenne par les Sciences Medicales et Pharmacologiques*, **14**, 53–61.

Cantani A, Lucenti P (1997) Natural history of soy allergy and/or intolerance in children, and clinical use of soy-protein formulas. *Pediatric Allergy and Immunology*, **8**, 59–74.

Carney MW, Barry S (1985) Clinical and subclinical thiamine deficiency in clinical practice. *Clinical Neuropharmacology*, **8**, 286–93.

Carter C (1994) The immune system. In: *Clinical Paediatric Dietetics* (eds. V Shaw, M Lawsons) Oxford: Blackwell Science.

Carter CM, Urbanowicz M, Hemsley R *et al.* (1993) Effects of a few food diet in attention deficit disorder. *Archives of Diseases in Childhood*, **69**, 564–8.

Casale TB, Bernstein IL, Busse W *et al.* (1997) Use of anti-IgE humanized monoclonal antibody in ragweed-induced allergic rhinitis. *Journal of Allergy and Clinical Immunology*, **100**, 100–10.

Castellanos FX (1997) Toward a pathophysiology of attention-deficit/hyperactivity disorder. *Clinical Pediatric (Philadelphia)*, **36**, 381–93.

Cataldo F, Lio D, Marino V, Picarelli A, Ventura A, Corazza GR (2000) IgG(1) antiendomysium and IgG anti-tissue transglutaminase (anti-tTG) antibodies in coeliac patients with selective IgA deficiency. Working Groups on coeliac disease of SIGEO and Club del Tenue. *Gut*, **47**, 366–9.

Cataldo F, Marino V, Ventura A, Bottaro G, Corazza GR (1998) Prevalence and clinical features of selective immunoglobulin A deficiency in coeliac disease: an Italian multi-centre study. *Gut*, **42**, 392–5.

Catassi C, Ratsch IM, Fabiani E *et al.* (1994) Coeliac disease in the year 2000: exploring the iceberg. *Lancet*, **343**, 200–203.

Caughey GE, Mantzioris E, Gibson RA, Cleland LG, James MJ (1996) The effect on human tumor necrosis factor alpha and interleukin 1 beta production of diets enriched in n-3 fatty acids from vegetable oil or fish oil. *American Journal of Clinical Nutrition*, **63**, 116–22.

Cavagni G, Paganelli R, Caffarelli C *et al.* (1988) Passage of food antigens into circulation of breast-fed infants with atopic dermatitis. *Annals of Allergy*, **61**, 361–5.

Champion RH, Roberts SO, Carpenter RG, Roger JH (1969) Urticaria and angio-oedema. A review of 554 patients. *British Journal of Dermatology*, **81**, 588 97.

Chandra RK (1975) Reduced secretory antibody response to live attenuated measles and poliovirus vaccines in malnourished children. *British Medical Journal*, **2**, 583–5.

Chandra RK (1979) Serum thymic hormone activity in protein-energy malnutrition. *Clinical and Experimental Immunology*, **38**, 228–30.

Chandra RK (1983) Numerical and functional deficiency in T helper cells in protein-energy malnutrition. *Clinical and Experimental Immunology*, **51**, 126–32.

Chandra RK (1984) Excessive intake of zinc impairs immune responses. *Journal of the American Medical Association*, **252**, 1443–6.

Chandra RK (1991) 1990 McCollum Award Lecture. Nutrition and immunity: lessons from the past and new insights into the future. *American Journal of Clinical Nutrition*, **53**, 1087–101.

Chandra RK (1992) Effect of vitamin and trace-element supplementation on immune responses and infection in elderly subjects. *Lancet*, **340**, 1124–7.

Chandra RK (1997a) Food hypersensitivity and allergic disease: selective review. *American Journal of Clinical Nutrition*, **66**, 526S–529S.

Chandra RK (1997b) Five-year follow-up of high-risk infants with family history of allergy who were exclusively breast-fed or fed partial whey hydrolysate, soy, and conventional cow's milk formulas. *Journal of Pediatric Gastroenterology and Nutrition*, **24**, 380–8.

Chandra RK, Chandra S, Gupta S (1984) Antibody affinity and immune complexes after immunization with tetanus toxoid in protein-energy malnutrition. *American Journal of Clinical Nutrition*, **40**, 131–4.

Chandra RK, Gupta S, Singh H (1982) Inducer and suppressor T cell subsets in protein-energy malnutrition. *Nutrition Research*, **2**, 21–6.

Chandra RK, Hamed A (1991) Cumulative incidence of atopic disorders in high risk infants fed whey hydrolysate, soy and conventional cow milk formulas. *Annals of Allergy*, **67**, 129–32.

Chandra RK, Puri S, Hamed A (1989) Influence of maternal diet during lactation and use of formula feeds on development of atopic eczema in high risk infants. *British Medical Journal*, **299**, 228–30.

Chandra RK, Puri S, Suraiya C, Cheema PS (1986) Influence of maternal food antigen avoidance during pregnancy and lactation on incidence of atopic eczema in infants. *Clinical Allergy*, **16**, 563–9.

Chavance M, Herbeth B, Fournier C, Janot C, Vernhes G (1989) Vitamin status, immunity and infections in an elderly population. *European Journal of Clinical Nutrition*, **43**, 827–35.

Chen Y, Inote J, Marks R, *et al.* (1995) Peripheral deletion of antigen-reactive T-cells in oral tolerance. *Nature*, **376**, 177–80.

Chiu JT, Haydik IB (1991) Sesame seed oil anaphylaxis. *Journal of Allergy and Clinical Immunology*, **88**, 414–15.

Ciclitira PJ, Evans DJ, Fagg NL, Lennox ES, Dowling RH (1984) Clinical testing of gliadin fractions in coeliac patients. *Clinical Science*, **66**, 357–64.

Ciclitira PJ, Sturgess RP (1992) Clinicopathogenic mechanisms in coeliac disease. *Current Opinion in Gastroenterology*, **8**, 262–7.

Clarke MC, Kilburn SA, Hourihane JO *et al.* (1998) Serological characteristics of peanut allergy. *Clinical and Experimental Allergy*, **28**, 1251–7.

Clough JB (1993) The effect of gender on the prevalence of atopy and asthma. *Clinical and Experimental Allergy*, **23**, 883–5.

Codex Alimentarius Commission (1981) Joint FAO/

WHO Food Standards Programme. Codex Standard 118, Rome.

Codex Alimentarius Commission (1998) Joint FAO/WHO Food Standards Programme. 21st Session, Berlin.

Codex Alimentarius Commission (2000) *Report of the 22nd session of the Codex Committee on Nutrition and Foods for Special Dietary Uses (Alinorm 01/26) CL2000/22 – NFSDU*. Rome: Codex.

Codex Committee on Food Labelling (1999) *Report of 26th Session, 26–29 May 1998, Alinorm 99/22*, Appendix III. Rome: Codex.

Cohen M, Splansky GL, Gallagher J, Bernstein DI, Bernstein IL (1985) Epidemiologic survey and validation of adverse food reactions in adult populations. *Journal of Allergy and Clinical Immunology*, **75**, 206 (abstract).

Collin P, Reunala T, Rasmussen M *et al.* (1997) High incidence and prevalence of adult coeliac disease. *Scandinavian Journal of Gastroenterology*, **32**, 1129–33.

Collins SM (1999) Current status of the irritable bowel syndrome. *Canadian Journal of Gastroenterology*, **13**, 7A.

Collins SM, Barbara G, Vallance B (1999) Stress, inflammation and the irritable bowel syndrome. *Canadian Journal of Gastroenterology*, **13**, 47A–49A.

Conners CK, Goyette CH, Newman LB (1980) Dose-time effect of artificial colors in hyperactive children. *Journal of Learning Disabilities*, **13**, 512–6.

Conners CK, Sitarenios G, Parker JD, Epstein JN (1998) The revised Conners Parent Rating Scale (CPRS-R): factor structure, reliability, and criterion validity. *Journal of Abnormal Child Psychology*, **26**, 257–68.

Conners CK, Wells KC, Parker JD *et al.* (1997) A new self-report scale for assessment of adolescent psychopathology: factor structure, reliability, validity, and diagnostic sensitivity. *Journal of Abnormal Child Psychology*, **25**, 487–97.

Connor DF, Fletcher KF, Swanson JM (1999) A meta-analysis of clonidine for symptoms of attention-deficit hyperactivity disorder. *Journal of the American Academy of Child and Adolescent Psychiatry*, **38**, 1551–9.

Cooke WT, Holmes GKI (1984) *Coeliac Disease*. Edinburgh: Churchill Livingstone.

Cookson JB (1987) Prevalence rates of asthma in developing countries and their comparison with those in Europe and North America. *Chest*, **91**, 97S–103S.

Coombs RR, Holgate ST (1990) Allergy and cot death: with special focus on allergic sensitivity to cows' milk and anaphylaxis. *Clinical and Experimental Allergy*, **20**, 359–66.

Corazza GR, Benati G, Di Sarioo A *et al.* (1995) Lactose intolerance and bone mass in postmenopausal Italian women. *British Journal of Nutrition*, **73**, 479–87.

Cosgrove M, Jenkins HR (1997) Experience of percutaneous endoscopic gastrostomy in children with Crohn's disease. *Archives of Diseases in Childhood*, **76**, 141–3.

Costa JJ, Weller PF, Galli SJ (1997) The cells of the allergic response. *Journal of the American Medical Association*, **78**, 1815–22.

Coutsoudis A, Bobat RA, Coovadia HM *et al.* (1995) The effects of vitamin A supplementation on the morbidity of childen born to HIV-infected women. *American Journal of Public Health*, **85**, 1076–81.

Coutsoudis A, Pillay K, Spooner E, Kuhn L, Coovadia HM (1999) Randomized trial testing the effect of vitamin A supplementation on pregnancy outcomes and early mother-to-child transmission in Durban, South Africa. South African Vitamin A Study Group. *AIDS*, **13**, 1517–24.

Crespo JF, Pascual C, Burks AW, Helm RM, Esteban MM (1995) Frequency of food allergy in a pediatric population from Spain. *Pediatric Allergy and Immunology*, **6**, 39–43.

Croner S, Kjellman NI (1992) Natural history of bronchial asthma in childhood. A prospective study from birth up to 12–14 years of age. *Allergy*, **47**, 150–57.

Croner S, Kjellman NI, Eriksson B, Roth A (1982) IgE screening in 1701 newborn infants and the development of atopic disease during infancy. *Archives of Diseases in Childhood*, **57**, 364–8.

Cronin CC, Jackson LM, Feighery C *et al.* (1998) Coeliac Disease and epilepsy. *Quarterly Journal of Medicine*, **91**, 303–8.

Cullen A, Kiberd B, McDonnell M *et al.* (2000) Sudden infant death syndrome – are parents getting the message? *Irish Journal of Medical Science*, **169**, 40–43.

Daly G, Hawi Z, Fitzgerald M, Gill M (1999) Mapping susceptibility loci in attention deficit hyperactivity disorder: preferential transmission of parental alleles at DAT1, DBH and DRD5 to affected children. *Molecular Psychiatry*, **4**, 192–6.

Daly JM, Reynolds JV, Thom A *et al.* (1988) Immune and metabolic effects of arginine in the surgical patient. *Annals of Surgery*, **208**, 512–23.

Dannaeus A, Inganas M (1981) A follow-up study of children with food allergy. Clinical course in relation to serum IgE- and IgG-antibody levels to milk, egg and fish. *Clinical Allergy*, **11**, 533–9.

Daroca P, Crespo JF, Reano M *et al.* (2000) Asthma and rhinitis induced by exposure to raw green beans and chards [in process citation]. *Annals of Allergy, Asthma and Immunology*, **85**, 215–18.

Davenport P (1996) Use your loaf and ignore the snobs. *Financial Times*, 9 March, xl.

David TJ (1984) Anaphylactic shock during elimination diets for severe atopic eczema. *Archives of Diseases in Childhood*, **59**, 983–6.

David TJ (1987) Unhelpful recent developments in the diagnosis and treatment of allergy and food intolerance in children. In: *Food Intolerance* (ed. J Dobing). London: Bailliere Tindall.

David TJ (1989) Short stature in children with atopic eczema. *Acta Dermalogia Venerologia*, **114**, S41–S44.

David TJ (1992) Extreme dietary measures in the management of atopic dermatitis in childhood. *Acta Dermato Venereologica Supplement (Stockholm)*, **176**, S113–116.

David TJ (ed.) (1993a) *Food and Food Additive Intolerance in Childhood*. Oxford: Blackwell Science.

David TJ (1993b) Soya protein intolerance. In: *Food and Food Additive Intolerance in Childhood* (ed. TJ David). Oxford: Blackwell Science.

Davidovits M, Levy Y, Avramovitz T, Eisenstein B (1993) Calcium-deficiency rickets in a four-year-old boy with milk allergy. *Journal of Pediatrics*, **122**, 249–51.

Dean TP, Adler BR, Ruge F, Warner JO (1993) In vitro allergenicity of cows' milk substitutes. *Clinical and Experimental Allergy*, **23**, 205–10.

Dearman RJ, Kimber I (2001) Determination of protein allergenicity: studies in mice. *Toxicology Letters*, **120**, 181–6.

Defrance T, Vanbervliet B, Briere F et al. (1992) Interleukin-10 and transforming growth factor beta cooperate to induce anti-CD40 activated naïve human B-cells to secrete immunoglobulin A. *Journal of Experimental Medicine*, **175**, 671–82.

Department of Health (1991) Dietary reference values for food energy and nutrients for the United Kingdom. *Report on Health and Social Subjects No. 41*. London: HMSO.

Department of Health (1994) Weaning and the weaning diet. *Report on Health and Social subjects No. 45*. London: HMSO.

Department of Health (1997) Peanut Allergy. Committee on Toxicity of Chemicals in Food, Consumer Products and the Environment. London: Department of Health.

D'Eufemia P, Celli M, Finocchiaro R et al. (1996) Abnormal intestinal permeability in children with autism. *Acta Paediatrica*, **85**, 1076–9.

Devereux G, Ayatollahi T, Ward R et al. (1996) Asthma and airway responsiveness in two Health Districts of Northern England. *Thorax*, **51**, 169–74.

Devey ME, Beckman S, Kemeny DM (1993) The functional affinities of antibodies of different IgG subclasses to dietary antigens in mothers and their babies. *Clinical Experimental Immunology*, **94**, 117–21.

Devlin J, David TJ (1992) Tartrazine in atopic eczema. *Archives of Diseases in Childhood*, **67**, 709–11.

Devlin J, David TJ, Stanton RH (1991) Six food diet for childhood atopic dermatitis. *Acta Dermato Venereologica*, **71**, 20–24.

Dhanjal MK, Towler AE, Tuft S et al. (1992) The detection of IgE-secreting cells in the peripheral blood of patients with atopic dermatitis. *Journal of Allergy and Clinical Immunology*, **89**, 895–904.

Dieterich W, Ehnis T, Bauer M et al. (1997) Identification of tissue transglutaminase as the autoantigen of coeliac disease. *Natural Medicine*, **3**, 797–801.

DiPalma JA, Collins MS (1989) Enzyme replacement for lactose malabsorption using a beta-D-galactosidase. *Journal of Clinical Gastroenterology*, **11**, 290–3.

DiPalma AM, DiPalma JA (1997) Recurrent abdominal pain and lactose maldigestion in school-aged children. *Gastroenterology Nursing*, **20**, 180–83.

Dodge RR, Burrows B (1980) The prevalence and incidence of asthma and asthma like symptoms in a general population sample. *American Review of Respiratory Diseases*, **122**, 567–75.

Dohan FC (1988) Genetic hypothesis of idiopathic schizophrenia: its exorphin connection. *Schizophrenia Bulletin*, **14**, 489–94.

Dolovich J, Hargreave FE, Chalmers R et al. (1973) Late cutaneous allergic responses in isolated IgE-dependent reactions. *Journal of Allergy and Clinical Immunology*, **52**, 38–46.

Douwes AC, Van Weert-Waltman ML, Folkerstma K, Fagel IFM, Verboom WSW (1988) Prevalentie van voedselallergie bij Amsterdamse zuigelingen. *Ned Tijdschr Geneesk*, **132**, 1392–6.

Dow L, Tracey M, Villar A et al. (1996) Does dietary intake of vitamins C and E influence lung function in older people? *American Journal of Respiratory and Critical Care Medicine*, **154**, 1401–404.

Dreborg S (on behalf of the Sub-Committee on Skin tests of the European Academy of Allergy and Clinical Immunology) (1989) Skin tests used in type I allergy testing. *Allergy*, **44**, Sl–59.

Ebner C, Hirchwehr R, Bauer L et al. (1995) Identification of allergens in fruits and vegetables: IgE cross-reactivities with the important birch pollen allergens Bet v 1 and Bet v 2 (birch profilin). *Journal of Allergy and Clinical Immunology*, **95**, 962–9.

Editorial (1994) Doubts about bran. *Lancet*, **3**, 334.

Editorial (2000) Occupational latex allergy: the magnitude of the problem and its prevention. *Clinical and Experimental Allergy*, **30**, 458–60.

Edston E, Gidlund F, Wickman M, Ribbing H, Van Hage-Hamsten M (1999) Increased mast cell tryptase in sudden infant death – anaphylaxis, hypoxia or artefact? *Clinical and Experimental Allergy*, **29**, 1648–54.

Egger J, Carter CM, Graham PJ, Gumley D, Soothill JF

(1985) Controlled trial of oligoantigenic treatment in the hyperkinetic syndrome. *Lancet*, **1**, 540–45.

Egger J, Carter CM, Soothill JF, Wilson J (1989) Oligoantigenic diet treatment of children with epilepsy and migraine. *Journal of Pediatrics*, **113**, 51–8.

Egger J, Carter CM, Wilson J, Turner MW, Soothill JF (1983) Is migraine food allergy? A double-blind controlled trial of oligoantigenic diet treatment. *Lancet*, **2**, 865–9.

Eigenmann PA, Calza AM (2000) Diagnosis of IgE-mediated food allergy among Swiss children with atopic dermatitis [in process citation]. *Pediatric Allergy and Immunology*, **11**, 95–100.

Eigenmann PA, Sampson HA (1998) Interpreting skin prick tests in the evaluation of food allergy in children [see comments]. *Pediatric Allergy and Immunology*, **9**, 186–91.

Elia M, Lunn PG (1997) The use of glutamine in the treatment of gastrointestinal disorders in man. *Nutrition*, **13**, 743–7.

Ellis HJ, Doyle AP, Wieser H, Day P, Ciclitira PJ (1994) Demonstration of the presence of coeliac activating gliadin-like epitopes in malted barley. *International Archives of Allergy and Immunology*, **104**, 308–10.

Ellis HJ, Frazer JS, Ciclitira PJ (2001) Markers of malabsorption: coeliac disease. In: *Biomarkers* (eds AK Trull, CP Price, DR Holt, A Johnston, JM Tredger, L Demers). Cambridge: Cambridge University Press (in press).

Ellis HJ, Freedman AR, Ciclitira PJ (1990) Detection and estimation of the barley prolamin content of beer and malt to assess their suitability for coeliac patients. *Clinica Chimica Acta*, **189**, 123–30.

Ellis HJ, Parnell ND, Ciclitira PJ (1998b) Cornflakes and coeliac disease. *Gut*, **42**, A35.

Ellis HJ, Rosen-Bronson S, O 'Reilly N, Ciclitira PJ (1998a) Measurement of gluten using a monoclonal antibody to a coeliac toxic peptide of A-gliadin. *Gut*, **43**, 190–5.

Emmett PM, Rogers IS (1997) Properties of human milk and their relationship with maternal nutrition. *Early Human Development*, **49**, S7–28.

Esteban M (1992) Advances in food reactions in childhood: concept, importance, and present problems. *Journal of Pediatrics*, **121**, S1–3.

Evans JM, Fleming KC, Talley NJ *et al.* (1998) Relation of colonic transit to functional bowel disease in older people: a population-based study. *Journal of the American Geriatric Society*, **46**, 83–7.

Evoy D, Lieberman MD, Fahey TJ, Daly JM (1998) Immunonutrition: the role of arginine. *Nutrition*, **14**, 611–17.

Ewan PW (1996) Clinical study of peanut and nut allergy in 62 consecutive patients: new features and associations. *British Medical Journal*, **27**, 1074–8.

Fahy JV, Fleming E, Wong HH *et al.* (1997) The effect of an anti-IgE monoclonal antibody on the early- and late-phase responses to allergen inhalation in asthmatic subjects. *American Journal of Respiratory and Critical Care Medicine*, **155**, 1828–34.

Falth-Magnusson K, Kjellman NI (1992) Allergy prevention by maternal elimination diet during late pregnancy – a 5-year follow-up of a randomized study. *Journal of Allergy and Clinical Immunology*, **89**, 709–13.

Falth-Magnusson K, Kjellman NI, Magnusson KE (1988) Antibodies IgG, IgA, and IgM to food antigens during the first 18 months of life in relation to feeding and development of atopic disease. *Journal of Allergy and Clinical Immunology*, **81**, 743–9.

Falth-Magnusson K, Kjellman NI, Odelram H, Sundqvist T, Magnusson KB (1986) Gastrointestinal permeability in children with cow's milk allergy: effect of milk challenge and sodium cromoglycate as assessed with polyethyleneglycols (PEG 400 and PEG 1000). *Clinical Allergy*, **16**, 543–51.

Falth-Magnusson K, Oman H, Kjellman NI (1987) Development of atopic disease in babies whose mothers were receiving exclusion diet during pregnancy – a randomized study. *Journal of Allergy and Clinical Immunology*, **80**, 868–75.

Fanning LJ, Connor AM, Wu GE (1996) Development of the immunoglobulin repertoire. *Clinical Immunology and Immunopathology*, **79**, 1–14.

Farah DA, Calder I, Benson L, Mackenzie JF (1985) Specific food intolerance: its place as a cause of gastrointestinal symptoms. *Gut*, **26**, 164–8.

Faraone SV, Seidman LJ, Kremen WS *et al.* (1999) Neuropsychological functioning among the nonpsychotic relatives of schizophrenic patients: a 4-year follow-up study. *Journal of Abnormal Psychology*, **108**, 176–81.

Faria AM, Weiner HL (1999) Oral tolerance: mechanisms and therapeutic applications. *Advanced Immunology*, **73**, 153–264.

Farooqi IS, Hopkin JM (1998) Early childhood infection and atopic disorder. *Thorax*, **53**, 927–32.

Farthing MJ (1998) New drugs in the management of the irritable bowel syndrome. *Drugs*, **56**, 11–21.

Fawzi WW, Msamanga GI, Spiegelman D *et al.* (1998) Randomised trial of effects of vitamin supplements on pregnancy outcomes and T cell counts in HIV-1-infected women in Tanzania. *Lancet*, **351**, 1477–82.

Fearon DT, Locksley RM (1996) The instructive role of innate immunity in the acquired immune response. *Science*, **272**, 50–53.

Feingold BF (1975) Hyperkinesis and learning disabilities linked to artificial food flavors and colors. *American Journal of Nursing*, **75**, 797–803.

Ferguson A (1999) The coeliac iceberg. *CME Journal Gastroenterology Hepatology and Nutrition*, **2**, 52–6.

Ferguson A, MacDonald DM, Brydon WG (1984) Prevalence of lactose deficiency in British adults. *Gut*, **25**, 163–7.

Ferguson A, Watret KC (1988) Cows' milk intolerance. *Nutrition Research Reviews*, **1**, 1–22.

Fergusson DM, Horwood LJ, Shannon FT (1990) Early solid feeding and recurrent childhood eczema: a 10-year longitudinal study. *Pediatrics*, **86**, 541–6.

Ferreira F, Ebner C, Kramer B *et al.* (1998) Modulation of IgE reactivity of allergens by site-directed mutagenesis: potential use of hypoallergenic variants for immunotherapy. *FASEB*, **12**, 231–42.

Fleming DM, Crombie DL (1987) Prevalence of asthma and hayfever in England and Wales. *British Medical Journal*, **294**, 279–83.

Florent B, Briet F, Leblond A *et al.* (1985) Influence of chronic lactulose ingestion on the colonic metabolism of lactulose in man (an in vivo study). *Journal of Clinical Investigation*, **75**, 6088–13.

Flourie B, Briet F, Florent C *et al.* (1993) Can diarrhoea induced by lactulose be reduced by prolonged ingestion of lactulose? *American Journal of Clinical Nutrition*, **58**, 369–75.

Fogarty A, Britton J (2000) The role of diet in aetiology of asthma. *Clinical and Experimental Allergy*, **30**, 615–27.

Food Standards Agency (2000) *Adverse Reactions to Food and Food Ingredients*. A report from the Committee on Toxicity of Chemicals in Food, Consumer Products and the Environment (COT). TSO, London.

Food Standards Agency (2001) *Be Allergy Aware: Advice for Catering Establishments*. FSA: London (Available from FSA, PO Box 369, Hayes, Middlesex, UB3 1UT.)

Food Standards Agency/Department of Health (2001) *Catering for Health*. London: FSA.

Ford RP, Schluter PJ, Taylor BJ, Mitchell EA, Scragg R (1996) Allergy and the risk of sudden infant death syndrome. The Members of the New Zealand Cot Death Study Group. *Clinical and Experimental Allergy*, **26**, 580–84.

Ford RP, Walker-Smith JA (1987) Paediatric gastrointestinal food allergic disease. In: *Food Allergy and Intolerance* (eds J Brostoff, SJ Challacombe). London: Bailliere Tindall.

Fossati G, Perri M, Careddu G, Mirra N, Camelli V (1992) Pulmonary hemosiderosis induced by cows milk proteins: a discussion of a clinical case. *Pediatrica Medicae Chirurgica*, **14**, 203–207.

Fotherby KJ, Hunter JO (1985) Symptoms of food allergy. *Clinical Gastroenterology*, **14**, 615–29.

Francis CY, Whorwell PJ (1994) Bran and the irritable bowel syndrome: time for a reappraisal. *Lancet*, **334**, 39–40.

Frank L, Marian A, Visser M, Weinberg E, Potter PC (1999) Exposure to peanuts in utero and in infancy and the development of sensitization to peanut allergens in young children. *Pediatric Allergy and Immunology*, **10**, 27–32.

Freeman J (1911) Further observations on the treatment of hay fever by hypodermic inoculations of pollen vaccine. *Lancet*, 16 September, 814–17.

Freeman J (1927) Modern technique in treatment. Treatment of hay-fever. *Lancet*, 30 April, 940–41.

Freeman J (1930) 'Rush' inoculation with special reference to hay-fever. *Lancet*, 5 April, 744.

Freigang B, Jadavji TP, Freigang DW (1994) Lack of adverse reactions to measles, mumps, and rubella vaccine in egg-allergic children. *Annals of Allergy*, **73**, 486–8.

Fremont DH, Rees WA, Kozono H (1996) Biophysical studies of T-cell receptors and their ligands. *Current Opinion in Immunology*, **8**, 93–100.

Friedman A, Sklan D (1993) Vitamin A and immunity. In: *Nutrition and Immunology* (ed. DM Klurfeld). New York and London: Plenum Press.

Fries JH (1982) Peanuts: allergic and other untoward reactions. *Annals of Allergy*, **48**, 220–26.

Fritsch R, Bohle B, Vollmann U *et al.* (1998) Bet v 1, the major birch pollen allergen, and Mal d 1, the major apple allergen, cross-react at the level of allergen-specific T helper cells. *Journal of Allergy and Clinical Immunology*, **102**, 679–86.

Fry L (1992) Dermatitis Herpetiformis. In: *Coeliac Disease* (ed. MN Marsh). Oxford: Blackwell Science.

Fuglsang G, Madsen C, Saval P, Osterballe O (1993) Prevalence of intolerance to food additives among Danish school children. *Pediatric Allergy Immunology*, **4**, 123–9.

Fukudome S, Jinsmaa Y, Matsukawa T, Sasaki R, Yoshikawa M (1997) Release of opioid peptides gluten exophins by the action of pancreatic elastase. *FEBS Letters*, **412**, 475–9.

Fukushima Y, Kawata Y, Onda T, Kitagawa M (1997) Long-term consumption of whey hydrolysate formula by lactating women reduces the transfer of beta-lactoglobulin into human milk. *Journal of Nutritional Science and Vitaminology (Tokyo)*, **43**, 673–8.

Fuller R (1992) History and development of probiotics. In: *Probiotics: The Scientific Basis* (ed. R Fuller). London: Chapman & Hall.

Gaby AR (1998) The role of hidden food allergy/intolerance in chronic disease. *Alternative Medicine Reviews*, **3**, 90–100.

Galant SP, Franz ML, Walher P, Wells ID, Lundak RL (1977) A potential diagnostic method for food allergy: clinical application and immunogenicity evaluation of an elemental diet. *American Journal of Clinical Nutrition*, **30**, 512–16.

Geha RS (2000) Allergy, a disease of the internal and the external environments. *Current Opinions in Immunology*, **12**, 615–17.

Genton C, Frei PC, Pecoud A (1985) Value of oral provocation tests to aspirin and food additives in the routine investigation of asthma and chronic urticaria. *Journal of Allergy and Clinical Immunology*, **76**, 40–45.

George EK, Mearin ML, Franken HC *et al.* (1997) Twenty years of childhood coeliac disease in The Netherlands: a rapidly increasing incidence. *Gut*, **40**, 61–6.

Germain RN (1994) MHC-dependent antigen processing and peptide presentation: providing ligands for T lymphocyte activation. *Cell*, **76**, 287–99.

Gerrard JW, MacKenzie JW, Goluboff N, Garson JZ, Maningas CS (1973) Cow's milk allergy: prevalence and manifestations in an unselected series of newborns. *Acta Paediatrica Scandinavia*, **234**, S1–21.

Geusens PP (1998) *n*-3 Fatty acids in the treatment of rheumatoid arthritis. In: *Medicinal Fatty Acids in Inflammation* (ed. J Kremer). Basel: Birkhauser Verlag.

Giampietro PG, Ragno V, Daniele S *et al.* (1992) Soy hypersensitivity in children with food allergy. *Annals of Allergy*, **69**, 143–6.

Gibney MJ, Hunter B (1993) The effects of short- and long-term supplementation with fish oil on the incorporation of *n*-3 polyunsaturated fatty acids into cells of the immune system in healthy volunteers. *European Journal of Clinical Nutrition*, **47**, 255–9.

Gillberg C (1995) Endogenous opioids and opiate antagonists in autism: brief review of empirical findings and implications for clinicians. *Developments of Medicine in Child Neurology*, **37**, 239–45.

Girodon F, Lombard M, Galan P *et al.* (1996) Effect of micronutrient supplementation on infection in institutionalised elderly subjects: a controlled trial. *Annals of Nutrition and Metabolism*, **41**, 98–107.

Gislason D, Bjornsson E, Gislason T *et al.* (1999) Sensitisation to airborne and food allergens in Reykjavik (Iceland) and Uppsala (Sweden) – a comparative study. *Allergy*, **54**, 1160–67.

Gjesing B, Osterballe O, Schwartz B, Wahn U, Lowenstein H (1986) Allergen-specific IgE antibodies against antigenic components in cow milk and milk substitutes. *Allergy*, **41**, 51–6.

Godfrey RC (1975) Asthma and IgE levels in rural and urban communities of the Gambia. *Clinical Allergy*, **5**, 201–207.

Goldin BR (1998) Health benefits of probiotics. *British Journal of Nutrition*, **80**, S203–207.

Golding DN (1990) Is there an allergic synovitis? *Journal of the Royal Society of Medicine*, **83**, 312–14.

Golding J, Emmett PM, Rogers IS (1997a) Gastroenteritis, diarrhoea and breast feeding. *Early Human Development*, **49**, S83–103.

Golding J, Emmett PM, Rogers IS (1997b) Does breast feeding protect against non-gastric infections? *Early Human Development*, **49**, S105–20.

Golding J, Emmett PM, Rogers IS (1997c) Breast feeding and infant mortality. *Early Human Development*, **49**, S143–55.

Goulet O, Ricour C (1995) Paediatric Enteral Nutrition. In: *Artificial Nutrition Support in Clinical Practice* (eds. J Payne-James, G Grimble, D Silk). London: Edward Arnold.

Grant EN, Daugherty SR, Moy JN *et al.* (1999) Prevalence and burden of illness for asthma and related symptoms among kindergartners in Chicago public schools. *Annals of Allergy Asthma and Immunology*, **83**, 113–20.

Gray J, Bentovim A (1996) Illness induction syndrome: paper I – a series of 41 children from 37 families identified at The Great Ormond Street Hospital for Children NHS Trust. *Child Abuse and Neglect*, **20**, 655–73.

Grazioli I, Melzi G, Balsamo V *et al.* (1993) Food intolerance and irritable bowel syndrome of childhood: clinical efficacy of oral sodium cromoglycate and elimination diet. *Minerva Pediatrica*, **45**, 253–8.

Greaves M, Lawlor F (1991) Angioedema: manifestations and management. *Journal of the American Academy of Dermatology*, **25**, 155–61; discussion 61–5.

Greaves MW (1995) Chronic urticaria [published erratum appears in *New England Journal of Medicine* 1995, **333**, 1091]. *New England Journal of Medicine*, **332**, 1767–72.

Greco L, Maki M, DiDonato F, Visakorpi JK (1992) Epidemiology of coeliac disease in Europe and the Mediterranean area. In: *Common Food Intolerances 1. Epidemiology of Coeliac Disease* (eds S Auricchio, JK Visakorpi). Basel: Karger.

Greden JF (1974) Anxiety or caffeinism: a diagnostic dilemma. *American Journal of Psychiatry*, **131**, 1089–92.

Greene LS (1995) Asthma and antioxidant stress – nutritional, environmental and genetic risk factors. *Journal of the American College of Nutrition*, **14**, 317–24.

Gribbin M, Walker-Smith J, Wood C (1976) Delayed

recovery following acute gastroenteritis. *Acta Paediatrica Belgica*, **29**, 167–76.

Gross RL, Newberne PM (1980) Role of nutrition in immunologic function. *Physiological Reviews*, **60**, 188–302.

Grulee CG, Sandford HN (1936) The influence of breast and artificial feeding on infantile eczema. *Journal of Pediatrics*, **9**, 223–5.

Gudzent F (1935) Testung und Geilbehhandlung von Rheumatismus und Gichtmit spezifischen Allergenen. *Dutch Medicine Wochenschr*, 61.

Gustafsson D, Lowhagen T, Andersson K (1992) Risk of developing atopic disease after early feeding with cows' milk based formula. *Archives of Diseases in Childhood*, **67**, 1008–10.

Hoby MM, Peat JK, Marks GB, Woolcock AJ, Leeder SR (2001) Asthma in preschool children: prevalence and risk factors. *Thorax*, **56**, 589–95.

Hadjivassilou M, Grunewald RA, Davies-Jones GA (1999) Gluten sensitivity: a many headed hydra. *British Medical Journal*, **318**, 1710–11.

Huffujee IE (1991) The pathophysiology, clinical features and management of rotavirus diarrhoea. *Quarterly Journal of Medicine*, **79**, 289–99.

Hagan LL, Goetz DW, Revercomb CH, Garriott J (1998) Sudden infant death syndrome: a search for allergen hypersensitivity. *Annals of Allergy Asthma Immunology*, **80**, 227–31.

Halken S, Hansen KS, Jacobsen HP *et al.* (2000) Comparison of a partially hydrolyzed infant formula with two extensively hydrolyzed formulas for allergy prevention: a prospective, randomized study. *Pediatric Allergy and Immunology*, **11**, 149–61.

Halken S, Jacobsen HP, Høst A, Holmenlund D (1995) The effect of hypo-allergenic formulas in infants at risk of allergic disease. *European Journal of Clinical Nutrition*, **49**, S77–83.

Hallert C (1998) The epidemiology of coeliac disease: a continuous enigma. In: *The Changing Features of Coeliac Disease* (eds S Lohiniemi, P Collin, M Maki). Tampere, Finland: The Finnish Coeliac Society.

Hallert C, Gotthard R, Jansson G, Norbrby K, Walan A (1983) Similar prevalence of coeliac disease in children and middle aged adults in a district of Sweden. *Gut*, **24**, 389–91.

Hammer HF, Petritsh W, Pristautz H, Krejs GJ (1996) Evaluation of the pathogenesis of flatulence and abdominal cramps in patients with lactose malabsorption. *Wien Klin Wochenschr*, **108**, 175–9.

Han SN, Meydani SN (1999) Vitamin E and infectious disease in the aged. *Proceedings of the Nutrition Society*, **58**, 697–705.

Hanifin JM (1987) Epidemiology of atopic dermatitis. *Monographs in Allergy*, **21**, 116–31.

Hanington E (1971) Migraine. *Trans Medical Society London*, **87**, 32–9.

Hankey GL, Holmes GK (1994) Coeliac disease in the elderly. *Gut*, **35**, 65–7.

Hannuksela M, Haahtela T (1987) Hypersensitivity reactions to food additives. *Allergy*, **42**, 561–75.

Hanson LA, Ahlstedt S, Andersson B *et al.* (1985) Protective factors in milk and the development of the immune system. *Pediatrics*, **75**, 172–6.

Hanson LA, Dahlman-Hoglund A, Lundin S *et al.* (1997) Early determinants of immunocompetence. *Nutrition Reviews*, **55**, S12–20.

Harris A, Twarog FJ, Geha RS (1983) Chronic urticaria in childhood: natural course and etiology. *Annals of Allergy*, **51**, 161–5.

Hasselmark L, Malmgren R, Zetterstrom O, Unge G (1993) Selenium supplementation in intrinsic asthma. *Allergy*, **48**, 30–36.

Hatch GE (1995) Asthma, inhaled oxidants and dietary antioxidants. *American Journal of Clinical Nutrition*, **61**, S625–30.

Hathaway MJ, Warner JO (1983) Compliance problems in the dietary management of eczema. *Archives of Diseases in Childhood*, **58**, 463–4.

Hattevig G, Kjellman B, Sigurs N, Bjorksten B, Kjellman NI (1989) Effect of maternal avoidance of eggs, cow's milk and fish during lactation upon allergic manifestations in infants. *Clinical and Experimental Allergy*, **19**, 27–32.

Hattevig G, Sigurs N, Kjellman B (1996) Maternal food antigen avoidance during lactation during the first 10 years of age. *Journal of Allergy and Clinical Immunology*, **97**, 241.

Healy D, Wallace FA, Miles EA, Calder PC, Newsholme P (2000) The effect of low to moderate amounts of dietary fish oil on neutrophil lipid composition and function. *Lipids*, **35**, 763–8.

Henz BM, Zuberbier T (1998) Most chronic urticaria is food-dependent, and not idiopathic. *Experimental Dermatology*, **7**, 139–42.

Hermans MM, Brummer R-JM, Ruijgers AM, Stockbrugger RW (1997) The relationship between lactose intolerance test results and symptoms of lactose intolerance. *American Journal of Gastroenterology*, **92**, 981–4.

Hertzler SR, Huynh BCL, Savaaiano DA (1996) How much lactose is low lactose? *Journal of the American Dietetic Association*, **96**, 243–6.

Hertzler SR, Savaiano DA (1996) Colonic adaptation to daily lactose feeding in lactose maldigesters reduces lactose intolerance. *American Journal of Clinical Nutrition*, **64**, 232–6.

Hewson DC (1984) Is there a role for gluten-free diets in multiple sclerosis? *Human Nutrition; Applied Nutrition*, **38**, 417–20.

Hide DW, Guyer BM (1985) Clinical manifestations of allergy related to breast- and cow's milk-feeding. *Pediatrics*, **76**, 973–5.

Hide DW, Matthews S, Matthews L *et al.* (1994) Effect of allergen avoidance in infancy on allergic manifestations at age two years. *Journal of Allergy and Clinical Immunology*, **93**, 842–6.

Hide DW, Warner JA (1997) *Allergy and Allergic Diseases*. Oxford: Blackwell Science.

Hijazi N, Abalkhail B, Seaton A (1998) Asthma and respiratory symptoms in urban and rural Saudi Arabia. *European Respiratory Journal*, **12**, 41–4.

Hill AS, Skerritt JH (1990) Determination of gluten in foods using a monoclonal antibody-based competition enzyme immunoassay. *Food and Agricultural Immunology*, **2**, 21–35.

Hill DJ, Ball G, Hosking CS (1988) Clinical manifestations of cows' milk allergy in childhood. I. Associations with in-vitro cellular immune responses. *Clinical Allergy*, **18**, 469–79.

Hill DJ, Bannister DG, Hosking CS, Kemp AS (1994) Cow milk allergy within the spectrum of atopic disorders. *Clinical and Experimental Allergy*, **24**, 1137–43.

Hill DJ, Ford RP, Shelton MJ, Hosking CS (1984) A study of 100 infants and young children with cow's milk allergy. *Clinical Review of Allergy*, **2**, 125–42.

Hill DJ, Heine RG, Cameron DJ, Francis DE, Bines JE (1999) The natural history of intolerance to soy and extensively hydrolyzed formula in infants with multiple food protein intolerance. *Journal of Pediatrics*, **135**, 118–21.

Hill DJ, Hudson IL, Sheffield U *et al.* (1995) A low allergen diet is a significant intervention in infantile colic: results of a community-based study. *Journal of Allergy and Clinical Immunology*, **96**, 886–92.

Hin H, Bird G, Fisher P, Mahy N, Jewell D (1999) Coeliac disease in primary care: a case finding study. *British Medical Journal*, **318**, 164–7.

Hodge L, Peat JK, Salome C (1994) Increased consumption of polyunsaturated oils may be a cause of increased prevalence of childhood asthma. *Australia and New Zealand Journal of Medicine*, **24**, 727.

Hodge L, Salome CE, Peat JK *et al.* (1996) Consumption of oily fish and childhood asthma risk. *Medical Journal of Australia*, **164**, 137–40.

Hoffenberg EJ, Haas J, Drescher A *et al.* (2000) A trial of oats in children with newly diagnosed celiac disease. *Journal of Pediatrics*, **137**, 361–6.

Hoffman DR, Collins-Williams C (1994) Cold pressed peanut oils may contain peanut allergens. *Journal of Allergy and Clinical Immunology*, **93**, 801–802.

Hoh J, Ott J (2000) Scan statistics to scan markers for susceptibility genes. *Proceedings of the National Academy of Science USA*, **97**, 9615–17.

Holgate ST, Walters C, Walls AF *et al.* (1994) The anaphylaxis hypothesis of sudden infant death syndrome (SIDS): mast cell degranulation in cot death revealed by elevated concentrations of tryptase in serum. *Clinical and Experimental Allergy*, **24**, 1115–22.

Holm K (1998) Markers of Latency. In: *The Changing Features of Coeliac Disease* (eds S Lohiniemi, P Collin, M. Maki). Tampere, Finland: The Finnish Coeliac Society.

Holmes GK (1998) Malignancy in coeliac disease. In: *The Changing Features of Coeliac Disease* (eds S Lohiniemi, P Collin, M. Maki). Tampere, Finland: The Finnish Coeliac Society.

Holmes GK, Thompson H (1992) Malignancy as a complication of coeliac disease. In: *Coeliac Disease* (ed. MN Marsh). Oxford: Blackwell Science.

Holt PG, O'Keeffe P, Holt BJ *et al.* (1995) T-cell 'priming' against environmental allergens in human neonates: sequential deletion of food antigen reactivity during infancy with concomitant expansion of responses to ubiquitous inhalant allergens. *Pediatric Allergy and Immunology*, **6**, 85–90.

Holtug K, Clausen MR, Hove H, Christiansen J, Mortensen PB (1992) The colon in carbohydrate malabsorption: short chain fatty acids, pH and osmotic diarrhoea. *Scandinavian Journal of Gastroenterology*, **27**, 545–52.

Høst A, Halken S (1990) A prospective study of cow milk allergy in Danish infants during the first 3 years of life. Clinical cause in relation to clinical and immunological type of hypersensitivity reaction. *Allergy*, **45**, 587–96.

Høst A, Husby S, Osterballe O (1988) A prospective study of cow's milk allergy in exclusively breast-fed infants. Incidence, pathogenetic role of early inadvertent exposure to cow's milk formula, and characterization of bovine milk protein in human milk. *Acta Paediatrica Scandinavia*, **77**, 663–70.

Høst A, Koletzko B, Dreborg S *et al.* (1999) Dietary products used in infants for treatment and prevention of food allergy. Joint Statement of the European Society for Paediatric Allergology and Clinical Immunology (ESPACI) Committee on Hypoallergenic Formulas and the European Society for Paediatric Gastroenterology, Hepatology and Nutrition (ESPGHAN) Committee on Nutrition. *Archives of Diseases in Childhood*, **81**, 80–84.

Hourihane JO (1997a) Peanut allergy and the peanut oil debate. In: *Food Allergy Issues for the Food Industry* (ed. M. Lessof). Leatherhead: Leatherhead Food Research Association.

Hourihane JO (1997b) Peanut allergy. Current status and future challenges. *Clinical and Experimental Allergy*, **27**, 1240–6.

Hourihane JO, Bedwani SJ, Dean TP, Warner JO (1997) Randomised, double blind, crossover challenge study of allergenicity of peanut oils in subjects allergic to peanuts. *British Medical Journal*, **314**, 1084–8.

Hourihane JO, Dean TP, Warner JO (1996) Peanut allergy in relation to heredity, maternal diet, and other atopic diseases: results of a questionnaire survey, skin prick testing, and food challenges. *British Medical Journal*, **313**, 518–21.

Hourihane JO, Kilburn SA, Dean P, Warner JO (1997b) Clinical characteristics of peanut allergy. *Clinical and Experimental Allergy*, **27**, 634–9.

Hourihane JO, Roberts SA, Warner JO (1998) Resolution of peanut allergy: case-control study. *British Medical Journal*, **316**, 1271–5.

Hourihane JO, Warner JO (1996) Allergy to peanut. *Lancet*, **348**, 1523.

Howarth PH (1998) Is allergy increasing? – early life influences. *Clinical and Experimental Allergy*, **28**, 2–7.

Howdle PD, Lowsowsky MS (1992) Coeliac disease in adults. In: *Coeliac Disease* (ed. MN Marsh). Oxford: Blackwell Science.

Howie PW, Forsyth JS, Ogston SA, Clark A, Florey CD (1990) Protective effect of breast feeding against infection. *British Medical Journal*, **300**, 11–16.

Hudson MJ (1995) Product development horizons – a view from industry. *European Journal of Clinical Nutrition*, **49**, S64–70.

Huebner FR, Lieberman KW, Rubino RP, Wall JS (1984) Demonstration of high opioid-like activity in isolated peptides from wheat gluten hydrolysates. *Peptides*, **5**, 1139–47.

Hughes DA (1999) Effects of carotenoids on human immune function. *Proceedings of the Nutrition Society*, **58**, 713–18.

Hughes EC (1978) Use of a chemically defined diet in the diagnosis of food sensitivities and the determination of offending foods. *Annals of Allergy*, **40**, 393–8.

Huijbers GB, Colen AA, Jansen JJ *et al.* (1994) Masking foods for food challenge: practical aspects of masking foods for a double-blind, placebo-controlled food challenge. *Journal of the American Dietetic Association*, **94**, 645–9.

Hunter AL, Rees BW, Jones LT (1984) Gluten antibodies in patients with multiple sclerosis. *Human Nutrition; Applied Nutrition*, **38**, 142–3.

Hunter JO, Alun Jones V, McLaughlan P (1982) Food intolerance: a major factor in the pathogenesis of irritable bowel syndrome. *Lancet*, **2**, 1116–17.

Huston DP (1997) The biology of the immune system. *Journal of the American Medical Association*, **278**, 1804–14.

Hyams JS, Treem WR, Etienne NL *et al.* (1995) Effect of infant formula on stool characteristics of young infants. *Pediatrics*, **95**, 50–54.

Iacono G, Carroccio A, Cavataio F *et al.* (1992) Use of

ass' milk in multiple food allergy. *Journal of Pediatric Gastroenterology and Nutrition*, **14**, 177–81.

Iacono G, Cavataio F, Montalto G *et al.* (1998) Intolerance of cow's milk and chronic constipation in children [see comments]. *New England Journal of Medicine*, **339**, 1100–1104.

ILSI (1998) *Scientific criteria and section of allergenic foodstuffs for labelling*. Brussels: International Life Sciences Institute.

Interstitial Cystitis Support Group (1998) Information leaflets, available from 76 High Street, Stony Stratford, Buckinghamshire, MK11 1AH, England.

Iqbal TH, Bradley R, Reilly HM, Lewis KO, Cooper BT (1996) Small intestinal lactase, frequency distribution of enzyme activity and milk intake in a multi-ethnic population. *Clinical Nutrition*, **15**, 297–302.

Isaacson PG, Spencer J, Connolly CE *et al.* (1985) Malignant histocytosis of the intestine: a T cell lymphoma. *Lancet* **ii**, 688–91.

Isolauri E (1995) The treatment of cow's milk allergy. *European Journal of Clinical Nutrition*, **49**, S49–55.

Isolauri E (1998) Elimination diet in cow's milk allergy: risk for impaired growth in young children. *Journal of Pediatrics*, **132**, 1004–1009.

Isolauri B, Turjanmaa K (1996) Combined skin prick and patch testing enhances identification of food allergy in infants with atopic dermatitis. *Journal of Allergy and Clinical Immunology*, **97**, 9–15.

Ivarsson A, Persson LA, Juto P *et al.* (1999) High prevalence of undiagnosed coeliac disease in adults: a Swedish population-based study. *Journal of International Medicine*, **245**, 63–8.

Jackson AA, Golden MH (1978) The human rumen. *Lancet* **ii**, 764–7.

Jacob RA, Kelley DS, Pianalto FS *et al.* (1991) Immunocompetence and oxidant defense during ascorbate depletion in healthy men. *American Journal of Clinical Nutrition*, **54**, 1302S–1309S.

Jakobsson I, Lindberg T (1979) A prospective study of cow's milk protein intolerance in Swedish infants. *Acta Paediatrica Scandinavia*, **68**, 853–9.

James MJ, Cleland LG (1997) Dietary *n*-3 fatty acids and therapy for rheumatoid arthritis. *Seminars in Arthritis and Rheumatism*, **27**, 85–97.

James JM, Bernhisel-Broadbent J, Sampson HA (1994) Respiratory reactions provoked by double-blind food challenges in children. *American Journal of Respiratory Critical Care Medicine*, **149**, 59–64.

James JM & Burks AW (1996) Food-associated gastrointestinal disease. *Current Opinion in Pediatrics*, **8**, 471–5.

James JM, Burks AW, Roberson PK, Sampson HA (1995) Safe administration of the measles vaccine to children allergic to eggs. *New England Journal of Medicine*, **11**, 332.

James JM, Eigenmann PA, Eggleston PA, Sampson HA (1996) Airway reactivity changes in asthmatic patients undergoing blinded food challenges. *American Journal of Respiratory Critical Care Medicine*, **153**, 597–603.

Janeway CA, Bottomly K (1994) Signals and signs for lymphocyte responses. *Cell*, **76**, 275–85.

Janeway CA, Travers P, Walport M, Capra JD (1999) *Immunology: The Immune System in Health and Disease*, 4th edn. London: Elsevier Science.

Janssen FW (1998) Codex Standards for gluten free products In: *The Changing Features of Coeliac Disease* (eds S Lohiniemi, P Collin, M Maki). Tampere, Finland: The Finnish Coeliac Society.

Janthuinen E, Pikkarainen P, Kemppainen T *et al.* (1995) A comparison of diets with and without oats in adults with coeliac disease. *New England Journal of Medicine*, **333**, 1033–7.

Jarisch R, Beringer K, Hemmer W (1999) Role of food allergy and food intolerance in recurrent urticaria. *Current Problems in Dermatology*, **28**, 64–73.

Jarvinen KM, Laine ST, Jarvenpaa AL, Suomalainen HK (2000) Does IgA in human milk predispose the infant to development of allergy? *Pediatric Research*, **48**, 457–62.

Jarvinen KM, Makinen-Kiljunen S, Suomalainen H (1999) Cow's milk challenge through human milk evokes immune responses in infants with cow's milk allergy. *Journal of Pediatrics*, **135**, 506–12.

Jeffery HE, Megevand A, Page H (1999) Why the prone position is a risk factor for sudden infant death syndrome. *Pediatrics*, **104**, 263–9.

Jiang T, Mustapha A, Savaiano DA (1996) Improvement of lactose digestion in humans by ingestion of unfermented milk containing *Bifidobacterium longum*. *Journal of Dairy Science*, **79**, 750–57.

Johansen BH, Gjertsen HA, Vartdal H *et al.* (1996) Binding of peptides from the N-terminal region of cx-gliadin to the celiac disease associated HLA-DQ2 molecule assessed in biochemical and T cell assays. *Clinical Immunology and Immunopathology*, **79**, 288–93.

Johnson AO, Semeeya JG, Buchowski MS, Enwonwu CO, Scrimshaw NS (1993) Correlation of lactose maldigestion, lactose intolerance and milk intolerance. *American Journal of Clinical Nutrition*, **57**, 399–401.

Johnston SD, Watson RG, McMillan SA, Sloan J, Love AH (1998). Coeliac disease detected by screening is not silent – simply unrecognised. *Quarterly Journal of Medicine*, **91**, 853–60.

Jones AC, Besley CR, Warner JA, Warner JO (1994) Variations in serum soluble IL-2 receptor concentration. *Pediatric Allergy and Immunology*, **5**, 230–34.

Jones PE, Pallis C, Peters TJ (1979) Morphological and biochemical findings in jejunal biopsies from patients with multiple sclerosis. *Journal of Neurology, Neurosurgery and Psychiatry*, **42**, 402–406.

de Jong MH, Scharp-van der Linden VT, Aalberse RC *et al.* (1998) Randomised controlled trial of brief neonatal exposure to cows' milk on the development of atopy. *Archives of Diseases in Childhood*, **79**, 126–30.

Juhlin L (1980) Incidence of intolerance to food additives. *International Journal of Dermatology*, **19**, 548–51.

Kahn A, Mozin MJ, Rebuffat E, Sottiaux M, Muller MF (1989) Milk intolerance in children with persistent sleeplessness: a prospective double-blind crossover evaluation. *Pediatrics*, **84**, 595–603.

Kajosaari M, Saarinen UM (1983) Prophylaxis of atopic disease by six months' total solid food elimination. Evaluation of 135 exclusively breast-fed infants of atopic families. *Acta Paediatrica Scandinavia*, **72**, 411–14.

Kanny G, Hatahet R, Moneret-Vautrin DA, Kohler C, Bellut A (1994) Allergy and intolerance to flavouring agents in atopic dermatitis in young children. *Allergy and Immunology (Paris)*, **26**, 204–6, 209–10.

Kaplan BJ, McNicol J, Conte RA, Moghadam HK (1989) Dietary replacement in preschool-aged hyperactive boys. *Pediatrics*, **83**, 7–17.

Kaukinen K, Collin P, Holm K *et al.* (1999) Wheat starch-containing gluten free flour products in the treatment of coeliac disease and dermatitis herpetiformis. *Scandinavian Journal of Gastroenterology*, **34**, 163–9.

Kauppinen K, Juntunen K, Lanki H (1984) Urticaria in children. Retrospective evaluation and follow-up. *Allergy*, **39**, 469–72.

Kay AB, Lessof MH (1992) Allergy: Conventional and alternative concepts. A report of the Royal College of Physicians Committee on Clinical Immunology and Allergy. *Clinical and Experimental Allergy*, **22**, Sl–44.

Keating MU, Jones RT, Worley NJ, Shively CA, Yunginger JW (1990) Immunoassay of peanut allergens in food-processing materials and finished foods. *Journal of Allergy and Clinical Immunology*, **86**, 41–4.

Kelley DS, Branch LB, Iacono JM (1989) Nutritional modulation of human immune status. *Nutrition Research*, **9**, 965–75.

Kelley DS, Branch LB, Love JE *et al.* (1991) Dietary alpha-linolenic acid and immunocompetence in humans. *American Journal of Clinical Nutrition*, **53**, 40–46.

Kelley DS, Daudu PA, Taylor PC, Mackey BE, Turnlund JR (1995) Effects of low-copper diets on human immune response. *American Journal of Clinical Nutrition*, **62**, 412–16.

Kelley DS, Dougherty RM, Branch LB, Taylor PC, Iacono JM (1992) Concentration of dietary n-6 polyunsaturated fatty acids and human immune status. *Clinical Immunology and Immunopathology*, **62**, 240–44.

Kemeny DM, Urbanek R, Amlot PL *et al.* (1986) Subclass of IgG in allergic disease. I. IgG sub-class antibodies in immediate and non-immediate food allergy. *Clinical Allergy*, **16**, 571–81.

Kenney RA (1986) The Chinese restaurant syndrome: an anecdote revisited. *Food Chemical Toxicology*, **24**, 351–4.

Kerner JA (1997) Use of infant formulas in preventing or postponing atopic manifestations. *Journal of Pediatric Gastroenterology and Nutrition*, **24**, 442–6.

Khoshoo V, Reifen R, Neuman MG, Griffiths A, Pencharz PB (1996) Effect of low- and high fat, peptide-based diets on body composition and disease activity in adolescents with active Crohn's disease. *Journal of Parenteral and Enteral Nutrition*, **20**, 401–405.

Kim TS, DeKruyff RH, Rupper R *et al.* (1997) Anovalbumin-Il-12 fusion protein is more effective than ovalbumin plus free recombinant IL-12 in inducing a T helper cell type-dominated immune response and inhibiting antigen-specific IgE production. *Journal of Immunology*, **158**, 4137–44.

Kim HS, Gilliland SE (1983) *Lactobacillus acidophilus* as dietary adjunct to aid lactose digestion in humans. *Journal of Dairy Science*, **66**, 959–66.

Kimber I, Dearman RJ (2001) Food allergy: what are the issues? *Toxicology Letters*, **120**, 165–70.

King AL, Yiannakou JY, Brett PM *et al.* (2001) A genome-wide family-based linkage study of coeliac disease. *Annals of Human Genetics*, **64**, part 6, 479–90.

King TS, Elia M, Hunter JO (1998) Abnormal colonic fermentation in irritable bowel syndrome [in process citation]. *Lancet*, **352**, 1187–9.

Kleinman RE (1998) *Pediatric Nutrition Handbook*. Elk Grove Village, Ill: American Academy of Pediatrics.

Klinkoski B, Leboeuf C (1990) A review of the research papers published by the International College of Applied Kinesiology from 1981 to 1987. *Journal of Manipulative Physiological Therapy*, **13**, 190–94.

Knights RJ (1985) Processing and evaluation antigenicity of protein hydolysates. In: *Nutrition for Special Needs in Infancy* (ed. F. Liftshitz). New York: Marcel Dekker.

Knutsen SF (1994) Lifestyle and the use of health services. *American Journal of Clinical Nutrition*, **59**, S1171–5.

Kolberg J, Sollid L (1985) Lectin activity of gluten identified as wheat germ agglutinin. *Biochemical and Biophysical Research Communications*, **130**, 867–72.

Kramer MS (1988) Does breast feeding help protect against atopic disease? Biology, methodology, and a golden jubilee of controversy. *Journal of Pediatrics*, **112**, 181–90.

Kramer MS (2000) Maternal antigen avoidance during pregnancy for preventing atopic disease in infants of women at high risk. *The Cochrane Library*, Issue 4, Oxford: Update Software.

Krause J, Kalrbeitzer, Schäfer R & Erckenbrecht JF (1997) Lactose malabsorption produces more symptoms in women as in men. Correlation of symptoms and the amount of malabsorbed carbohyrates. *Gastroenterology*, **112**, A377.

Kuitunen P, Visakorpi JK, Savilahti E, Pelkonen P (1975) Malabsorption syndrome with cow's milk intolerance. Clinical findings and course in 54 cases. *Archives of Diseases in Childhood*, **50**, 351–6.

Kuvibidila S, Yu L, Ode D, Warrier RP (1993) The immune response in protein-energy malnutrition and single nutrient deficiencies. In: *Nutrition and Immunology* (ed. DM Klurfeld). New York and London: Plenum Press.

Labib M, Gama R, Wright J, Marks V, Robins D (1989) Dietary maladvice as a cause of hypothyroidism and short stature. *British Medical Journal*, **298**, 232–3.

Lacey JM, Wilmore DW (1990) Is glutamine a conditionally essential amino acid? *Nutrition Reviews*, **48**, 297–309.

Lack G, Bradley KL, Hamelmann E *et al.* (1996) Nebulized IFN-γ inhibits the development of secondary allergic responses in mice. *Journal of Immunology*, **157**, 1432–9.

Lack G, Nelson HS, Amran D *et al.* (1997) Rush immunotherapy results in allergen-specific alterations in lymphocyte function and interferon-gramma production in CD4+ T cells. *Journal of Allergy and Clinical Immunology*, **99**, 530–38.

Lack G, Renz H, Saloga J *et al.* (1994) Nebulized but not parenteral IFN-gamma decreases IgE production and normalizes airways function in a murine model of allergen sensitization. *Journal of Immunology*, **152**, 2546–54

Lahti A, Bjorksten F, Hannuksela M (1980) Allergy to birch and apple, and cross-reactivity of the allergens studied with the RAST. *Allergy*, **35**, 297–300.

Lambris JD, Reid KB, Volanakis JE (1999) The evolution, structure, biology and pathophysiology of complement. *Immunology Today*, **20**, 207–11.

Lee M-F, Krasinski SD (1998) Human adult onset lactase decline: an update *Nutrition Reviews*, **56**, 1–8.

Lee SK, Kniker WT, Cook CD, Heiner DC (1978) Cow's milk-induced pulmonary disease in children. *Advanced Pediatrics*, **25**, 39–57.

Lessof MH (1995) Reactions to food additives. *Clinical and Experimental Allergy*, **25**, (Suppl 1), 27–8.

Lessof MH, Buisseret PD, Merrett, J, Merrett TG, Wraith DG (1980a) Assessing the value of skin prick tests. *Clinical Allergy*, **10**, 115–20.

Lessof MH, Kemeny DM, Price JF (1991) IgG antibodies to food in health and disease. *Allergy Proceedings*, **12**, 305–307.

Lessof MH, Wraith DG, Merrett J, Biusseret PD (1980b)

Food allergy and intolerance in 100 patients: Local and systemic effects. *Quarterly Journal of Medicine*, **49**, 259–71.

Lever R, MacDonald C, Waugh P, Aitchison T (1998) Randomised controlled trial of advice on an egg exclusion diet in young children with atopic eczema and sensitivity to eggs. *Pediatric Allergy and Immunology*, **9**, 13–19.

Levitt MD, Bereggren T, Hastings J (1974) Hydrogen ($H_2$) catabolism in the colon of the rat. *Journal of Laboratory and Clinical Medicine*, **84**, 163–7.

Levy J (1998) Immunonutrition: the pediatric experience. *Nutrition*, **14**, 641–7.

Lewin P, Taub SJ (1936) Allergic synovitis due to ingestion of English walnuts. *Journal of the American Medical Association*, **106**, 21–44.

Li JT, Yunginger JW, Reed CE *et al.* (1990) Lack of suppression of IgE production by recombinant interferon gamma: a controlled trial in patients with allergic rhinitis. *Journal of Allergy and Clinical Immunology*, **85**, 934–40.

Li XM, Huang CK, Schofield B *et al.* (1999) Strain-dependent induction of allergic sensitization caused by peanut allergen DNA immunization in mice. *Journal of Immunology*, **162**, 3045–52.

Li X-M, Serebrisky D, Lee S-Y *et al.* (2000) A murine model of peanut anaphylaxis: T- and B-cell responses to a major peanut allergen mimic human responses. *Journal of Allergy and Clinical Immunology*, **106**, 150–58.

Lifschitz CH, Hawkins HK, Guerra C, Byrd N (1988) Anaphylactic shock due to cow's milk protein hypersensitivity in a breast-fed infant. *Journal of Pediatric Gastroenterology and Nutrition*, **7**, 141–4.

Lilja G, Dannaeus A, Falth-Magnusson K *et al.* (1988) Immune response of the atopic woman and foetus: effects of high- and low-dose food allergen intake during late pregnancy. *Clinical Allergy*, **18**, 131–42.

Lin MY, DiPalma JA, Martini MC *et al.* (1993) Comparative effects of exogenous lactase (beta-galactosidase on in vivo lactose digestion. *Digestive Diseases and Sciences*, **38**, 2022–7.

Lindfors A, Enocksson E (1988) Development of atopic disease after early administration of cow milk formula. *Allergy*, **43**, 11–16.

Lira PI, Ashworth A, Morris SS (1998) Effect of zinc supplementation on the morbidity, immune function and growth of low birth weight full-term infants in northeast Brazil. *American Journal of Clinical Nutrition*, **69**, 418S–424S.

Littleton RH, Farah RN, Cerny JC (1982) Eosinophilic cystitis: an uncommon form of cystitis. *Journal of Urology*, **127**, 132–3.

Littlewood JM, MacDonald A (1987) Food intolerance. *Our Practice, Nutrition and Health*, **5**, 119–35.

Littlewood JT, Gibb C, Glover V *et al.* (1988) Red wine as a cause of migraine. *Lancet*, **1**, 558–9.

Lloyd-Still JD (1979) Chronic diarrhoea of childhood and the misuse of elimination diets. *Journal of Pediatrics*, **95**, 10–13.

Lo CW (1997) Human milk: nutritional properties. In: *Nutrition* (eds AW Walker, JB Watkins), pp. 436–48. Hamilton: BC Deker.

Locke GR, III (1999) Nonulcer dyspepsia: what it is and what it is not. *Mayo Clinical Proceedings*, **74**, 1011–14; quiz 5.

Logan RF (1992a) Epidemiology of coeliac disease. In: *Coeliac Disease* (ed. MN Marsh). Oxford: Blackwell Science.

Logan RF (1992b) Problems and pitfalls in epidemiological studies of coeliac disease. In: *Common Food Intolerances 1: Epidemiology of Coeliac Disease* (eds S Auricchio, JK Visakorpi). Basel: Karger.

Lopez-Rubio A, Rodriguez J, Crespo JF *et al.* (1998) Occupational asthma caused by exposure to asparagus: detection of allergens by immunoblotting. *Allergy*, **53**, 1216–20.

Lothe L, Lindberg T (1989) Cow's milk whey protein elicits symptoms of infantile colic in colicky formula-fed infants: A double-blind crossover study. *Pediatrics*, **83**, 262–6.

Lucarelli S, Frediani T, Zingoni AM *et al.* (1995) Food Allergy and infantile autism. *Panminerva Medicine*, **37**, 137–41.

Lucas A, Brooke OG, Morley R, Cole TJ, Bamford MF (1990) Early diet of preterm infants and development of allergic or atopic disease: randomised prospective study. *British Medical Journal*, **300**, 837–40.

Lucassen PL, Assendelft WJ, Gubbels JW *et al.* (1998) Effectiveness of treatments for infantile colic: systematic review [published erratum appears in *British Medical Journal*, 1998 **317**, 171] [see comments]. *British Medical Journal*, **316**, 1563–9.

Lundeberg T, Liedberg H, Nordling L *et al.* (1993) Interstitial cystitis: correlation with nerve fibres, mast cells and histamine. *British Journal of Urology*, **71**, 427–9.

Lundin KE, Scott H, Hansen T *et al.* (1993) Gliadin specific, HLA-DQ restricted, small intestinal T cells isolated from the small intestinal mucosa of celiac disease patients. *Journal of Experimental Medicine*, **178**, 187–96.

Mabin DC, Sykes AE, David TJ (1995a) Controlled trial of a few foods diet in severe atopic dermatitis. *Archives of Diseases in Childhood*, **73**, 202–207.

Mabin DC, Sykes AE, David TJ (1995b) Nutritional content of few foods diet in atopic dermatitis. *Archives of Diseases in Childhood*, **73**, 208–10.

McAlister L, Pollard G, Carter C (1997) Peanut allergy and sensitisation. *Health Visitor*, **70**, 116.

McCarthy DM, Coleman M (1979) Response of intestinal mucosa to gluten challenge in autistic subjects. *Lancet*, **ii**, 877–8.

MacDonald A, Forsythe WI (1986) The cost of nutrition and diet therapy for low-income families. *Human Nutrition; Applied Nutrition*, **40A**, 87–96.

MacDonald A, Forsyth I, Wall C (1989) Dietary treatment of migraine. In: *Headache in Children and Adolescents* (eds L Lanzig, U Balottin, A Cernibori). Amsterdam: Elsevier Science Publishers BV (Biomedical Division).

MacDonald TT (1992) T cell mediated intestinal injury. In: *Coeliac Disease* (ed. MN Marsh), pp. 238–304. Oxford: Blackwell Science.

MacGlashan DW, Bochner BS, Adelman DC *et al.* (1997) Down-regulation of Fc(epsilon)RI expression on human basophils during in vivo treatment of atopic patients with anti-IgE antibody. *Journal of Immunology*, **158**, 1438–45.

McGowan M, Gibney MJ (1993) Calcium intakes in individuals on diets for the management of cows' milk allergy: a case control study. *European Journal of Clinical Nutrition*, **47**, 609–16.

McKee AM, Prior A, Whorwell PJ (1988) Exclusion diets in irritable bowel syndrome: Are they worthwhile? *Journal of Clinical Gastroenterology*, **10**, 526–8.

McLeish CM, MacDonald A, Booth IW (1995) Comparison of an elemental with a hydrolysed whey formula in intolerance to cows' milk. *Archives of Diseases in Childhood*, **73**, 211–15.

McNeil D, Strauss RH (1988) Exercise-induced anaphylaxis related to food intake. *Annals of Allergy*, **61**, 440–42.

Magnusson CG, Masson PL (1985) Immunoglobulin F assayed after pepsin digestion by an automated and highly sensitive particle counting immunoassay: application to human cord blood. *Journal of Allergy and Clinical Immunology*, **75**, 513–24.

Mahler V, Fischer S, Fuchs T *et al.* (2000) Prevention of allergy by selection of low-allergen gloves. *Clinical and Experimental Allergy*, **30**, 509–20.

Majamaa H, Isolauri E (1997) Probiotics: a novel approach in the management of food allergy. *Journal of Allergy and Clinical Immunology*, **99**, 179–85.

Maki M (1998) Changing features of coeliac disease. In: *The Changing Features of Coeliac Disease* (eds S Lohiniemi, P Collin, M Maki). Tampere, Finland: The Finnish Coeliac Society.

Malek A, Sager R, Kuhn P, Nicolaides KH, Schneider H (1996) Evolution of maternofetal transport of immunoglobulins during human pregnancy. *American Journal of Reproductive Immunology*, **36**, 248–55.

Mandallaz MM, de Weck AL, Dahinden CA (1988) Bird-egg syndrome. Cross-reactivity between bird antigens and egg-yolk livetins in IgE-mediated hypersensitivity. *International Archives of Allergy and Applied Immunology*, **87**, 143–50.

Mannino DM (2000) How much asthma is occupationally related? *Occupational Medicine*, **15**, 359–68.

Mansfield LE, Vaughan TR, Waller SF, Haverly RW, Ting S (1985) Food allergy and adult migraine: double-blind and mediator confirmation of an allergic etiology. *Annals of Allergy*, **55**, 126–9.

Mariani P, Viti MG, Montuori M *et al.* (1998) The gluten-free diet: a nutritional risk factor for adolescents with celiac disease? *Journal of Pediatric Gastroenterology and Nutrition*, **27**, 519–23.

Marini A, Agosti M, Motta G, Mosca F (1996) Effects of a dietary and environmental prevention programme on the incidence of allergic symptoms in high atopic risk infants: 3 years follow-up. *Acta Paediatrica Supplement*, **414**, 1–22.

Marsh MN (1992) Mucosal pathology in gluten sensitivity. In: *Coeliac Disease* (ed. MN Marsh). Oxford: Blackwell Science.

Marteau P, Florie B, Pochart P *et al.* (1990) Effect of the microbial lactase (EC3.2.1.23) activity in yogurt on the intestinal absorption of lactose: an in vivo study in lactase-deficient humans. *British Journal of Nutrition*, **64**, 71–9.

Mason D (1996) The role of B-cells in the programming of T-cells for IL-4 synthesis. *Journal of Experimental Medicine*, **183**, 717–19.

Mata LJ, Kromal RA, Urrutia JJ, Garcia B (1977) Effect of infection on food intake and the nutritional state: perspectives as viewed from the village. *American Journal of Clinical Nutrition*, **30**, 1215–27.

Mattes JA, Gittelman R (1981) Effects of artificial food colorings in children with hyperactive symptoms. A critical review and results of a controlled study. *Archives of General Psychiatry*, **38**, 714–18.

Matthew DJ, Taylor B, Norman AP, Turner MW (1977) Prevention of eczema. *Lancet*, **12**, 321–4.

Maulitz RM, Pratt DS, Shocket AL (1979) Exercise-induced anaphylactic reaction to shellfish. *Journal of Allergy and Clinical Immunology*, **63**, 433–4.

Mecheri S, David B (1997) Unravelling the mast cell dilemma: culprit or victim of its generosity. *Immunology Today*, **18**, 213–16.

Medina JL, Diamond S (1978) The role of diet in migraine. *Headache*, **18**, 31–4.

Medzhitov R, Janeway CA (1997) Innate immunity: the virtues of a nonclonal system of recognition. *Cell*, **91**, 295–8.

Mehanni M, Kiberd B, McDonnell M, O'Regan M, Mathews T (1999) Reduce the risk of cot death guidelines. The effect of a revised intervention programme. National Sudden Infant Death Register, Dublin. *Irish Medical Journal*, **92**, 266–9.

Meydani SN, Barklund MP, Liu S *et al.* (1990) Vitamin E supplementation enhances cell-mediated immunity in healthy elderly subjects. *American Journal of Clinical Nutrition*, **52**, 557–63.

Meydani SN, Beharka AA (1998) Recent developments in vitamin E and immune response. *Nutrition Reviews*, **56**, S49–58.

Meydani SN, Lichtenstein AH, Cornwall S *et al.* (1993) Immunologic effects of national cholesterol education panel step-2 diets with and without fish-derived *n*-3 fatty acid enrichment. *Journal of Clinical Investigation*, **92**, 105–13.

Meydani SN, Meydani M, Blumberg JB *et al.* (1997) Vitamin E supplementation and in vivo immune response in healthy subjects. *Journal of the American Medical Association*, **277**, 1380–86.

Meydani SN, Ribaya-Mercado JD, Russell RM *et al.* (1991) Vitamin B6 deficiency impairs interleukin-2 production and lymphocyte proliferation in elderly adults. *American Journal of Clinical Nutrition*, **53**, 1275–80.

Midhagen G, Jarnerot G, Kraaz W (1988) Adult coeliac disease within a defined geographic area of Sweden. A study of prevalence and associated diseases. *Scandinavian Journal of Gastroenterology*, **23**, 1000–1004.

Milgrom H, Fick RB, Su JQ *et al.* (1999) Treatment of allergic asthma with monoclonal anti-IgE antibody. *New England Journal of Medicine*, **341**, 1968–73.

Min KU, Metcalfe DD (1991) Eosinophilic gastroenteritis. *Immunology and Allergy Clinics of North America*, **11**, 799–813.

Ministry of Agriculture, Fisheries and Food (2000) *National Food Survey 1999*. London: The Stationery Office.

Mirchandani HG, Mirchandani IH, House D (1984) Sudden infant death syndrome: measurement of total and specific serum immunoglobulin F (IgE). *Journal of Forensic Science*, **29**, 425–9.

Moffett A, Swash M, Scott DF (1972) Effect of tyramine in migraine: a double-blind study. *Journal of Neurology, Neurosurgery and Psychiatry*, **35**, 496–9.

Moffett AM, Swash M, Scott DF (1974) Effect of chocolate in migraine: a double-blind study. *Journal of Neurology Neurosurgery and Psychiatry*, **37**, 445–8.

Mølberg O, Kett K, Scott H *et al.* (1997) Gliadin specific, HLA DQ2-restricted T cells are commonly found in small intestinal biopsies from coeliac disease patients, but not from controls. *Scandinavian Journal of Immunology*, **46**, 103–108.

Moller C (1989) Effect of pollen immunotherapy on food hypersensitivity in children with birch pollinosis. *Annals of Allergy*, **62**, 343–5.

Mond JJ, Lees A, Snapper CM (1995) T-cell independent antigens type 2. *Annals of Reviews of Immunology*, **13**, 655–92.

Moneret-Vautrin DA, Hatahet R, Kanny G, Ait-Djafer Z (1991) Allergenic peanut oil in milk formulas. *Lancet*, **338**, 1149.

Moneret-Vautrin DA, Kanny G (1995) L'anaphylaxie alimentaire. Nouvelle conquete multicentrique francaise. *Bulletin of Academic Medicine*, **179**, 161–84.

Moneret-Vautrin DA, Kanny G, Halpem G (1993) Detection of antifood IgE by in vitro tests and diagnosis of food allergy. *Allergy and Immunology (Paris)*, **25**, 198–204.

Moneret-Vautrin DA, Kanny G, Thevenin F (1996) Asthma caused by food allergy. *Revue de Medecine Interne*, **17**, 551–7.

Moon A, Kleinman RE (1995) Allergic gastroenteropathy in children. *Annals of Allergy*, **74**, 5–12

Morris M-A, Yiannakou KY, King AL *et al.* (2000) Coeliac disease and Down syndrome: associations not due to genetic linkage on chromosome 21. *Scandinavian Journal of Gastroenterology*, **35**, 177–80.

Mosmann TR, Coffman RL (1989) Th1 and Th2 cells: different patterns of lymphokine secretion lead to different functional properties. *Annals of Reviews of Immunology*, **7**, 145–73.

Mosmann TR, Sad S (1996) The expanding universe of T-cell subsets: Th1, Th2 and more. *Immunology Today*, **17**, 139–45.

Mudde G, Bheekha R, Bruijnzeel-Koomen C (1995) Consequences of IgE/CD23-mediated antigen presentation in allergy. *Immunology Today*, **16**, 380–83.

Munkvad M, Danielsen L, Hoj L *et al.* (1984) Antigen-free diet in adult patients with atopic dermatitis. A double-blind controlled study. *Acta Dermato Venereologica*, **64**, 524–8.

Murray JS (1998) How the MHC selects Th1/Th2 immunity. *Immunology Today*, **19**, 157–63.

Naidu AS, Bidlack WR, Clemens RA (1999) Robiotic spectra of lactic acid bacteria (LAB). *Critical Reviews in Food Science and Nutrition*, **38**, 13–126.

Nanda R, James R, Smith H, Dudley CR, Jewell DP (1989) Food intolerance and irritable bowel syndrome. *Gut*, **30**, 1099–104.

Negro Alvarez JM, Martinez Arrieta F, Miralles Lopez JC, Sarrio Amoros F, Hernandez Garcia J (1994) [Techniques for determining case mix and their application to allergology. 1]. *Allergologia Immunopathologia (Madrid)*, **22**, 60–69.

Neuberger MS, Milstein C (1995) Somatic hypermutation. *Current Opinion in Immunology*, **7**, 248–54.

Newsholme EA, Calder PC (1997) The proposed role of glutamine in some cells of the immune system and speculative consequences for the whole animal. *Nutrition*, **13**, 728–30.

Nickel R, Kulig M, Forster J *et al.* (1997) Sensitization to hen's egg at the age of twelve months is predictive for allergic sensitisation to common indoor and outdoor allergens at the age of three years. *Journal of Allergy and Clinical Immunology*, **99**, 613–17.

Nicolai T, Bellach B, Von Mutius E, Thefeld W, Hoffmeister H (1997) Increased prevalence of sensitisation against aeroallergens in adults in West compared to East Germany. *Clinical and Experimental Allergy*, **27**, 886–92.

Niec AM, Frankum B, Talley NJ (1998) Are adverse reactions to food linked to irritable bowel syndrome? *American Journal of Gastroenterology*, **93**, 2184–90.

Niestijil Jansen JJ, Kardinaal AF, Huijbers G *et al.* (1994) Prevalence of food allergy and intolerance in the adult Dutch population. *Journal of Allergy and Clinical Immunology*, **93**, 446–56.

Niggemann B, Binder C, Klettke U, Wahn U (1999) In vivo and in vitro studies on the residual allergenicity of partially hydrolysed infant formulac. *Acta Paediatrica*, **88**, 394–8.

Ninan TK, Russell G (1992) Respiratory symptoms and atopy in Aberdeen schoolchildren: evidence from two surveys 25 years apart. *British Medical Journal*, **304**, 873–5.

Noon L (1911) Prophylactic inoculation against hay fever. *Lancet*, 10 June, 1572–3.

Not T, Horvath K, Hill ID *et al.* (1998) Coeliac disease risk in the USA: high prevalence of antiendomysium antibodies in healthy blood donors. *Scandinavian Journal of Gastroenterology*, **33**, 494–8.

Novembre E, de Martino M, Vierucci A (1988) Foods and respiratory allergy. *Journal of Allergy and Clinical Immunology*, **81**, 1059–65.

Novembre E, Veneruso G, Sabatini C *et al.* (1987) Incidence of asthma caused by food allergy in childhood. *Pediatrica Medica e Chirurgica*, **9**, 399–404.

Nsouli TM, Nsouli SM, Linde RE *et al.* (1994) Role of food allergy in serous otitis media [see comments]. *Annals of Allergy*, **73**, 215–19.

O'Banion D, Armstrong B, Cummings RA, Stange J. (1978) Disruptive behaviour: a dietary approach. *Journal of Autism and Childhood Schizophrenia*, **8**, 325–37.

Oehling A, Baena Cagnani CE (1980) Food allergy and child asthma. *Allergologia et Immunopathologia (Madrid)*, **8**, 7–14.

Oehling A, Garcia B, Santos F *et al.* (1992) Food allergy as a cause of rhinitis and/or asthma. *Journal of Investigations in Allergology and Clinical Immunology*, **2**, 78–83.

Oldaeus G, Anjou K, Bjorksten B, Moran JR, Kjellman NI (1997) Extensively and partially hydrolysed infant formulas for allergy prophylaxis. *Archives of Diseases in Childhood*, **77**, 4–10.

Oldaeus G, Björksten B, Einarsson R, Kjellman NI (1991) Antigenicity and allergenicity of cow milk hydrolysates intended for infant feeding. *Pediatric Allergy and Immunology*, **4**, 156–64.

O'Leary MP, Sant GR, Fowler FJ, Jr, Whitmore KE, Spolarich-Kroll J (1997) The interstitial cystitis symptom index and problem index. *Urology*, **49**, 58–63.

O'Mahony S, Howdle PD, Losowsky MS (1996) Review article: managment of patients with non-responsive coeliac disease. *Alimentary, Pharmacology and Therapeutics*, **10**, 671–80.

O'Mahony S, Vesley JP, Fergusson A (1990) Similarities in intestinal humoral immunity in dermatitis herpetiformis without enteropathy and in coeliac disease. *Lancet*, **335**, 1487–90.

Omran M, Russell G (1996) Continuing increase in respiratory symptoms and asthma in Aberdeen schoolchildren. *British Medical Journal*, **312**, 34.

Onorata J, Merland N, Terral C, Michel FB, Bousquet J (1986) Placebo-controlled double-blind food challenge in asthma. *Journal of Allergy and Clinical Immunology*, **78**, 1139–46.

Ortolani C, Pastorello EA, Farioli L *et al.* (1993) IgE mediated allergy from vegetable allergens. *Annals of Allergy*, **83**, 683–90.

Osbourne T (1907) *The Proteins of the Wheat Kernel.* Washington DC: Carnegie Institute.

Palosuo K, Alenius H, Varjonen E *et al.* (1999) A novel wheat gliadin as a cause of exercise-induced anaphylaxis. *Journal of Allergy and Clinical Immunology*, **103**, 912–17.

Panush RS, Stroud RM, Webster EM (1986) Food-induced (allergic) arthritis. Inflammatory arthritis exacerbated by milk. *Arthritis Rheumatology*, **29**, 220–26.

Parker SL, Sussman, GL, Krondl M (1988) Dietary aspects of adverse reactions to foods in adults. *Canadian Medical Association Journals*, **139**, 711–18.

Pavone L, Fiumara A, Bottaro G, Mazzone D, Coleman M (1997) Autism and coeliac disease: failure to validate the hypothesis that a link might exist. *Biological Psychiatry*, **42**, 72–5.

Pearson DJ, Rix KJ, Bentley SJ (1983) Food allergy: how much in the mind? A clinical and psychiatric study of suspected food hypersensitivity. *Lancet* **i**, 1259–61.

Peat JK (1996) The epidemiology of asthma. *Current Opinion in Pulmonary Medicine*, **2**, 7–15.

Peatfield RC (1995) Relationships between food, wine, and beer-precipitated migrainous headaches. *Headache*, **35**, 355–7.

Pelikan Z, Pelikan-Filipek M (1987) Bronchial response

to the food ingestion challenge. *Annals of Allergy*, **58**, 164–72.

Pelto L, Isolauri E, Lilius EM, Nuutila J, Salminen S (1998) Probiotic bacteria down-regulate the milk-induced inflammatory response in milk-hypersensitive subjects but have an immunostimulatory effect in healthy subjects. *Clinical and Experimental Allergy*, **28**, 1474–9.

Pelto L, Laitinen I, Lilius E-M (1999) Current perspectives on milk hypersensitivity. *Trends in Food Science and Technology*, **10**, 229–33.

Pene J, Rousett F, Briere F *et al.* (1988) IgE by normal human lymphocytes is induced by interleukin-4 and suppressed by interferons gamma and alpha and prostaglandin E2. *Proceedings of the National Academy of Sciences of the USA*, **85**, 6880–84.

Perman JA, Modler S, Olson AC (1981) Role of pH in production of hydrogen from carbohydrates form colonic bacterial flora. *Journal of Clinical Investigation*, **67**, 6433–50.

Peters TJ, Bjarnason I (1984) Coeliac disease: biochemical mechanisms and the missing peptidase hypothesis re-visited. *Gut*, **25**, 913–18.

Peterson JD, Herzenberg LA, Vasquez K, Waltenbaugh C (1998) Glutathione levels in antigen-presenting cells modulate Th1 versus Th2 response patterns. *Proceedings of the National Academy of Sciences of the USA*, **95**, 3071–6.

Pfaffenbach B, Adamek RJ, Bethke B, Stolte M, Wegener M (1996) Eosinophilic gastroenteritis in food allergy. *Zeitschrift fuer Gastroenterologie*, **34**, 490–93.

Phillips VL, Goodrich MA, Sullivan TJ (1999) Health care worker disability due to latex allergy and asthma: a cost analysis. *American Journal of Public Health*, **89**, 1024–8.

Pike MG, Carter CM, Boulton P *et al.* (1989) Few foods diet in the treatment of atopic eczema. *Archives of Diseases of Childhood*, **64**, 1691–8.

Pinnock CB, Arney WK (1993) The milk-mucus belief: sensory analysis comparing cow's milk and a soy placebo. *Appetite*, **20**, 61–70.

Pocino M, Baute L, Malave I (1991) Influence of oral administration of excess copper on the immune response. *Fundamentals of Applied Toxicology*, **15**, 249–56.

Pollock I, Warner JO (1990) Effect of artificial food colours on childhood behaviour. *Archives of Diseases in Childhood*, **65**, 74–7.

Potkin SG, Weinberger D, Kleinman J *et al.* (1981) Wheat gluten challenge in schizophrenic patients. *American Journal of Psychiatry*, **138**, 1208–11.

Pribila BA, Hertzler SR, Martin BR, Weaver CM, Savaiano DA (2000) Improved lactose digestion and intolerance among African-American adolescent girls fed a dairy-rich diet. *Journal of the American Dietetic Association*, **100**, 524–8.

Price CE, Rona RJ, Chinn S (1988). Height of primary school children and parents' perceptions of food intolerance. *British Medical Journal*, **296**, 1696–9.

Primeau M-N, Kagan R, Joseph L *et al.* (2000) The psychological burden of peanut allergy as perceived by adults with peanut allergy and the parents of peanut-allergic children. *Clinical and Experimental Allergy*, **30**, 1129–34.

Prohaska JR, Failla ML (1993) Copper and immunity. In: *Nutrition and Immunology* (ed. DM Klurfeld). New York and London: Plenum Press.

Propert KJ, Schaeffer AJ, Brensinger CM *et al.* (2000) A prospective study of interstitial cystitis: results of longitudinal follow up of the interstitial cystitis data base cohort. The Interstitial Cystitis Data Base Study Group. *Journal of Urology*, **163**, 1434–9.

Przemioslo RT, Lundin KE, Sollid LM, Nelufer JM, Ciclitira PJ (1995) Histological changes in small bowel mucosa induced by gliadin sensitive T lymphocytes can be blocked by anti-interferon antibody. *Gut*, **36**, 874–9.

Rahman I, Morrison D, Donaldson K, MacNee W (1996) Systemic oxidative stress in asthma, COPD, and smokers. *American Journal of Respiratory and Critical Care Medicine*, **154**, 1055–60.

Ramirez FC, Lee K, Graham DY (1994) All lactase preparations are not the same: results of a prospective, randomized, placebo-control led trial. *American Journal of Gastroenterology*, **89**, 566–70.

Rance F, Dutau G (1999) Peanut hypersensitivity in children. *Pediatric Pulmonology*, **18S**, 165–7.

Rance F, Kanny G, Dutau G, Moneret-Vautrin DA (1999) Food hypersensitivity in children: clinical aspects and distribution of allergens. *Pediatric Allergy and Immunology*, **10**, 33–8.

Raz E, Tighe H, Sato Y *et al.* (1996) Preferential induction of a Th1 immune response and inhibition of specific IgE antibody formation by plasmid DNA immunization. *Proceedings of the National Academy of Science of the USA*, **93**, 5141–5.

Rea F, Polito C, Marotta A *et al.* (1996) Restoration of body composition in celiac children after one year of gluten-free diet. *Journal of Pediatric Gastroenterology and Nutrition*, **23**, 408–12.

Redmond HP, Daly JM (1993) Arginine. In: *Nutrition and Immunology* (ed. DM Klurfeld). New York and London: Plenum Press.

Repine JE, Bast A, Lankhorst I and the Oxidative Stress Study Group (1999) Oxidative stress in chronic obstructive pulmonary disease. *American Journal of Respiratory and Critical Care Medicine*, **156**, 341–57.

Ricci M, Matucci A & Rossi O (1997) Source of IL-4 able

to induce the development of TH2 like cells. *Clinical and Experimental Allergy*, **27**, 488–500.

Rings EH, Grand RJ, Buller HA (1994) Lactose intolerance and lactase deficiency in children. *Current Opinions in Pediatrics*, **6**, 562–7.

Riordan AM, Hunter JO, Cowan RE *et al.*(1993) Treatment of active Crohn's disease by exclusion diet: East Anglian multicentre controlled trial. *Lancet*, **342**, 1131–4.

Riordan AR, Cotterell JC, Pickerdgill CS, Workman EM, Hunter JO (1990) Evaluating an exclusion diet in the treatment of patients with irritable bowel syndrome. *Journal of Human Nutrition and Dietetics*, **3**, 362–3.

Rivera J, Habicht J-P, Torres N *et al.* (1986) Decreased cellular immune response in wasted but not in stunted children. *Nutrition Research*, **6**, 1161–70.

Rodgers JB (1998) *n*-3 Fatty acids in the treatment of ulcerative colitis. In: *Medicinal Fatty Acids in Inflammation* (ed. J Kremer). Basel: Birkhauser Verlag.

Rodriguez J, Crespo IF, Lopez-Rubio A *et al.* (2000) Clinical cross-reactivity among foods of the Rosaceae family. *Journal of Allergy and Clinical Immunology*, **106**, 183–9.

Roe DA & Fuller CJ (1993) Carotenoids and immune function. In: *Nutrition and Immunology* (ed. DM Klurfeld). New York and London: Plenum Press.

Roesler TA, Barry PC, Bock SA (1994) Factitious food allergy and failure to thrive. *Archives of Pediatric and Adolescent Medicine*, **148**, 1150–55.

Roger A, Pena M, Botey J, Eseverri JL, Mann A (1994) The prick test and specific 1gB (RAST and MAST-CLA) compared with the oral challenge test with milk, eggs and nuts. *Journal of Investigative Allergology and Clinical Immunology*, **4**, 178–81.

de Roos NM, Katan MB (2000) Effects of probiotic bacteria on diarrhoea, lipid metabolism and carcinogenesis: a review of papers published between 1988 and 1988. *American Journal of Clinical Nutrition*, **71**, 405–11.

Rosado JL (1997) Lactose digestion and maldigestion: implications for dietary habits in developing countries. *Nutrition Research Reviews*, **10**, 137–49.

Rosado JL, Solomons NW, Allen LH (1992) Lactose digestion from unmodified, low fat and lactose hydrolysed yogurt in adult lactose maldigesters. *European Journal of Clinical Nutrition*, **46**, 61–7.

Rosenthal E, Schlesinger Y, Bimbaum Y *et al.* (1991) Intolerance to casein hydrolysate formula. Clinical aspects. *Acta Paediatrica Scandinavia*, **80**, 958–60.

Ross DJ, Keynes HL, McDonald JC (1998) SWORD '97: surveillance of work-related and occupational respiratory disease in the UK. *Occupational Medicine (London)*, **48**, 481–5.

Rostami K, Mulder CJ, Were JM *et al.* (1999) High prevalence of celiac disease in apparently healthy blood donors suggests a high prevalence of undiagnosed celiac disease in the Dutch population. *Scandinavian Journal of Gastroenterology*, **34**, 276–9.

Rowe AH (1928) Food allergy: its manifestations, diagnosis and treatment. *Journal of the American Medical Association*, **91**, 1623–31.

Rowe KS (1988) Synthetic food colourings and 'hyperactivity': a double-blind crossover study. *Australian Paediatric Journal*, **24**, 143–7.

Rowntree S, Cogswell JJ, Platts-Mills TA, Mitchell EB (1985) Development of IgE and IgG antibodies to food and inhalant allergens in children at risk of allergic disease. *Archives of Diseases in Childhood*, **60**, 727–35.

Royal College of Paediatrics and Child Health (1999) *Medicines for Children*. London: RCPCH Publications.

Rugo E, Wahl R, Wahn U (1992) How allergenic are hypoallergenic infant formulae? *Clinical and Experimental Allergy*, **22**, 635–9.

Ruhrah J (1909) The soybean in infant feeding. Preliminary report. *Archives of Pediatrics*, **26**, 496–501.

Ruiz RG, Kemeny DM, Price JF (1992) Higher risk of eczema from maternal atopy than from paternal atopy. *Clinical and Experimental Allergy*, **22**, 762–6.

Ruiz RG, Richards D, Kemeny DM, Price JE (1990) Low prevalence of elevated neonatal IgE in atopic infants. *Lancet*, **ii**, 808.

Ruiz RG, Richards D, Kemeny DM, Price JF (1991) Neonatal IgE: A poor screen for atopic disease. *Clinical and Experimental Allergy*, **21**, 467–72.

Saarinen KM, Savilahti E (2000) Infant feeding patterns affect the subsequent immunological features in cow's milk allergy. *Clinical and Experimental Allergy*, **30**, 400–406.

Saarinen UM, Kajosaari M (1995) Breastfeeding as prophylaxis against atopic disease: prospective follow-up study until 17 years old. *Lancet*, **346**, 1065–9.

Sahi T (1994) Genetics and epidemiology of adult-type hypolactasia. *Scandinavian Journal of Gastroenterology*, **29**, 7–20.

Salfield SA, Wardley BL, Houlsby WT *et al.* (1987) Controlled study of exclusion of dietary vasoactive amines in migraine. *Archives of Diseases in Childhood*, **62**, 458–60.

Saltmarsh M (ed.) (2000) *Essential Guide to Food Additives*. Leatherhead: Leatherhead Food RA Publishing.

Saltzman JR, Russell RM, Golner B *et al.* (1999) A randomized trial of *Lactobacillus acidophilus* BG2FO4 to treat lactose intolerance. *American Journal of Clinical Nutrition*, **69**, 140–46.

Sampson HA (1988) The role of food hypersensitivity and mediator release in atopic dermatitis. *Journal of Allergy and Clinical Immunology*, **81**, 635–45.

Sampson HA (1992) Atopic dermatitis. *Allergy*, **69**, 469–81.

Sampson HA (1996a) Epidemiology of food allergy. *Pediatric Allergy and Immunology*, **7**, 42–50.

Sampson HA (1996b) Managing peanut allergy. *British Medical Journal*, **312**, 1050–51.

Sampson HA (1997) Food allergy. *Journal of American Medical Association*, **278**, 1888–94.

Sampson HA (1999) Food allergy. Part 1: Immunopathogenesis and clinical disorders. *Journal of Allergy and Clinical Immunology*, **103**, 717–28.

Sampson HA, Albergo R (1984) Comparison of skin tests, RAST, and double-blind, placebo controlled food challenges in children with atopic dermatitis. *Journal of Allergy and Clinical Immunology*, **74**, 26–33.

Sampson HA, James JM, Bernhisel-Broadbent J (1992b) Safety of an amino acid-derived formula in children allergic to cow milk. *Paediatrics*, **90**, 463–5.

Sampson HA, Mendelson LM, Rosen JP (1992a) Fatal and near-fatal anaphylactic reactions to food in children and adolesecnts. *New England Journal of Medicine*, **327**, 380–84.

Sampson HA, Scanlon SM (1989) Natural history of food hypersensitivity in children with atopic dermatitis. *Journal of Pediatrics*, **115**, 23–7.

Sandler M, Carter SB, Goodwin BL *et al.* (1974) Multiple forms of monoamine oxidase: some in vivo correlations. *Advanced Biochemistry and Psychopharmacology*, **12**, 3–10.

Savaiano DA, ElAnouar AA, Smith DE, Levitt MD (1984) Lactose malabsorption from yogurt, pasteurised yogurt, sweet acidophilus milk, and cultured milk in lactase deficient subjects. *American Journal of Clinical Nutrition*, **40**, 1219–23.

Savilahti E, Launiala K, Kuitunen P (1983) Congenital lactase deficiency. *Archives of Diseases in Childhood*, **58**, 246–52.

Savilahti E, Tainio VM, Salmenpera L, Siimes MA, Perheentupa J (1987) Prolonged exclusive breast feeding and heredity as determinants in infantile atopy. *Archives of Diseases in Childhood*, **62**, 269–73.

Saylor JD, Bahna SL (1991) Anaphylaxis to casein hydrolysate formula. *Journal of Pediatrics*, **118**, 71–4.

Scadding G, Bjamason I, BrostoffJ, Levi AJ, Peters TJ (1989) Intestinal permeability to 51Cr-labelled ethylenediaminetetraacetate in food-intolerant subjects. *Digestion*, **42**, 104–109.

Schaumburg HH, Byck R, Gerstl R, Mashman JH (1969) Monosodium L-glutamate: its pharmacology and role in the Chinese restaurant syndrome. *Science*, **163**, 826–8.

Schloss QM (1912) A case of allergy to common foods. *American Journal of Diseases in Childhood*, **3**, 341–62.

Schmitz J (1992) Coeliac disease in childhood. In: *Coeliac Disease* (ed. MN Marsh). Oxford: Blackwell Science.

Schoenthaler SJ (1994) Sugar and children's behavior [letter; comment]. *New England Journal of Medicine*, **330**, 1901, discussion 3.

Schoenthaler SJ, Bier ID (2000) The effect of vitamin-mineral supplementation on juvenile delinquency among American schoolchildren: a randomized, double-blind placebo-controlled trial [see comments]. *Journal of Alternative and Complementary Medicine*, **6**, 7–17.

Schoenthaler SJ, Bier ID, Young K, Nichols D, Jansenns S (2000) The effect of vitamin-mineral supplementation on the intelligence of American schoolchildren: a randomized, double-blind placebo-controlled trial [see comments]. *Journal of Alternative and Complementary Medicine*, **6**, 19–29.

Schofield AT (1908) A case of egg poisoning. *Lancet*, **1**, 716.

Schorah CJ, Morgan DB, Hullin RP (1983) Plasma vitamin C concentrations in patients in a psychiatric hospital. *Human Nutrition Clinical Nutrition*, **37**, 447–52.

Schrander JJ, Van den Bogart JP, Forget PP *et al.* (1993) Cows' milk protein intolerance in infants under 1 year of age: a prospective epidemiological study. *European Journal of Pediatrics*, **152**, 640–44.

Schwartz HJ (1997) Asthma and food additives. In: *Food allergy: Adverse Reactions to Food and Food Additives* (eds DD Metcalfe, HA Sampson, RA Simon) 2nd edn, pp. 414–15. Cambridge, Mass: Blackwell Science.

Schwartz J, Weiss ST (1990) Dietary factors and their relation to respiratory symptoms. Second National Health and Nutrition Examination Survey. *American Journal of Epidemiology*, **132**, 67–76.

Schwartz J, Weiss ST (1994a) Relationship between dietary vitamin C intake and pulmonary function in the First National Health and Nutrition Examination Survey (NHANES-I). *American Journal of Clinical Nutrition*, **59**, 110–14.

Schwartz J, Weiss ST (1994b) The relationship of dietary fish intake to level of pulmonary-function in the First National Health and Nutrition Survey. *European Respiratory Journal*, **7**, 1821–4.

Schwartz RH, Amonette MS (1991) Cow milk protein hydrolysate infant formulas not always 'hypoallergenic'. *Journal of Pediatrics*, **119**, 839–40.

Schweitzer JW, Friedhoff AJ, Schwartz R (1975) Letter: Chocolate, beta-phenethylamine and migraine reexamined. *Nature*, **257**, 256.

Scrimshaw NS, Murray EB (1988) The acceptability of milk and milk products in populations with a high prevalence of lactose intolerance. *American Journal of Clinical Nutrition*, **48**, 1086S–1098S.

Scrimshaw NS, SanGiovanni JP (1997) Synergism of

nutrition, infection and immunity: an overview. *American Journal of Clinical Nutrition*, **66**, 464S–477S.

Scriver CR, Beaudet AC, Sly WS *et al.* (2001) *The Metabolic and Molecular Bases of Inherited Disease*, New York: McGraw-Hill.

Sears MR, Burrows B, Flannery EM, Herbison GP, Holdaway MD (1993) Atopy in childhood. I. Gender and allergen related risks for development of hayfever and asthma. *Clinical and Experimental Allergy*, **23**, 941–8.

Seaton A, Godden DJ, Brown KM (1994) Increase in asthma: a more toxic environment or a more susceptible population? *Thorax*, **49**, 171–4.

Selner JC, Staudenmayer H (1997) Food allergy: psychological considerations. In: *Food Allergy: Adverse Reactions to Foods and Food Additives* (eds DD Metcalfe, HA Sampson, RA Simon) 2nd edn. Cambridge, Mass: Blackwell Science.

Semba RD (1998) The role of vitamin A and related retinoids in immune function. *Nutrition Reviews*, **56**, S38–48.

Semba RD (1999) Vitamin A and immunity to viral, bacterial and protozoan infections. *Proceedings of the Nutrition Society*, **58**, 719–27.

Semba RD, Tang AM (1999) Micronutrients and the pathogenesis of human immundeficiency virus infection. *British Journal of Nutrition*, **81**, 181–9.

Sethi TJ, Lessof MH, Kemeny DM *et al.* (1987) How reliable are commercial allergy tests? *Lancet*, **i**, 92–4.

Shaheen S (1997) Discovering the causes of atopy. *British Medical Journal*, **314**, 987–8.

Shankar AH, Prasad AS (1998) Zinc and immune function: the biological basis of altered resistance to infection. *American Journal of Clinical Nutrition*, **68**, 447S–463S.

Shaw AD, Brooks JL, Dickerson JW, Davies GJ (1998) Dietary triggers in irritable bowel syndrome. *Nutrition Research Reviews*, **11**, 279–309.

Sher KS, Fraser RC, Wickes AC, Mayberry JF (1993) High risk of coeliac disease in Punjabis. Epidemiological study in south Asian and European populations of Leicestershire. *Digestion*, **54**, 178–82.

Sheridan MS (1999) Risk reduction to prevent sudden infant death syndrome: knowledge and opinions of Hawaii physicians. *Hawaii Medical Journal*, **58**, 207–8.

Shermak MA, Saavedra JM, Jackson TL *et al.* (1995) Effect of yogurt on symptoms and kinetics of hydrogen production in lactose malabsorbing children. *American Journal of Clinical Nutrition*, **62**, 1003–1006.

Sherman AR, Spear AT (1993) Iron and immunity. In: *Nutrition and Immunology* (ed. DM Klurfeld). New York and London: Plenum Press.

Shewry PR, Tatham AS, Kasarda DD (1992) Cereal proteins in coeliac disease. In: *Coeliac Disease* (ed. MN Marsh). Oxford: Blackwell Science.

Shidrawi RG, Day P, Przemioslo R *et al.* (1995) *In vitro* activity of gluten peptides assessed by organ culture. *Scandinavian Journal of Gastroenterology*, **30**, 758–63.

Shidrawi RG, Parnell ND, Ciclitira PJ *et al.* (1998) Binding of gluten derived peptides to the HLA DQ (alpha*050l, beta*0201) molecule assessed in a cellular assay. *Clinical and Experimental Immunology*, **111**, 158–65.

Sicherer SH (1999) Manifestations of food allergy: evaluation and management [see comments]. *American Family Physician*, **59**, 415–24.

Sicherer SH, Morrow EH, Sampson HA (2000) Dose-response in double-blind, placebo-controlled oral food challenges in children with atopic dermatitis. *Journal of Allergy and Clinical Immunology*, **105**, 582–6.

Sicherer SH, Munoz-Furlong A, Burks AW, Sampson HA (1999) Prevalence of peanut and tree nut allergy in the US determined by a random digit telephone survey. *Journal of Allergy and Clinical Immunology*, **103**, 559–62.

Siegel BV (1993) Vitamin C and the immune response in health and disease. In: *Nutrition and Immunology* (ed. DM Klurfeld). New York and London: Plenum Press.

Siemensma AD, Wicher JW, Bak HJ (1993) The importance of peptide lengths in hypoallergenic infant formulae. *Trends in Food Science and Technology*, **4**, 16–21.

Sigurs N, Hattevig G, Kjellman B (1992) Maternal avoidance of eggs, cow's milk, and fish during lactation: effect on allergic manifestations, skin-prick tests, and specific IgE antibodies in children at age 4 years. *Pediatrics*, **89**, 735–9.

Singh MM, Kay SR (1976) Wheat gluten as a pathogenic factor in schizophrenia. *Science*, **191**, 401–402.

Singh MM, Kay SR (1983) The problem of type II error in the 'gluten hypothesis' [letter]. *American Journal of Psychiatry*, **140**, 644–5.

Sjoberg K, Eriksson S (1999) Regional differences in coeliac disease prevalence in Scandinavia. *Scandinavian Journal of Gastroenterology*, **34**, 41–5.

Skerritt JH, Hill AS (1991a) Self-management of dietary compliance in coeliac disease by means of ELISA 'home test' to detect gluten. *Lancet*, **337**, 379–81.

Skerritt JH, Hill AS (1991b) Enzyme-immunoassay for determination of gluten in foods; collaborative study. *Journal of the Association of Official Analytical Chemists*, **74**, 257–64.

Skerritt JH, Hill AS (1992) How 'free' is 'gluten free'? Relationship between Kjeldahl nitrogen values and gluten protein for wheat starches. *Cereal Chemistry*, **69**, 110–12.

Sladden MJ, Dure-Smith B, Berth-Jones J, Graham-

Brown RA (1991) Ethnic differences in the pattern of skin disease seen in a dermatology department – atopic dermatitis is more common among Asian referrals in Leicestershire. *Clinical and Experimental Dermatology*, **16**, 348–9.

Sloper KS, Wadswirth J, Brostoff J (1991) Children with atopic eczema. I: Clinical response to food elimination and subsequent double-blind food challenge. *Quarterly Journal of Medicine*, **80**, 677–93.

Smecuol E, Gonzalez D, Matutalen C et al. (1997) Longitudinal study on the effect of treatment on body composition and antropometry of celiac disease patients. *American Journal of Gastroenterology*, **92**, 639–43.

Sollid LM, Molberg O, McAdam S et al. (1997) Auto-antibodies in coeliac disease: tissue transglutaminase-guilt by association? *Gut*, **41**, 851–2.

Sorell L, Lopez JA, Valdes I et al. (1998) An innovative sandwich ELISA system based on an antibody cocktail for gluten analysis. *FEBS Letters*, **439**, 46–50.

Sorva R, Makinen-Kiljunen S, Juntunen-Backman K (1994) Beta-lactoglobulin secretion in human milk varies widely after cow's milk ingestion in mothers of infants with cows' milk allergy. *Journal of Allergy and Clinical Immunology*, **93**, 787–92.

Soutar A, Seaton A, Brown K (1997) Bronchial reactivity and dietary antioxidants. *Thorax*, **52**, 166–70.

Sponheim E (1991) Gluten free diet in infantile autism. A therapeutic trial. *Tidsskr Nor Laegeforen*, **111**, 704–707.

Sprikkelman AB, Heymans HAS, van Aaleren WMC (2000) Development of allergic disorders in children with cows' milk protein allergy or intolerance in infancy. *Clinical and Experimental Allergy*, **30**, 1358–63.

Stallings VA, Oddleifson NW, Negrini BY, Zemel BS, Wellens R (1994) Bone mineral content and dietary calcium intake in children prescribed a low-lactose diet. *Journal of Pediatric Gastroenterology and Nutrition*, **18**, 440–45.

Stavnezer J (1996) Immunoglobulin class switching. *Current Opinion in Immunology*, **8**, 199–205.

Stefanini GF, Saggioro A, Alvisi V et al. (1995) Oral cromlyn sodium in comparison with elimination diet in the irritable bowel syndrome, diarrheic type. Multi-center study of 428 patients. *Scandinavian Journal of Gastroenterology*, **30**, 535–41.

Stern M (2000) Comparative evaluation of serological tests for celiac disease: a European initiative towards standardization. *Journal of Pediatric Gastroenterology and Nutrition*, **31**, 513–19.

Stoker TW, Castle JL (1996) Special diets. In: *Nutrition in Pediatrics* (eds WA Walker, JB Watkins). Ontario: BC Decker.

Storms LH, Clopton JM, Wright C (1982) Effects of gluten on schizophrenics. *Archives of General Psychiatry*, **39**, 323–7.

Stout R, Bottomly K (1989) Antigen-specific activation of effector macrophages by interferon-γ producing (Th1) T-cell clones: failure of IL-4 producing (Th2) T-cell clones to activate effector functions in macrophages. *Journal of Immunology*, **142**, 760–68.

Strobel S, Brydon WG, Ferguson A (1984) Cellobiose/mannitol sugar permeability test complements biopsy histopathology in clinical investigation of the jejunum. *Gut*, **25**, 1241–6.

Strobel S, Mowat AM (1998) Immune responses to dietary antigens: oral tolerance. *Immunology Today*, **19**, 173–81.

Stuart HC (1923) The excretion of foreign protein in human milk. *American Journal of Diseases in Childhood*, **25**, 135–8.

Sturgess RP, Day P, Ellis HJ et al. (1994) Wheat peptide challenge in coeliac disease. *Lancet*, **343**, 758–76.

Suarez FL, Savaiano DA, Arbisi P, Levitt MD (1997) Tolerance to the daily ingestion of two cups of milk by individuals claiming lactose intolerance. *American Journal of Clinical Nutrition*, **65**, 1502–506.

Suarez FL, Savaiano DA, Levitt MD (1995) A comparison of symptoms with self-reported severe lactose intolerance after drinking milk or lactose-hydrolysed milk. *New England Journal of Medicine*, **333**, 1–4.

Sulkanen S, Halttunen T, Laurila K et al. (1998) Tissue transglutaminase autoantibody enzyme-linked immunosorbent assay in detecting celiac disease. *Gastroenterology*, **115**, 1322–8.

Sur S, Camara M, Buchmeier A, Morgan S, Nelson HS (1993) Double-blind trial of pyridoxine (vitamin B6) in the treatment of steroid resistant asthma. *Annals of Allergy*, **70**, 147–52.

Swanson JM, Flodman P, Kennedy J et al. (2000) Dopamine genes and ADHD. *Neuroscience and Biobehaviour Review*, **24**, 1–5.

Szepfalusi Z, Nentwich I, Gersimayr M et al. (1997) Prenatal allergen contact with milk proteins [see comments]. *Clinical and Experimental Allergy*, **27**, 28–35.

Tappia PS, Troughton KL, Langley-Evans SC, Grimble RF (1995) Cigarette smoking influences cytokine production and antioxidant defences. *Clinical Science*, **88**, 485–9.

Tariq SM, Stevens M, Mathews S et al. (1996) Cohort study of peanut and tree nut sensitisation by age 4 years. *British Medical Journal*, **313**, 514–17.

Taylor B, Wadsworth J, Wadsworth M, Peckham C (1984) Changes in the reported prevalence of childhood eczema since the 1939–45 war. *Lancet*, **2**, 1255–7.

Taylor CJ, Jenkins P & Manning D (1988) Evaluation of a

peptide formula (milk) in the management of multiple GIT intolerance. *Clinical Nutrition*, **7**, 183–90.

Taylor DC (1992) Outlandish factitious illness. In: *Recent Advances in Paediatrics* (ed. TJ David). London: Churchill Livingstone.

Taylor MA (1999) Attention-deficit hyperactivity disorder on the frontlines: management in the primary care office. *Comprehensive Therapy*, **25**, 313–25.

Taylor SL, Bush RK, Nordless JA (1997) Sulfites. In: *Food Allergy: Adverse Reactions to Food and Food Additives*, 2nd edn (eds DD Metcalfe, HA Sampson, RA Simon) pp. 339–57. Cambridge, Mass: Blackwell Science.

Taylor SL, Busse WW, Sachs MI, Parker JL, Yunginger JW (1981) Peanut oil is not allergenic to peanut sensitive individuals. *Journal of Allergy and Clinical Immunology*, **68**, 372–5.

Thies F, Nebe-von-Caron G, Powell JR *et al.* (2001) Dietary supplementation with eicosapentaenoic acid, but not with other long chain *n*-3 or *n*-6 polyunsaturated fatty acids, decreases natural killer cell activity in healthy subjects aged >55 y. *American Journal of Clinical Nutrition*, **73**(3), 539–48.

Thomas B (Ed.) (1988) *Manual of Dietetic Practice*. Oxford: Blackwell Science.

Thompson WG & Heaton KW (1980) Functional bowel disorders in apparently healthy people. *Gastroenterology*, **79**, 283–8.

Tiainen JM, Nuutinen OM, Kalavainen MP (1995) Diet and nutritional status in children with cow's milk allergy. *European Journal of Clinical Nutrition*, **49**, 605–12.

Tighe MR, Ciclitira PJ (1995) Molecular biology of coeliac disease. *Archives of Diseases in Childhood*, **73**, 189–91.

Trinchieri G, Gerosa F (1996) Immunoregulation by Interleukin-12. *Journal of Leukocyte Biology*, **59**, 505–11.

Troelsen JT, Mitchelmore C, Spondsberg N *et al.* (1997) Regulation of lactase-phlorizin hydrolase gene expression by the caudal-related homeodomain protein Cdx-2. *Biochemical Journal*, **322**, 833–8.

Troisi RJ, Willett WC, Weiss ST *et al.* (1995) A prospective study of diet and adult onset asthma. *American Journal of Respiratory and Critical Care Medicine*, **151**, 1401–408.

Trounce JQ, Walker-Smith JA (1985) Sugar intolerance complicating acute gastroenteritis. *Archives of Diseases in Childhood*, **60**, 986–90.

Tryphonas H, Trites R (1979) Food allergy in children with hyperactivity, learning disabilities and/or minimal brain distinction. *Annals of Allergy*, **42**, 22–7.

Tucker P, Boehler SD, Dickson W, Lensgraf SJ, Jones D (1999) Mental health response to the Oklahoma City bombing. *Journal of Oklahoma State Medical Association*, **92**, 168–71.

Tuft I, Blumstein GI (1942) Studies in food allergy. II. Sensitization to fresh fruits: clinical and experimental observations. *Journal of Allergy*, **13**, 574–81.

Turnbull JA (1944) Changes in sensitivity to allergenic foods in arthritis. *American Journal of Digestive Diseases*, **11**, 182–90.

Turner KJ, Baldo BA, Carter RF, Kerr HR (1975) Sudden infant death syndrome in South Australia. Measurement of serum IgE antibodies to three common allergens. *Medical Journal of Australia*, **2**, 855–9.

Urbanek R, Kemeny DM, Richards D (1986) Sub-class of IgG anti-bee venom antibody produced during bee venom immunotherapy and its relationship to long-term protection from bee stings and following termination of venom immunotherapy. *Clinical Allergy*, **16**, 317–22.

Valyasevi MA, Maddox DE, Li JT (1999) Systemic reactions to allergy skin tests. *Annals of Allergy, Asthma and Immunology*, **83**, 132–6.

Van Bever HP, Docx M, Stevens WJ (1989) Food and food additives in severe atopic dermatitis. *Allergy*, **44**, 588–94.

van der Hulst RRW, van Kreel BK, von Meyenfeldt MF *et al.* (1993) Glutamine and the preservation of gut integrity. *Lancet*, **341**, 1363–5.

Van de Laar MF, Van der Korst JK (1992) Food intolerance in rheumatoid arthritis. I. A double blind, controlled trial of the clinical effects of elimination of milk allergens and azo dyes. *Annals of Rheumatic Disease*, **51**, 298–302.

Vandenplas Y, Hauser B, Van den Borre C *et al.* (1995) The long-term effect of a partial whey hydrolysate formula on the prophylaxis of atopic disease. *European Journal of Pediatrics*, **154**, 488–94.

Ventura A, Magazzu G, Greco L (1999) Duration of exposure to gluten and risk for autoimmune disorders in patients with celiac disease. *Gastroenterology*, **117**, 297–303.

Vesa TH, Korpela RA, Sahi T (1996a) Tolerance of small amounts of lactose in lactose maldigesters. *American Journal of Clinical Nutrition*, **64**, 197–201.

Vesa TH, Lember M, Korpela R (1997) Tolerance of high fat milk and fat free milk in lactose intolerant subjects. *European Journal of Clinical Nutrition*, **51**, 633–6.

Vesa TH, Marteau P, Zidi S *et al.* (1996b) Digestion and tolerance of lactose from yogurt and different semi-solid fermented dairy products containing *Lactobacillus acidophilus* and bifidobacteria in lactose maldigesters – is bacterial lactase important? *European Journal of Clinical Nutrition*, **50**, 730–33.

Vesa TH, Seppo LM, Mateau PR, Sahi T, Korpela R (1998) Role of irritable bowel syndrome in subjective lactose intolerance. *American Journal of Clinical Nutrition*, **67**, 710–5.

Vila L, Barbarin E, Sanz ML (1998) Chicken meat induces oral allergy syndrome: a case report. *Annals of Allergy Asthma and Immunology*, **80**, 195–6.

Vlissides DN, Venulet A, Jenner LA (1986) A double-blind gluten-free/gluten-load controlled trial in a secure ward population. *British Journal of Psychiatry*, **148**, 447–52.

Volker D, Garg M (1996) Dietary *n*-3 fatty acid supplementation in rheumatoid arthritis – mechanisms, clinical outcomes, controversies, and future directions. *Journal of Clinical Biochemistry and Nutrition*, **20**, 83–97.

Von Mutius E, Fritzsch C, Weiland SK, Roell G, Magnusson H (1992) Prevalence of asthma and allergic disorders among children in united Germany: a descriptive comparison. *British Medical Journal*, **305**, 1395–9.

Von Mutius E, Martinez FD, Fritzsch C *et al.* (1994) Prevalence of asthma and atopy in two areas of West and East Germany. *American Journal of Respiratory Critical Care Medicine*, **149**, 358–64.

Von Mutius E, Weiland SK, Fritzsch C, Duhme H, Keil U (1998) Increasing prevalence of hayfever and atopy in Leipzig, East Germany. *Lancet*, **351**, 826–66.

Walker-Smith J (1994) Food sensitive enteropathy: overview and update. *Acta Paediatrica Japan*, **36**, 545–9.

Walker-Smith JA (1988) *Diseases of the Small Intestine in Childhood*, 3rd edn. London: Butterworths.

Walker-Smith JA (1995) Diagnostic criteria for gastro-intestinal food allergy in childhood. *Clinical and Experimental Allergy*, **1**, 20–22.

Walker-Smith JA (1997) Therapy of Crohn's disease in childhood. *Baillieres Clinical Gastroenterology*, **11**, 593–610.

Walker-Smith JA, Ford RP, Phillips AD (1984) The spectrum of gastrointestinal allergies to food. *Annals of Allergy*, **53**, 629–36.

Walker-Smith JA, Guandalini S, Schmitz J, Shmerling DH, Visakorpi JK (1990) Revised criteria for diagnosis of coeliac disease. *Archives of Diseases in Childhood*, **65**, 909–11.

Walker-Smith JA, Harrison M, Kilby A, Phillips A, France NE (1978) Cows' milk sensitive enteropathy. *Archives of Diseases in Childhood*, **53**, 375–82.

Wantke F, Gotz M, Jarisch R (1993) The histamine-free diet. *Hautarzt*, **44**, 512–16.

Warner JA, Jones CA, Jones AC *et al.* (1997) Immune responses during pregnancy and the development of allergic disease. *Pediatric Allergy and Immunology*, **8**, S5–10.

Warner JA, Miles EA, Jones AC *et al.* (1994) Is defi-ciency of interferon gamma production by allergen triggered cord blood cells a predictor of atopic eczema? [see comments]. *Clinical and Experimental Allergy*, **24**, 423–30.

Warner JO (1999) Peanut allergy: a major public health issue. *Pediatric Allergy and Immunology*, **10**, 14–20.

Warner JO, Hathaway MJ (1984) Allergic form of Meadow's syndrome (Munchausen by proxy). *Archives of Diseases in Childhood*, **59**, 151–6.

Weaver S, Robertson D (1999) Osteoporosis and coeliac disease. *CME Journal of Gastroenterology, Hepatology and Nutrition*, **2**, 9–11.

Webster AD, Slavin G, Shiner M, Platts-Mills TA, Asherson GL (1981) Coeliac disease with severe hypogammaglobulinaemia. *Gut*, **22**, 153–7.

Weisselberg B, Dayal Y, Thompson JF *et al.* (1996) A lamb-meat-based formula for infants allergic to casein hydrolysate formulas. *Clinical Pediatrics*, **35**, 491–5.

Wieser H (1998) Prolamins in coeliac disease. In: *The Changing Features of Coeliac Disease* (eds S Lohiniemi, P Collin, M Maki). Tampere, Finland: The Finnish Coeliac Society.

Wieser H, Seilmeier W, Belitz H-D (1994) Quantitative determination of gliadin subgroups from different wheat varieties. *Journal of Cereal Science*, **19**, 149–55.

Williams HC, Pembroke AC, Forsdyke H *et al.* (1995) London-born black Caribbean children are at increased risk of atopic dermatitis. *Journal of the American Academy of Dermatology*, **32**, 212–17.

Williams TJ, Jones CA, Miles FA, Warner JO, Warner JA (2000) Fetal and neonatal IL-13 production during pregnancy and at birth and subsequent development of atopic symptoms. *Journal of Allergy and Clinical Immunology*, **105**, 951–9.

Wilmore DW, Shabert JK (1998) Role of glutamine in immunologic responses. *Nutrition*, **14**, 618–26.

Wilson AC, Forsyth JS, Greene SA, Irvine L, Hau C, Howie PW (1998) Relation of infant diet to childhood health: seven year follow of cohort of children in Dundee infant feeding study. *British Medical Journal*, **316**, 21–5.

Wilson N, Silverman M (1985) Diagnosis of food sensitivity in childhood asthma. *Journal of the Royal Society of Medicine*, **78**, 11–16.

Wilson NM (1988) Bronchial hyperreactivity in food and drink intolerance. *Annals of Allergy*, **61**, 75–9.

Wilson NW, Self TW, Hamburger RN (1990) Severe cow's milk induced colitis in an exclusively breast-fed neonate. Case report and clinical review of cow's milk allergy. *Clinical Pediatrics (Philadelphia)*, **29**, 77–80.

Witkin SS (1993) Immunology of the vagina. *Clinical Obstetrics and Gynecology*, **36**, 122–8.

Wolfe SP (1995) 'Prevention programmes' – a dietetic

minefield. *European Journal of Clinical Nutrition*, **49**, S92–9.

Woodward B (1998) Protein, calories and immune defences. *Nutrition Reviews*, **56**, S84–92.

Woodward B (2000) The effect of protein-energy malnutrition on immune competence. In: *Nutrition, Immunity and Infectious Diseases in Infants and Children* (eds RM Suskind & K. Tontisirin). Lippincott Williams and Wilkins, Philadelphia pp 89–120.

Wüthrich B (1998) Food-induced cutaneous adverse reactions. *Allergy*, **53**, 131–5.

Yaqoob P, Pala HS, Cortina-Borja M, Newsholme EA, Calder PC (2000) Encapsulated fish oil enriched in alpha-tocopherol alters plasma phospholipid and mononuclear cell fatty acid compositions but not mononuclear cell functions. *European Journal of Clinical Investigation*, **30**, 260–74.

Yeung VP, Gieni RS, Umetsu DT, DeKruyff RH (1998) Heat-killed *Listeria monocytogenes* as an adjuvant converts established murine Th-2-dominated immune responses into Th1-dominated responses. *Journal of Immunology*, **161**, 4146–52.

Ylitalo L, Makinen-Kiljunen S, Turjanmaa K, Palosuo T, Reunala T (1999) Cow's milk casein, a hidden allergen in natural rubber latex gloves. *Journal of Allergy and Clinical Immunology*, **104**, 177–80.

Young E, Patel S, Stoneham M, Rona R, Wilkinson JD (1987) The prevalence of reaction to food additives in a population survey. *Journal of the Royal College of Physicians London*, **21**, 241–7.

Young E, Stoneham MD, Petruckevitch A, Barton J, Rona R (1994) A population study of food intolerance. *Lancet*, **343**, 1127–30.

Yunginger JW, Sweeney KG, Sturner WQ *et al.* (1988) Fatal food induced anaphylaxis. *Journal of the American Medical Association*, **260**, 1450–52.

Zeiger RS (1997) Prevention of food allergy and atopic disease. *Journal of the Royal Society of Medicine*, **90**, S21–33.

Zeiger RS, Heller S (1995) The development and prediction of atopy in high-risk children: follow-up at age seven years in a prospective randomized study of combined maternal and infant food allergen avoidance. *Journal of Allergy and Clinical Immunology*, **95**, 1179–90.

Zeiger RS, Heller S, Mellon MH *et al.* (1989) Effect of combined maternal and infant food-allergen avoidance on development of atopy in early infancy: a randomised study. *Journal of Allergy and Clinical Immunology*, **84**, 72–89.

Zeiger RS, Sampson HA, Bock SA *et al.* (1999) Soy allergy in infants and children with IgE-associated cow's milk allergy. *Journal of Pediatrics*, **134**, 614–22.

Ziboh VA (1998) The role of *n*-3 fatty acids in psoriasis. In: *Medicinal Fatty Acids in Inflammation* (ed J Kremer). Basel: Birkhauser Verlag.

Ziegler DK, Stewart R (1977) Failure of tyramine to induce migraine. *Neurology*, **27**, 725–6.

Zimmerman B, Forsyth S, Gold M (1989) Highly atopic children: formation of IgE antibody to food protein, especially peanut. *Journal of Allergy and Clinical Immunology*, **83**, 764–70.

Zioudrou C, Streaty RA, Klee WA (1979) Opioid peptides derived from food proteins. The exorphins. *Journal of Biological Chemistry*, **254**, 2446–9.

Zuberbier T, Ifflander J, Semmier C, Henz BM (1996) Acute urticaria: clinical aspects and therapeutic responsiveness. *Acta Dermato Venereologica*, **76**, 295–7.

# Index

Abbreviations used in the index: ADHD = attention deficit hyperactivity disorder; Task Force = British Nutrition Foundation Task Force; DBPCFC = double-blind placebo-controlled food challenge; HACCP = hazard analysis critical control point; Ig = immunoglobulin; Th = T helper.